Abnormal Psychology

Abnormal Psychology

Jafar Mahmud
Former Academic Counsellor,
Indira Gandhi National Open University

A.P.H. Publishing Corporation
Ansari Road, Darya Ganj,
New Delhi-110002

Published by
S.B. Nangia
A P H Publishing Corporation
4435-36/7, Ansari Road, Daryaganj
New Delhi 110002
Ph.: 23274050
E-mail : aphbooks@gmail.com

2026

₹2995/-

Printed at
Balaji Offset
Navin Shahdara, Delhi 110032

Dedicated to

my beloved

for her patience,

love & support

CONTENTS

PREFACE

Virtually al of us have at least some interest in abnormalities of behaviour, and probably a large majority of readers of this text will have had at least some direct experience with persons whose behaviour they considered to be abnormal. Abnormal behaivour is thus a part of our common experience. It is the main purpose of this book to help you gain a better understanding of the variety of psychlogical problems that any of us may experience. The book deals with Classification, Diagnosis and Assessment, Disorders of Psychophysiology, Stress related disorders, the Anxiety, Somotoform and Dissociative disorders, Sexual dysfunctions adisorders, Personality Disorder. It also covers Schizophrennic Disorders, Paranoid Disorders, Affective Disorders, Organic Brain Disorders, Disorders of Childhood and Adolescence.

I am greatly beholden to Hon'ble Mrs. Sonia Gandhi for being a great source of inspiration to me to write. I would like to thank Mrs. A.H. Laljee, Ms. Sonali Bhagwati, Mrs. Atia Abedi, and Mrs. Mehar Jahan Begum for their support and encouragement and enthusiasm for this project.

I am also thankful to the following persons: Professor A. Rahman, Former Chairman of the International Council of Science Policy; Prof. Mohd. Farooque, Former HOD AIIMS; Mr. Asif Anwar Alig; Mr. Abbas Mahdi; Dr. C.S. Nanda, Asstt. Divisional Medical Officer, Northern Railway & Former Secretary, Indian Medical Associations (SDB); Dr. Fatima Abbas Husainy; S. Khursheed Musanna; Dr. Ranjana Nanda, Consultant, Gynacologist, Consultant Damodar Valley Corporation, Govt. of India; Mr. Syed Masood Husain, Director CWC, Govt. of India; Dr. K.B. Nangia; Mr. Aniq Husain, Managing Director, Gallium Industries Ltd.; Ms. Shahida Haider. I am also thankful to Mohd. Hasan Zaidi and Abbas Kazim. This work would not have been possible without the inspiration of my niece and my friend Mohd Ali Ansari to whom I am deeply indepted. I would also like to thank Tajinder Singh and Jitender Pal Singh for the painstaking secretarial assistance.

Most of all, I would like to thank my beloved, for her thoughts and suggestions and for bearing through the long months of writing. I can never thank her enough for her patience, love and support.

New Delhi
India

Jafar Mahmud

1

Classification, Diagnosis and Assessment

Classification, assessment and diagnosis of abnormal behaviour are important and necessary part of abnormal and clinical psychology classification helps us to understand and study. The assessment and diagnosis of abnormal behaviour are necessary to understand not only the type of disorder and its etiology but also plays an important role in deciding about the therapeutic technique to be used and the prognostic course of the disorder.

In clinical practice a particular disorder is rarely manifested in its pure form with classic symptoms. Very often, disorder may have multiple symptoms. Two or more disorders may appear at the same time. Under such condition it becomes necessary to arrive at the diagnosis and determine what type of disorder it is. Such a decision is necessary to plan appropriate treatment.

We would define classification and discuss the different type of classification systems. The two most well known classification systems are the Diagnostic and Statistical Manual of Mental Disorders, 3rd edition, 1980 (DSM-III) and the International Classification of Diseases. We would discuss the salient features of these two classification system, stimulated simultaneous efforts to construct effective and reliable techniques for the assessment of abnormal behaviour. The techniques developed have been quite diverse. We would discuss the various assessment techniques. Some of these techniques are the clinical interview, Intelligence tests, projective techniques, personality inventories and tests of organic impairment.

CLASSIFICATION IN ABNORMAL PSYCHOLOGY

The terms classification, diagnosis and assessment are, very often used interchangeably to refer to one and the same aspect.

Classification is an important characteristic of almost all scientific disciplines. Classification involves categorization. Through the process of classification we categorize certain information into different categories on some predetermined criteria. This helps us to understand the area of our operation.

Diagnosis is the process of categorization too. By the process of diagnosis we categorize the person into certain fixed categories which helps us to understand individuals and their problems in better manner.

Assessment refers to collection of information through wide variety of means. The proper word is psychological assessment. Psychological assessment, according to Sundberg & Tyler is defined as the systematic collection, organization and interpretation of information about a person and his situation.

Hippocrates 'personality types were an early effort in this direction, and Emil Kraepelin's identification of specific disorders in the late 1800s formed the basis for modern classification systems. In the past few decades, investigators concerned with abnormal behaviour have developed classification systems of quite complex natures. For most students of abnormal behaviours, classification of the immense range of abnormal behaviour promises to simplify their task of understanding its causes, character and treatment.

The specific procedure, focus, and goal of classification, however, have been the subjects of intense criticism. Some critics question whether we should attempt to classify at all. Others think that classification can be useful, but the current approach to the classification of abnormal behaviour is so flawed that it hinders, rather than helps, our attempt to understand and deal with disturbed functioning.

When a classification system is developed and used, its utility is partly dependent upon the collection of information. This process of information collection, or assessment, provides the information needed in order to classify disorders into their appropriate categories. Assessment, however, does not have to be used only to classify. It may be used to gain greater understanding of an individual's assets, deficits, and potentials, without assigning a label to the person.

ESSENTIAL REQUIREMENTS OF AN IDEAL CLASSIFICATION SYSTEM

Following are the characteristics of an ideal classification system.

1. There must be reasonable homogeneity within categories and heterogeneity between categories:
2. The system must yield reliable differentiations;
3. The categories should be relatively stable; and
4. The categories should have validity.

1. Homogeneity/Heterogeneity: Each diagnostic category should be composed of elements which do not appear in other categories: the category should have homogeneity. When elements appear in more than one class, there is heterogeneity. The elements should allow one to discriminate between categories. Most classification systems vary significantly from the ideal. Some studies have demonstrated a broad overlap of many characteristics among the categories of the Diagnostic and Statistical Manual of the American Psychiatric Association, the classification system used by many mental health professionals. Though this system has recently been revised, a study conducted prior to the revision illustrates the problem. In a study of 793 patients diagnosed as either manic-depressive, neurotic, schizophrenic, or as having a character disorder. Zigler and Phillips (1969), found the hallucinations were reported in 11 percent of manic-depressive patients, 4 percent of neurotic, 35 percent of schizophrenic patients, and 12 percent of patients with character disorders. The overlap of hallucinatory behaviour in these categories indicates that the categories are not homogeneous. Ideally, we would not want such a situation to exist in a classification system. But overlap compromises the system's usefulness.

Psychologist Nacy Cantor and Colleagues (1980) have suggested that diagnosis (or categorization) of abnormal behaviour should be viewed as an approach in which "prototypes" are developed. From their perspective, an absolute lack of overlap among categories is not necessary. In prototype classification, a disorder such as depression is described by a cluster of behaviours (a prototype) which can be used to define the disorder, even though some of the behaviours may appear as part of another disorder. Cantor et al. illustrate this concept with the following example: The features that make up the category of birds include "feathered", "winged", "flies", and "sings". Feathered and winged are necessary features (all birds are feathered and winged). But while most birds fly and sing, many do no. These features are only correlated with the category of birds. In DSM-III (1980), a common current classification system, the categories are similar to this prototype system of classification: Some features of a category are necessary, others are correlated, and the defining characteristics are clusters of behaviours.

2. **Reliability:** An adequate classification system must result in reliable categorization. A diagnostician should classify an individual in the same category at different times (assuming that the subject's behaviours have not changed). In addition, different diagnosticians who have access to the same data should agree on the category in which a subject should be placed. Most studies have indicated that this level of agreement is relatively low when standard diagnostic categories are used (J. Greemberg, 1977). A study by A.T. Beck et al., (1962), for example, indicates that inter diagnostician agreement on diagnoses of patients varied from 63 percent on neurotic depression to 38 percent on specific personality trait disturbances. However, when the categories were more general and induced only psychosis, neurosis, and character disorder, the agreement reached 70 percent.

Recent revision of the diagnostic categories, that Beck and colleagues studied, promise to increase agreement levels by increasing the exactness of each category's criteria. The more inexact the criteria, the less likely two individuals are to agree whether a specific behaviour meets the definition (Winoker, 1977). Other factors also influence the accuracy of diagnosis and inter rater (between examiners) reliability. Subjects may give different date to different examiners, either on purpose, because of the setting, because they have changed, or because of differences in the examiners. Examiners must be trained differently, or may have different levels of competence. However, Kendall (1973) in reviewing studies of DSM-II (1968), a diagnostic classification system used until 1968 concluded that 60 percent of the disagreements between diagnosticians were due to the internal problems of the classification system, rather than to problems of the person making the diagnosis.

3. **Stability:** Categories must be stable over time. Of course, diagnoses of individuals may change over time with treatment or because of other factors. However, if diagnostic categories change in prevalence over historical periods, this may indicate that they reflect more about society's perception of behaviour than about disorder itself. Infact, to some extent, this seems to occur. J.D. Blum (1978) for example found major changes in the diagnosed incidence of affective disorders (threefold increase), neurotic disorders (major decrease) and schizophrenia (significant increase) from 1954 to 1974. He discovered that changes in symptoms or behaviour could not fully explain the different, and concluded that interpretation of behaviour was relative to the historical period. Such studies raise questions about the validity of diagnostic categories. If the disorder's behaviours or symptoms do not change significantly, but the diagnosis does, does the diagnostic category really exist outside of the perception of the diag-

nostician?

4. Validity: In the context of a classification of diagnostic system, we can view the issue of validity from two perspectives: Do the categories really exist? Are they useful? No one seriously rejects the notion that the behaviours that make up the symptoms of the various categories exist. However, some individuals feel that to call these behaviours "Disorder", illnesses", or "disease", misrepresents reality. Thomas Szasz (1961, 1970), for example, says these behaviours are "problems in living" that do not fall into discrete categories. The more radical behaviourists takes a similar view, arguing that each behaviour has a unique learning history, so that traditional categorization can add little to our understanding. Most clinicians, however, would argu that clusters of behaviours exist, whether or not one calls them diseases.

Certainly, categories can be useful. The benefits of classification in organizing information, making generalizations, and facilitation communication have let most clinicians to accept the necessity of classification system. At the same time, most clinicians are painfully aware of the shortcomings of current classification systems. Although the potential benefits of an accurate, valid classification system have not been fully achieved, it seems better to try to improve classification systems than to dispense with them.

BENEFITS OF CLASSIFICATION

The use of a system for classifying abnormal behaviour must be of some worth if time and energy are to be invested in it. Mental health professional expect to gain positive benefits from effective assessment and classification, inspite of the inadequacies of the systems available.

(a) Organization of Information: The use of classification system allows information and data to be organized so that they are easier to understand. And classification is a necessary aspect of sound research: when one uses research methodology to study abnormal behaviour, the behaviour must be clearly specified, since individuals and groups are contrasted on specific variables.

(b) Generalization: An effective classification system allows us to generalize. Suppose a grouping of behaviours are found to consistently appear together. For example, perhaps almost every individual encountered who is depressed also has difficulty sleeping, has a poor self-concept, and has few social contents. As confidence is gained that this pattern of behaviours is usually seen in depressed individuals, conclusions can be generalized from the group studied to other people who are depressed. We may be able to generalization about the causes of depression, the best treatments, and the likely outcomes. Our ability to generalize from our limited samples may allow us to predict behaviour. If an individual is depressed, has a poor self-concept, and few social contacts, we can predict that sleeping difficulty is also likely. However, generalization is a two-edged sword. If a classification system is inaccurate, the generalizations may be in error.

(c) Shorthand Communication: If an individual can be identified as belonging to a specific category for which other professional know the characteristics necessary for membership, then a great deal of information can be communicated in a few words. If a psychologist states the "Raju manifests paranoid behaviours," something quite different is being communicated about is consensus about the features of depression and paranoid behaviour, it is not necessary to list and describe each behaviour in order to communicate them to another person.

PROBLEMS OF CLASSIFICATION

The process of classification in not free of problems. Some commonly encountered problems in the process of classification are as follows:

1. Biases: Classification assists us in organization our thinking. However, since classification systems are often based on specific models of behaviours, the organization of the system may bias our thinking. For example, if our classification system assumes that disturbed behaviour is a disease, we are not likely to look for alternative conceptualizations of abnormal behaviours. We may become locked into viewing problems as diseases, conceptualizing behaviours as symptoms, clustering symptoms into syndromes, searching for underlying causes, and applying a medical model of treatment.

2. Loss of Information: While classification assists the process of generalization, generalization may result in the loss of information. The uniqueness of the individual is lost, for example, when a diagnosis such as paranoid schizophrenia is made. Such a diagnosis tells much about some characteristics, but little about others. We would not know that the person is a loving parent, bright, a good golfer, a doctor, personable, or concerned for the welfare of spouse-facts that may be relevant to an understanding of the problems the person is experiencing. Our process of shorthand communication may be short on some information.

In addition to these potentially negative consequences of classification, discrete categories may tend to obscure the range of human behaviour. People are often seen as either belonging or not belonging to a specific category. One is either a schizophrenic or depressive, disturbed or normal. Most clinicians are well aware of the range of human behaviour. However, once a clinician has placed a person into a specific category, the diagnostic label can result in undesirable secondary effects.

3. **Damaging Effects of Labeling:** When an individual is "labeled", or receives a classification or diagnosis, there may be effects that are not intended. For example, consider the label "schizophrenic". Each of us has many preconceptions about people who are so labeled. We might expect that such a person has bizarre behaviours, is unable to maintain a job or care for a family, is dangerous, and needs to be locked up for his or her "own good". In any individual case or in most cases, such expectations may not be valid; but they are likely to influence how we perceived and react to the individual. Our expectations may also influence the labeled person's behaviour. If we expect individuals to be bizarre, and we respond according to our expectations, these persons are more likely to behave in a way that conforms to our expectations – they are more likely to be bizarre!

Thomas Szasz (1961, 1970), a psychiatrist, and Nicholas Kittrie (1971), a professor of law, have both criticized the diagnostic system because of its stigmatizing effects. Once labeled with a category of severe mental disturbance, people may have difficulty finding jobs and places to live; their civil right may be violated in the name of treatment. The stigmatization because of a psychiatric label appears to be sometimes used purposely to destroy the credibility of political dissenters. In 1979, a Russian Army general was found mentally ill after he began to dissent with the political powers in the Soviet Union. The Russian psychiatrists who examined him found that he was suffering from "choice paranoia"; three United State psychiatrists found him to be "perfectly sane". Psychiatrist Alan Stone, of Harvard, concluded that this case confirms that psychiatry (and by extension, psychology) is sometimes used as a tool of political repression.

SALIENT FEATURES OF DSM-III

The German Psychiatrist Emil Kraepelin is credited with developing the first systematic and widely accepted classification scheme for mental disorder.

He noted that certain symptom patterns occurred with sufficient regularity to be used as a basis for identifying and classifying mental disorders. The classification scheme he developed is the basis of our present day diagnostic system.

A guiding philosophy behind Kraepelin's works was the belief that once various forms of mental illness were successfully distinguished and classified, then one presumably would be able to predict the outcome of a specific type of disorder. Classification, according to Kraepelin, would also provide a framework within which medical research could begin to look for agents responsible for the disease and treatment methods for curing it. The nosological system be developed greatly influenced the field of psychiatry for many years during which time great emphasis was put on the description and classification of disorders.

The present day classification system had its beginning in the diagnostic structure of the Association of Medical Superintendents of American Institutions for the Insane (1914). However, this early diagnostic system did not include many important disorders and the categories used were not easy to agree upon. Efforts to develop a more comprehensive and reliable system continued throughout the twentieth century. In 1939, the World Health Organization (WHO) developed a diagnostic system that was revised in 1948 and again in 1978. Partly because of differences of opinion regarding certain diagnostic classifications such as homosexuality, the WHO system has not been widely used in the United States, and other countries.

In 1952, the American Psychiatric Association published its first Diagnostic and Statistical Manual (DSM-I). Though it was one of the first system to be accepted among most mental health disciplines, it was flawed. The authors had difficulty agreeing on the system's central organizing principles, and this resulted in a hodgepodge of classification that was often applied inconsistently.

DSM-II (1968) represented an attempt to respond to the shortcomings of DSM-I by using symptoms as the central organizing factors in the determination of diagnostic categories. Its authors sought to delineate "clusters" of symptoms in hopes of making diagnosis more reliable. However, because the system depended heavily on human judgment to identify the symptoms, there continued to be a low level of agreement among psychiatric diagnosticians (Spitzer & Wilson 1975). Further there was little attempt to deal with how the disorders came about (etiology) so that unlike physical disorder diagnoses which direct treatments, the DSM-II diagnoses often did not provide clear therapeutic guidance.

The valid criticisms and dissatisfactions expressed about DSM-II led finally to a major revision of the system. In 1974, the American Psychiatric Association began development of the third edition, DSM-III. The task force and advisory committees which worked on the revision were large, totaling almost 200 members. Although these groups were composed mainly of psychiatrists, a significant number of representative from psychology, social work, and the other mental health clinical and research fields were also involved. Many professional organizations acted as reviewers of prepublication drafts. From late 1977 to late 1979, a series of field trails used the new materials, and subsequent modifications were made. The final product was completed and published in 1980.

The Diagnostic and Statistical Manual, third edition (DSM-III, 1980), lists and describes over 200 specific diagnostic categories or disorders. Its descriptive approach does not assume that sharp boundaries must exist among diagnostic entities. The manual's designers assume that individuals identified as belonging in a particulars category will manifest a least the defining criteria of the category. DSM-III is a prototype classification approach, similar to that described by Cantor and colleagues (1980). While there are many similarities in the categories of DSM-II and DSM-III, there also are some significant differences. Some disorders listed in DSM-II are no longer included, and some new categories have been added to DSM-III.

Thus, we see that, DSM-III differs from DSM-II in many specific details some disorders have been renamed, some added, some dropped, some subdivided in new ways, in keeping with recent research findings. The new edition also differs from its predecessor in three important general respects.

(a) **Specific Diagnostic Criteria:** First, the criteria for diagnosis have been made much more specific. In contrast to DSM-II's brief and rather general descriptions, DSM-III offers extensive and highly detailed descriptions for the different diagnostic categories. These description include:

1. Essential features of the disorder, those that "define" it.

2. Association features, those that are usually present.

3. Diagnostic criteria, a list of symptoms (taken from the lists of essential and association features) that must be present for the patient to be give this diagnostic label.

4. Information on differential diagnosis-that is, how to distinguish this disorder from other disorders with which it might be confused.

In addition, the descriptions offer information on the course of the disorder, age at onset, degree of impairment, complications involved, predisposing factors, prevalence, sex ratio, and family pattern (that is, whether the disorder tends to run in families). However, the most important feature of the descriptions is the highly specific quality of the diagnostic criteria.

(b) **Five Axes of Diagnosis:** A second important change is that DSM-III requires that much more information be given about the patient in the process of diagnosis. DSM-II called for nothing more than a simple diagnostic label. DSM-III, in contrast, instructs the diagnostician to evaluate the patient on five different "axes", or areas of functioning:

Axis I: Clinical psychiatric syndrome: the diagnostic label for the patient's most serious psychological problem, the problem for which he or she is being diagnosed.

(This is the only information that DSM-II required)

Axis II: Personality disorders (adults) or specific developmental disorders (children and adolescents): any accompanying adjustment disorders not covered by the Axis I label.

Axis III: Physical disorders: any medical problems that may be relevant to the psychological problem.

Axis IV: Psychosocial stressors: current sources of stress (e.g., divorce, retirement, miscarriage) that may have contributed to the patient's psychological problem.

Axis V: Highest level of adaptive functioning during the past year: a rating of the patient's adjustment – occupational functioning, social relationships, use of leisure time – within the past year.

Thus, whereas with DSM-II a patient's diagnosis might have been simply "alcohol addiction", under the new system he might be diagnosed as follows:

Axis I	:	Alcohol dependence
Axis II	:	Avoidant personality disorder
Axis III	:	Diabetes
Axis IV	:	Loss of Job.
		One child moved out of house
		Marital conflict.
Axis V	:	Fair.

Needless to say, this offers a good deal more information about the patient-information that may be useful in devising a treatment program. Furthermore, such five-part diagnoses may be extremely helpful to researchers trying to discover connections between psychological disorders and other factors, such as stress and physical illness.

(c) **Unspecified Etiology-** A final important difference between DSM-II and DSM-III is that the latter avoids any suggestion as to the cause of disorder unless the cause has been definitely established. This new policy has necessitated some substantial changes in the classification system. For example, the term "neurosis" has been dropped altogether, since it implies a Freudian interpretation (i.e., that the disorder is due to anxiety over repressed wishes or conflicts). Likewise, whereas DSM-II subdivided severe depression according to whether it was caused by environmental stress or by some presumed biological dysfunction, unsupported by research, is no longer made in DSM-III. In other words, DSM-III aims simply to name the disorders and to describe them as clearly and specifically as possible their causes, if they are not known, are not speculated upon.

The major goal of the DSM-III revision is to solve the problem mentioned above and that diagnostic groups created according to the earlier DSM categories were too heterogeneous to aid researchers in locating causes and treatments for the various disorders. To put it in the vocabulary of psychological assessment, what the new edition attempts to do is improve the reliability and validity of psychiatric diagnosis.

GENERAL CRITICISMS OF DSM-III

Although DSM-III has attempted to consider the concerns of critics (e.g. Feighner, 1979 M.A. Taylor & Heiser, 1979) who have argued for a descriptive a theoretical approach to the classification of disturbed human functioning, many criticisms applicable to DSM-I and DSM-II still apply. For example, the fact that DSM-III has redefined several disorders raise the question whether the categories describe stable entities. Gergen (1973) argues that classification should focus on the enduring phenomena such as behaviours, rather than on conceptual entities such as "diseases", which may be considered pathological only because of a prevailing cultural belief at a particular time. As a case in point, we can consider homosexuality. In early editions of DSM, published at a time when sexual attitudes were very constricted, homosexuality was considered a mental disorder. Today sexual attitudes are more liberal, and homosexuality is diagnosed in DSM-III as a mental disorder only if the homosexual persistently desires to be heterosexual.

McLemore and Benjamin (1979) have described the shortcomings of DSM-III. Some of these are a continued reliance on impressionistic clinical judgment, continued use of an implicit illness model, and what they consider to be almost total neglect of social-psychological variables and interpersonal behaviour. They argue that abnormal behaviour is primarily as issue of problematic interactions, rather than on the internal pathology of the individual. While DSM-III tries to include issues off psychosocial functioning and adaptation, it seems to ignore the fact that problems may occur in a relationship between two people, rather than be vested within an individual.

Impressionistic clinical judgment still remains a primary problem in the use of DSM-III. The types of ratings used on Axes Iv to V are extremely global and sensitive to a great deal of subjective judgement. This subjectivity is likely to result in a lack of reliability. The DSM-III system still lacks a process for the rigorous and systematic description of social behaviour that many feel is critical for the effective definition and treatment of disordered functioning.

The diagnostic reliability of DSM-III appears more adequate than that of previous editions. In early field trails (Spitzer & Forman, 1979; Spitzer, Forman, & Nee, 1979), 274 clinicians were paired and made diagnoses of a total of 281 patients. Most clinicians assessed 2 patients each. A prepublication draft of DSM-I and DSM-II. However, other studies have been less positive. Mezzich and Mezzich (1979) found a poor degree of agreement between clinicians using DSM-III criteria on diagnoses of childhood and adolescent behaviour disorders. At best, only 4 out of 10 clinicians agreed on the diagnoses of childhood disorders using the DSM-III criteria. DSM-III has not totally solved the problem of the lack of reliability of diagnoses. However, studies conducted after DSM-III has been more widely used and clinicians have gained experience, may indicate greater reliability (Scheftner, 1980).

PSYCHOLOGICALASSESSMENT

Psychological assessment, according to Sundberg and Tyler is "The Systematic collection, organization and interpretation of information about a person and his situation".

Psychological assessment is also sometimes called as clinical assessment. Such an assessment is concerned with identifying and nature and severity of maladaptive behaviour on the part of the individual or group and with understanding the conditions that have caused and/or are maintaining the maladaptive behaviour.

Psychological assessment has wide variety of uses. Some of which are as follows:

(1) To identify the nature and severity of the individual's maladaptive behaviour.

(2) Provide a basis for discussing the problem with the individual, his family of the group.

(3) Detect pathological trends before a disorder becomes acute or to anticipate possible problems and help the person prevent them.

(4) Plan an appropriate treatment programme and make needed modifications as therapy progresses

(5) Evaluate given treatment procedures and outcomes.

(6) In many, instances, clinical assessment data can also be used to increase self understanding. For e.g., helping the individual better understand his motives, feelings, attitudes and maladaptive coping patterns.

Psychological Assessment is a great source of information, a wide variety of methods are used to yield a wide variety of information from the subjects. Table 3.1 lists the various sources or methods of psychological assessment.

Table 3.1

Sources of information in psychological assessment

Source	**Variants**	**Information Yield**
Observation	1. Direct observation (natural setting)	1. Reactions to everyday situations. Scars, Tattoos. Expressive behaviours. Characteristic modes of responding to specific persons. Ratings of any of these.
	2. Direct observation (laboratory)	2. Reactions to "rigged" stimuli. Information about specific behaviours under controlled conditions. Ratings of any of these.
	3. Indirect observation	3. Reports or ratings by others who remember (or do not) the subject.
Interview	1. Employment of personal interview 2. Diagnostic interview 3. Stress interview	1. Information for and about job candidate. Generally, the interview yields data about content of individual's thinking. 2. In medicine, the past history of the patient. In psychological assessment, the mental status of the respondent. 3. Reactions of persons under unusual or stressful conditions.
Psychological tests	1. Self-report inventories	1. Responses about personal habits, attitudes, beliefs, or fantasies.
	2. Projective tests	2. Responses to ambiguous or unstructured situation. These responses are assumed to reflect inner states of the person.

Thus from the above table we see that following are important techniques or methods of assessment.

1. Interview or clinical interview.

2. Psychological tests

3. Observation

CHARACTERISTICS OF EFFECTIVE ASSESSMENT

To be useful to clinical evaluator, assessment procedures should possess certain attributes: validity, reliability, standardization, and norms. These published by joint committee of the American Psychological Association, the American Education Research Association, and the National Council on Measurement in Education in 1974. the first and foremost attribute of an assessment procedure established by the joint commission is its validity.

(a) **Validity:** if an assessment procedure measures what it is supposed to it is said to be valid. For example, for the Scholastic Aptitude Test (SAT), a test purporting to measure knowledge necessary for college achievement, to be valid, students who do well on the SAT should also do well in college. If this correlation occurs, then the SAT is said to possess some amount of predictive validity. Predictive validity is also important in the area of abnormal behaviour. Often professional are asked to predict the future behaviour of their patients. Known as "making the prognosis," such predictions re usually based on information obtained from a variety of assessment procedures. The more accurate the predictions, the higher the predictive validity.

(b) **Reliability:** If an assessment procedure measures something in a consistent fashion, it possesses reliability. It is possible for an assessment procedure to measure some characteristic consistently but still not be valid because the characteristic may not be what the test is supposed to measure. For example, if a test of anxiety has items that are so obviously related to anxiety that, rather than admit to anxiety, people consistently answer items to put themselves in a "good light", the test would be reliable but not valid. Perhaps the best way to describe the relationship between reliability and validity is to say that reliability is a necessary but not sufficient attribute of an assessment procedure, but validity is essential.

There are to major kinds of reliability that are of great interest to students of abnormal psychology: test-retest and inter judge reliabilities. Test-retest reliability is assessed by calculating how similar results are when administering the same assessment procedure twice. The more similar t he results, the higher the test-retest reliability.

While test-retest reliability refers to consistency over test and time, interjudge reliability refers to consistency of opinions among judge. There are many times in the study of abnormal behaviours, when people are asked to judge the behaviour of others. Nowhere is the process more important than when judges are asked to decide whether or not someone belongs in a particular diagnostic category. Should two or more people observe the behaviour of a patient and be asked to diagnose the patient, interjudge reliability would be high if all judges agree on particular diagnosis.

However as is too often the case in field of abnormal psychology, here may be some disagreement among the judges which leads to a lowered interjudge reliability. For example, in many instances the interjudge reliability of DSM-II was low (Blashfield, 1973). The development of operational criteria in DSM-III was one attempt to increase diagnostic interjudge reliability, and data presented by Spitzer et al.,, (1979) suggest that the attempt has been successful.

(d) **Standardization:** The concept of standardizing assessment procedures is an intuitively obvious one. It simply means making sure that all materials and instructions given to the test takers are identical so that all administrations of the assessment procedure are the same for all subjects. Without standardization, results between various administrations of the assessment procedures are not comparable.

(e) **Norms:** in addition to assessment procedures being valid, reliable, and standardized, they need to have acceptable norms. Scores obtained as a result of an assessment procedure receive their meaning by being compared with normative groups. Normative groups help to answer such questions as: "Is a person's score higher of lower than average?" To know that a person's score on a test of anxiety is, for example, 60, is virtually meaningless until it is also known that the average score of a group of people possessing similar characteristics to that of the test taker is 40. if it also known that only 2 people of 100 in the normative group scored 60 or above, then the subject's score of 60 suggests strongly that he or she may be quite anxious.

The composition of the normative group is critical to making generalization about test scores. For example, if the person being assessed is very different from those people composing the normative group, then although they are difficult to obtain, representative norms are very important to the development of adequate assessment procedures.

PROBLEMS OF ASSESSMENT

Various assessment techniques pose a wide variety of problems. Many experts as well as general public view assessment with suspicious and hostility. The development of such an attitude is due to he invasion of privacy and over the possible misuse of test information.

Additional impetus has derived from concern over the cultural bias of many psychological tests, and over the use of such tests for arbitrarily labeling people and assigning them to psychiatric categories-often with damaging consequences of their general well-being, career opportunities, and total life situation.

We would discuss the following problems of assessment in brief:

1. **Confidentiality and Informed Consent:** Psychological tests and other assessment procedures often elicit very personal information. The implicit or explicit agreements of the professional clinician to keep this information confidential is a basic component in the client-professional relationship. In fact, the loss of confidentiality seriously endangers the very relationship on which professional mental health personnel must rely if they are to render effective service.

The problem of safeguarding assessment data initially appears to be a simple one; in the field of law any information supplied by the client to his attorney is held inviolate unless the client consents to its release. In the mental health field, however, ii is not so simple. For one thing, it may be advisable to share such information with parents, teachers, or other personnel who will be involved in planning and carrying out treatment. In addition, there are a number of special circumstances in which the disturbed person's right to confidentiality may be abridge, as when there is reason to believe that he may be dangerous to himself or others, or when legal authorities request such information. In fact, under some circumstances, professional mental health personnel are obligated to reveal information to legal authorities and are themselves subject to fine or imprisonment for failure to do so.

Most authorities agree that getting free and informed consent from the client is the safest method of preventing invasion of privacy. It is recommended that before assessment is undertaken, the client should be informed of the limits of confidentiality; then, if he takes part in assessment, his participation is presumably based on free and informed consent.

The two most important concepts associated with privacy and confidentiality of test results are, relevance of the information that is elicited from the subject and informed consent. During testing we must only use those tests that will give us information about he subjects behaviour relevant for our present or future purpose. No attempt should be made to seek information which is not related to our purpose, eliciting information from the subject through psychological testing, not relevant to our stated purposes, constitutes a breach of his privacy and is against the code of ethics.

By informed consent we mean that the examinee is not forced to testing. He is informed about the purpose of testing, the kind of data sought and the use that will be made of his scores.

One of the fundamental questions with regards to confidentiality of test results is that who shall have access to the test results of an examinee and for that purposes. Of course, and examinee has full right not only to know his test results but also to comment on the contents of his reports and if necessary to clarify or correct factual information. However, when an individual is a minor-his parents or guardians has a right to have access to his ward's test results, but this should not be the case with adults.

Generally the discussion of confidentiality of test results has usually dealt with accessibility to a third person, other than the individual tested (or parent of a minor) and the examiner. The underlying principle is that such records should not be released without the knowledge and consent of the individual.

2. **The issue of cultural bias:** Most psychological tests have been designed by Middle-class psychologists for prediction of performance valued by middle-class people, and many have been standardized on white subjects from predominantly middle or upper socio-economic levels. It would be expected that persons from other backgrounds might be handicapped in taking such tests and that their scores would not be a fair measure of their potential.

Most of the psychological tests that we use in India, has not been standardized on Indian population or Indian conditions. These tests are mere adaptations of tests developed on other culture. Hence their use in India is of doubtful validity.

The issue of cultural bias in tests has been of special concern in the movement toward greater equality or opportunity for racial minorities during the last decade. In 1971 the U.S. Supreme Court ruled the employers could not require individuals to pass a standardized intelligence test as a condition of employment unless such a test could be shown to be directly related to job performance. It is widely believed that in the past such test have, in effect, been used as a means of excluding minority-group individuals from certain jobs where employers have traditionally given preference to whites.

As yet, no completely culture-free psychological test has been developed. Such tests must have content of some kind, and the meaning any content will have for the person being tested depends partly on his previous experience. Even nonverbal psychological test are not completely free of this dependence on past experience. A great deal of research effort, however, has gone into attempts to develop tests of intelligence and other abilities that are "culture fair". Unfortunately, serious questions remain concerning the actual validity and "bias free" nature of such tests.

Minority groups sometimes charge cultural bias in testing on still other grounds. A test on which a ghetoo resident does poorly may, in fact, give an accurate prediction of how he will perform on a job requiring middle-class behaviour and attitudes, while failing to reveal many skills and abilities that he does have. Is he therefore to be rejected unless he can be taught to show the middle-class behaviour and attitudes? The problem here is in what the objectives of tested should be – whether they should be for screening out those who do not conform to the current accepted mold or for identifying more diverse kinds of talents. Many persons who have been denied equal opportunity in the past see tests as a way of continuing to exclude them, a way of maintaining to status-quo.

3. **Criticism of Psychological test theory:** As even more basic challenge to the use of psychological tests in clinical assessment has stemmed from psychologist's own questioning of the long-accepted assumption that maladjustive behaviour can best be understood by looking within the individual at his traits and characteristics. The whole concept of putting a person in a category and giving him a label places the emphasis on internal causation of his behaviour. The development of tests to assess these continuing inner characteristic was a logical extension of this concept. Although the contributing influence of he environment was never denied, more or less stable traits within the individual were assumed to account for the consistency in his behaviour.

Evidence from two sources has been altering this view:

(a) The study of groups as social systems has repeatedly shown the extent to which social goals, role requirements, and other group conditions determine the feelings, behaviours, and even abilities of individual members, although their behaviour may remain consistent so long as their social setting remains the same.

(b) The dramatic changes in behaviour brought about by changes in reinforcement contingencies have demonstrated how inconstant many supposed "inner characteristics" may be.

Both these development call into question the concept of entities within the individual. Although they do not demonstrate that internal conditions can be disregarded, their net effect has been to lower clinicians' expectations of what test will be able to predict. Of the time now allotted to the psychosocial assessment of the individual, a far higher proportion is given to assessment of his transaction with his social environment. Much of the behaviour observed does not fit anywhere in the established classification scheme, and result is a further disenchantment with classification and labeling in general.

4. **Communication Test Result:** Another major problem of assessment of testing is with respect to communication.

The language of psychological testing is highly scientific and it makes use of certain technical terms which is unique to this field. Such a technical or scientific language, many a times, creates difficulties because often an examiner has to communicate test results to persons who are either laymen or who don't know much about this field. Under such circumstances, communication not only becomes difficult but at times it can be misinterpreted and misunderstood. Hence, psychologists have devoted much attention to communication of test results in a form that will be meaningful, useful and unlikely to be misinterpreted.

Many are of the view that the information should not be transmitted routinely but should be accompanied by interpretive explanations in simple non-technical terms by a trained professional. It should be remembered that report should not just merely be handed over to the subject but a discussion should be accompanied while handing over the report to an individual (in case of minors with their parents or guardians) so that clarifications are made, if any, and at the same time the examiner will come to know about the discrepancies that exist between the subject's self-perception and the test result. It is desirable to take into account an individual's general personality characteristic and his socio-cultural background. This helps not only in communicating factual information but also makes the communicated information much more meaningful.

PSYCHOLOGICAL ASSESSMENT THROUGH PSYCHOLOGICAL TESTS

The primary purpose of using psychological tests is to obtain information that will aid the clinician and the client. Tests are often used in conjunction with the clinical interviews, because of the belief that the tests will provide a more detailed assessment of the client's assets, deficits and potentials. In contrast to most interviews, tests are more structured and quantifiable. In addition, tests are efficient and can provide a great deal of information with less expenditure of time and effort than many other assessment approaches.

The following are some of the most frequently used tests as observed by Lubin et.al. (1985).

1. Wechsler Adult Intelligence Scale.
2. Minnesota Multiphasic Personality Inventory.
3. Bender-Gestalt Visual Motor Test.
4. Rorschach.
5. Thermatic Apperception Test.
6. Wechsler Intelligence Scale for Children.

7. Peabody Picture Vocabulary Test.

8. Sentence Completion Test.

9. House Tree – Persons

10. Draw A Person

We would discussed some of the commonly used tests. These include-

I. Personality tests, or Inventories.

II. Projective Techniques.

III. Intelligence tests.

I. Personality Tests or Inventories

Some clinicians use "objective" tests such as personality inventories to measure personality and clinical variables. These inventories usually have people respond to a series of written statements (Such as "I like fast cars") by answering either "true", "false", or indicating that they are unsure. The tests are considered objective, partly because the statements are much less ambiguous than the stimuli in a projective test. In addition, the process through which the tests are developed is much less reliant upon the speculative theorizing and clinical inference which characterizes the early development of the projective technique.

Although many objective personality tests have been developed, the Minnesota Multiphasic Personality Inventory (MMPTI) remains among the most popular in clinical and research settings (J.R. Graham, 1978). For example, Dahlstrom (1974) reports that at least 11000 studies using this instrument had been published by the mid 1970s.

Minnesota Multiphasic Personality Inventory: The 566 – item MMPI was developed in 1943 (Hathaway & Mackinley, 1943). The test constructors gathered many items that could be answered "true", "false", or "cannot say". These items were grouped into clinical scales, depending on how well responses to the item distinguished various groups of patients identified as belonging to a particular diagnostic category from patient groups and people who were not psychiatric patients. The items cover a wide range of areas including fears, social interests, sexual behaviour, and physical health. Some sample items are the following: "I am likely not to speak to people unit they speak to me", "I loved may father". The result of this effort was the identification of nine clinical scales, each related to a different disorder.

Four additional scales were developed – some what differently. The lie scale (L) contains 15 items which measure the subject' denial of common frailties; for example, one item is "I never tell a lie". A "true" response to this item raises suspicion about the openness of the subject's self report. The Frequency Scale (F) contains items which, if endorsed, indicate that the subject was careless or confused about taking the test. The Correction Scale (K) measures defensiveness, and the Question Scale (?) measures evasiveness. The complete list of scales and the original interpretation of elevated scores appear in Table 3.2.

Table 3.2 MMPI scales and original interpretations of elevated scores

Title	Abbre viation	Scale number	Interpretation
Lie	L	-	Denial of common frailties
Question	?	-	Evasiveness
Frequency	F	-	Invalidity of profile
Correction	K	-	Defensive, evasive
Hypochondriasis	Hs	1	Emphasis on physical complaints
Depression	D	2	Unhappy, depressed.
Hysteria	Hy	3	Hysterical symptomatology
Psychopathic	Pd	4	Lack of social conformity often in trouble with law.
Masculinity tion Femininity	Mf	5	Effeminate (males); mesculine orienta- (females)
Paranoia	Pa	6	Suspicious
Psychasthenia	Pt	7	Worried, arodous
Schizophrenia	Sc	8	Withdrawn; bizarre thinking
Hypomania	Ma	9	Impulsive; expansive
Social intro Version-extroversion	Si	0	Interoverted, Shy

The MMPI has several clinical uses, like other psychological tests, it is used to identify the appropriate categorization of clients. It may also be used for treatment planning and the development of recommendations. In clinical research the MMPI is particularly useful because of its standardization, ease of administration, and reputation for reliability. The MMPI is highly efficient in terms of human labour and costs, particularly when the assessments are scored, interpreted, and typed by a computer.

The MMPI is not without problems. The sampling procedures used in its development have been sharply criticized. Norman (1972) has pointed out that the sample of patients and the nonpatient controls did not represent a broad crossection of either group. In addition, the definition of the diagnostic categories used as reference groups were vague and may have contained subjects who were not representative of the specific disorders.

In spite of these criticisms, the MMPI remains one of the more reliable and useful personality tests. A recent study found considerable stability in MMPI profiles of individuals tested repeatedly over a 30-year period while they aged from an average of 49 to 77 years. (Lenon et al. 1979). Changes in scores were consistent with changes that would be expected in people as they aged. The clinical validity of the MMPI has also been found to be high. For example, H.A. Skinner and Jackson (1978) have found thar the MMPI was accurate 76 percent of the time in differentiating between severely and moderately disturbed clinical groups. Hathaway (1972), one of the test's originators, has pointed out that the MMPI's primary utility lies in obtaining a large amount of data with a minimal expenditure of energy.

II Projective Techniques

Unlike self-report tests of personality that generally consist of straight forward verbal statements the require a fixed kind of response, projective techniques consist of ambiguous stimuli to which a person can rêplay in limitless ways. The projective approach is based on the belief that, if people are given amorphous stimuli such as inkblots or vague pictures to look at, they will tend to project onto these amorphous stimuli their inner feelings, drives, and needs. Leonardo da Vinci reportedly used images seen in clouds and fireplace ashes to test the creativity of his students and to again some insight into their personalities (Exner, 1976). Projective techniques can be less susceptible to "faking" than self-report inventories. Test takers usually have a difficult time figuring out how their responses will be scored, thus making it difficult time figuring out how their responses will be scored, thus making it difficult for them to make the test "come out" in any certain way. For instance, what does it mean to see fog in an inkblot? Does it suggest anxiety, depression, or perhaps something else?

Some of the most commonly used projective techniques are as follows:

(A) Rorschach Inkblot Test, and

(B) TAT

(A) Rorschach Inkblot Test: The Rorschach test consist of 10 cards having bilateral symmetrical Inkblots. Half of the cards are achromatic and other five share one or more colours. The cares are presented to the subjects in a definite sequence. Rorschach did not impose any time limit on this test nor do present users. There is also freedom to give any type of responses and as many type of responses that are possible.

Administration of Rorschach: While administering the test, the examiner notes various aspects of subject's behaviour. He keeps a verbatim record of the responses, notes the time elapsed between the presentation of each card and the first response to it (called as initial reaction time) length of the pauses between responses, total time required for each card and the subject's extraneous movements, spontaneous remarks, emotional expressions and any other specific behaviours which appear significant to the examiner.

After all the 10 cards have been presented in a sequential order another phase called as the inquiry phase starts in which the examiner questions the individual systematically regarding the parts and aspects of each blot to which the associations were given. The two most important purposes of the inquiry are:

(1) First, to determine which aspects of blot initiated and sustained the association process,

(2) Second, the inquiry gives the subject an opportunity to add, elaborate or to clarify his original response, but if this is done it must completely spontaneous on the part of the subject and without any suggestions from the examiners.

Several scoring categories for Rorschach test have developed but the most commonly scored categories are location, determinant, content, originals and popular and the form quality i.e. accuracy of perception.

(i) **Location:** Location responses refer to the area of the blot which has been perceived by the subject as the basis of his response. The subject many respond to entire blot to a large or small portion of it or to small minute detail and sometimes even to the white background. The location responses can be very well defined or only vaguely defined. The location response to the test are categorized into following classes: 'W' (responses to the Whole blot). 'D' (responses to large usual details), 'Dd' (responses to small unusual details) and 'S' (responses to white space of the card). The location responses can be given by combining some of the above categories for e.g. D and S also be perceived together.

The location responses and the subject's ability to delineate them are regarded as indicative of subject's organizing process and the ability to analyze and articulate the part of every day experience. The analysis of the subject's location response is made in the light of norms prepared by the test author.

(ii) **Determinants:** Determinants refer to the characteristics of the inkblot as perceived by the subject. They are those qualities of the blot that have produced the response to it, four such determinants are form, shading, colour and movement. Although there is of coursed no movement in the blot itself, the respondent's perception of the blot as a representation of a moving object is scored in this category. Further differentiations are made within these categories. Movement (FM) or inanimate movement (M). Similarly, form may be perceived with ordinary accuracy (F), with unusual accuracy (F+) or in a very poor accuracy (F). Shading may be perceived as representing depth (V) or texture (T) which can be perceived in its pure form (V to T) or it can be combined with form (FV, VE, FT, TF). Colour can be perceived along with form being dominant (PC) or colour being dominant (CF). Colour can be perceived all by itself also (C). These are some of the commonly scored categories of determinants as developed by Rorschach and various other systematizes.

Determinants reveal a lot of information about a wide variety of personality characteristics. They tell us about one's & emotionality, imagination, fantasy life, an individual's ability to indulge in creative and conceptual thinking, about ego strength, conflicts, oppositional tendency etc.

(iii) **Content-**The treatment of content varies from one scoring system to another, some emphasizing it heavily whereas others ignoring it altogether. Some of the commonly scored content categories are Human (H), Animal (A), Human detail (Hd), Animal detail (Ad), Clouds (Cl), Botany (Bt), blood (BL), Sexual materials (Sx), X-Rays, Anatomy (At) etc. Content categories help us to discover many important aspects of subjects behaviour. Content analysis is a source of ascertaining the subject's personal meanings. Attitudes, interests and even complexes. Content responses are supposed to possess psychiatric and psychoanalytic interpretations often pointing towards pathological tendencies present in the subject.

(iv) **Originals and Popular:** This scoring category tells us whether subject's responses are common or original. A popularity score is often found on the basis of the relative frequency of different responses among people in general. However, there is often differences of opinions among specialties as to which responses should be regarded as original and which as popular. Popular responses help us to know about an individuals interpersonal behaviour. It also tells us whether an individual is socially confirming or conventional in this approach or not.

(v) Total number of Responses and Rejection: Besides these four scoring categories, discussed above, we also take into account the total number of responses (R) given by the subject and rejections if there are any i.e., a subject may not give any response to a particular card. These two scoring categories also provide us with important information about many aspects of subject's personality.

The nature of the Roischach test makes it an important tool which can be used with any age group, any cultural group and which docs not make any demand on the part of the subject. It can, very easily, be used with illiterates and culturally backward groups.

The normative data on Rorschach was originally derived in large part from adult groups. In recent years normative data has also been prepared for younger and older age groups. Ames and her coworkers and also Exner have published Rorschach norms for children as young as 2 years and other persons upto even above 70 years.

Rorschach is a continuously developing test. Recent research has some what modified, clarified and contradicted some of the earlier Rorschach hypothesis and studies demonstrating their refutations, clarifications and modifications.

(B) Thematic Apperception Test: The only other projective technique that has approached the Rorschach method in amount of use and volume of research is the T.A.T. which was introduced by C.D. Morgan and Henry A. Murray in 1935 as a method to explore the unconscious thoughts and fantasies.

Murray found that T. A. T. enabled the trained examiner to interpret and to reconstruct on the basis of subjects stories, his dominant drives, emotions, sentiments, complexes and conflicts. Although the TAT was at first slow in gaining wide acceptance, it is now a test that approximates the Rorschach in popularity and in amount of research it has stimulated.

At first it gained popularity only among clinical psychologists, but gradually, it became a research tool in developmental, social and personality psychology- and in the cross cultural studies in Anthropology. It is also used for

personality assessment in the fields of counseling and Industrial Psychology.

In contrast to the Inkblot techniques, which we discussed above, the Thematic Apperception Test (T.A.T) presents more highly structured stimuli and requires more complex and meaningfully organized verbal responses.

Interpretation of the responses by the examiner is usually based on content analysis of a rather qualitative nature. Murray's system for scoring TAT is largely qualitative whereas Mcclelland and Eron has developed a highly quantitative system for scoring and interpreting TAT responses.

Administration of TAT : The third revision of TAT consists of 30 pictures and blank card. The pictures have been selected and marked in such a way that there are four sets of 20 cards each, one for boys, one for girls, one for males and one for females, over 14 years. The testing process is divided into two sessions and for each of these it is suggested that no more than 10 TAT cards be administered with at least one day intervening between the two sessions. More recently practical consideration have led to reduction in the number of cards administered. Most testers now present the subject with 8 to 12 cards and use only single session. The cards are presented individually and the respondent is instructed to provide a story about the picture that described the depicted scene, what led up to it, what the characters in the picture are thinking and what the outcome will be.

Although typically administered as an oral test in clinical situation, the TAT may also be administered in writing and as a group test.

Scoring of TAT: Like Rorschach the TAT also has multiple scoring system. Murray's lack of detailed scoring instructions in his manual and the relative case with which the TAT can be administered have been cited as factors contributing to the multiplicity of scoring system (Murstein 1963). Furthermore, the non-technical nature of the TAT and the simple verbal contents of stories have encouraged clinicians to invent their own system of analysis. Some important TAT scoring systems arc as follows :

(a) Murray's Scoring System (Non quantitative),

(b) Mcclelland's system (Quantitative), and

(c) Eron's System (Quantitative).

Here we will examine Murray's Scoring system in brief. Although amenable to quantification, Murray's recommended system of analysis is highly content oriented and relies heavily on the qualitative characteristics of the stories.

(i) **The Hero:** The first step in the analysis of the story is to distinguish the hero or the character with whom the subject seemed to have identified in principle. This would be the character in whom the story teller is most interested and the individual who mostly resembles him. The tester must be aware to the fact that the hero of the story may shift from one story character to another or that there may be no hero in the story. The interpreter should direct his attention to following aspects of the hero's personality. His intelligence achievement ability, conflicts, leadership qualities, feeling etc.

(ii) **Needs of the Hero:** After the identification of the hero heroes the interpreter must formulate the reactions of the hero to various forces. These formulations are usually influenced by the theoretical orientations of the test interpreter. However, Murray recommends that this may be accomplished within a classification of the needs of the hero. The needs can be either primary or secondary.

(iii) **Environmental:** Forces are categorized according to their effect on the hero. Murray's system consists of a comprehensive list of environmental forces or presses. These presses could be real or imaginary and include aggression in which the hero's property and or possessions are destroyed. Dominance, where the hero is exposed to commands, order or forceful arguments and rejection in which persons reject, repudiate, are indifferent or leave the hero.

(iv) **Outcomes:** Outcome refers to the results of the story. It refers to the relative strength of the forces emitting from the hero and the strengths of these. The amount of frustration and hero ships experienced and the relative degree of success and failure of the hero must be assessed.

(v) **Themes or themas:** Themes or themas refer to the interplay within the story of the hero's needs, presses and successful or unsuccessful resolutions of his conflicts. Themes represent need-press combination, it can be simple or complex.

(vi) **Interests, sentiments and relationship:** These are the last category to be scored. In this a note is made of the various interests, sentiments and interpersonal relationship as expressed in the stones by the subject.

A great deal of normative information is available regarding the most frequent responses characteristic of each card including the way each card is perceived, the themes developed, the roles ascribed to the characters, emotional tones expressed, speed of responses, length of responses, length of stories etc. (Atkinson 1956, Herin 1956, Murstein 1972). These available normative studies provide a general framework for interpreting individual responses, however, most clinicians "rely heavily on subjective norms' which they have developed as a result of their experience with the test.

III. **Intelligence:** Tests are another widely used group of test. Beginning from the pioneering works of Alfred Binet, Intelligence testing movement has developed to a massive extent. Today there are wise variety of intelligence tests which can be used individually and in group setting also.

Some of the commonly used tests of intelligence tests are as follows:

(a) **Binet tests** developed in 1905, 1908 and 1911.

(b) **Stanford Binet** Scales: After Binet's death in 1911, Binet tests underwent more and more revision, especially in America. The most widely used revision of this test come to be called as Stanford Binet revision or test, because these tests were revised under the direction of Prof. L.M. Terman at Stanford University.

The following are the important revisions of this test.

1. 1916 Stanford Binet Scale.

2. 1937 Revision of the Stanford Binct Scales which had two form called as form L and M.

3. 1960revisionoftheStanford--Binct Scales.

4. Thel972revisionofStanfordBinet Scales.

(c) Wcchsler Scales were originally developed to measure adult intelligence. Today there are Wechsler Scales or children and infants too.

We will now discuss the Wechsler Adult Intelligence Scale as it is the most widely used intelligence test in a clinical set up.

Wechsler Adult Intelligence Scale : David Whechsler developed an intelligence test to measure intelligence of an adult individual. Wechsler Scales differ from intelligence Scale like Stanford-Binet and Binet Simon scale in many ways. It is a point scale rather than age scales. In this scale all the items of a given type are grouped into subtests and arranged in an increasing order of difficulty within each subtest. Another characteristics of this scale is that they include verbal as well as performance items from whi6h separate verbal and performance IQS can be computed.

Besides being used for determining the intelligence, it is also useful in psychiatric diagnosis in cases of brain damage, psychosis, emotional difficulties and such other clinical varieties. It was the contention of Wechsler that analysis of the intelligence with his test should reveal psychiatric disorders.

The first Wechsler Scale, called as the Wechsler Bellrue scale was constructed in the year 193910 measure adult intelligence. However, this scale had a number of technical difficulties which were corrected in the 1955 scale which has become famous as WAIS. The 1955 WAIS was revised in 1981 and is called as WAIS-R.

WAIS comprises of II subtests, six subtests are grouped into verbal scale and five into performance scale; which are as follows :

Verbal Subtests:

1. Information: 29 questions covering a wide variety of information that adults have an opportunity to gather in American culture.

2. **Comprehension:** 14 problems similar to those encountered in elementary school arithmetic.

3. Similarities: 13 items requiring the subject to say in what ways two things are similar.

4. Digit Span-Orally presented list of 3 to 9 digit are to be orally reproduced.

5. Vocabulary-*40* words of increasing difficulty are presented both orally and visually, the subject is asked to give the meaning.

Performance Subtests

6. Digit Symbol: this version is similar to Petersons Rational Learning test. The key contains 9 symbols paired with 9 digits. The subject's score is the number of symbols correctly written in 1-1/2 minutes (ie. 90 second).

7. Picture Completion21 cards, each containing a picture born which some part is missing, subject must tell what is missing in each picture.

8. Block Design: Similar to Khos block design test. The subject produces the design by placing the blocks which are coloured in white, red or half 'red and half white.

9. Picture Arrangement: each item consists of a set of cards containing pictures to be arranged in proper sequence so as to tell a story.

10. Object Assembly: Similar to Marikin profile described earlier.

Both speed and accuracy of performance are taken into account for scoring.

Standardization Sample: The WAIS standardization sample was chosen with exceptional care to ensure its representative ness. It consisted of 1700 cases, half men and half women distributed over the age range from 161C64. The subjects were selected to match as closely as possible the proportions of 1950 US census with regard to the part of the country, urban, rural residence, race, occupational level and education. At each stage level, one mentally defective woman and man was included.

Scoring of WAIS: All parts of this scale are scored on a point basis, for some subjects earned raw score is simply the number correct, items each item being scored either as plus or minus. Is some tests the earned raw score is based on the time taken to solve the item. This is specially so of the non-verbal subtests.

The raw score for each subtest is first obtained by addition of the credits on the items in that part and then this score is converted into weighted score by means of a conversion table. The purpose of the conversion is to place all the subjects scores on comparable basis. The weighted scores of all the tests are then added to obtain the full score of the test.

Raw scores of WAIS are transmitted into standard scores with mean of 10 and SD of 3.

By reference to appropriate tables in the manual of the test these scores can be expressed in as Deviation I.Q. (DIQ) with mean of 100 and SD of 15. These IQS are found with individual's own age group and show individual's standing in comparison with persons of his own age.

Wechsler Scales as Diagnostic Instrument; Whechsler scales besides their use as a measure of general intelligence have been investigated as a possible aid in psychiatric diagnosis. Beginning with the observation that brain damage, psychotic disorder and other emotional difficulties may effect some intellectual functions more than others. Wechsler and other clinical psychologists argued that an analysis of the individual's relative performance on different subtests should reveal specific psychiatric disorders.

The diagnostic use of this test is discussed by Wechsler in the 1958 edition of his test manual, the use is further elaborated and discussed by Rapaport. Three important measures are useful in diagnosis made from WAIS.

These three measures areas follows :

1. Measuring the amount of scatter (or scatter analysis).
2. Analysing score patterns (pattern analysis)
3. Computing a deterioration Index.

We will discuss these measures in brief.

1. **Scatter analysis:** Scatter is simply the extent of variation among the individuals score or all the subtest. Wechsler proposes that it be measured by finding the average deviation (A.D.) of the subtest scores around the individuals own mean. The underlying rationale of scatter indicates that the A.D. should be larger in pathological cases then in normal.

Wechsler illustrates this hypothesis, with data on small method groups of schizophrenics and formals, the former showing significantly greater A.D.

2. **Score Pattern** or Pattern Analysis:; Both Wechsler and Rapaport have described what they consider characteristic score patterns for various clinical syndromes Wechsler provides such a pattern for organic brain

syndromes. Schizophrenia anxiety states, juvenile delinquency and mental deficiency. Each pattern is expressed in terms of the portion of each subtest with reference to the individuals mean on all subtests. These patterns are supplemented with various diagnostic signs associated with each syndrome.

Wechsler lists the following for schizophrenia.

(1) Sum pf picture arrangement and picture completion much less than information and block design.

(2) Object assembly much below block design.

(3) Very long similarities with high Vocabulary and Information.

The important question that arises pertains to the minimum score difference required for statistical significance. Wechsler has given table of sum differences in the manual. The minimum difference values found in his table for different test pairs vary from 2 to 4, most comparison requiring 3 points for significant difference.

3. **Deterioration Index:** Another type of interest comparison proposed by Wechsler requires computation of deterioration Index. The administration of these tests on various groups showed that the tests requiring utilization of past experience showed less decline in their scores than those involving speed, new learning and perceptions of new relations in Verbal or Spatial content. On the basis of such findings Wechsler made distinction between his eleven subjects. He called one group of test as "Hold tests" exhibiting no decline due to age and "Don't hold tests" manifesting very step decline. These are listed below :

	Hold tests		**Don't Hold tests**
1.	Vocabulary	(1)	Digit Span
2.	Tnfonnatioii	(2)	Similarities
3.	Object Assembly	(3)	Digit symbol
4.	Picture completion	(4)	Block design.

Deterioration Index is calculated by the following formula:

Deterioration Index = Hold Tests – Don't Tests/Hold Test.

Wechsler maintains that at any stage individuals with mental disorder " show same differential loss on WAIS Subtests found in general population with advancing age. The WAIS manual gives scaled scores used in computing the DI. Such scores arc based on individual's relative performance on each subtests by comparing it with that of his age peers.

(A) THEORETICAL PERSPECTIVES ON ASSESSMENT

There definitely exists a relationship between examiner's theoretical orientation and his/her assessment conclusions.

The evidence that the clinician gets is determined by their assessment methods, and their assessment methods are determined by their theoretical orientations. While acknowledging that abnormal behaviour may have many different kinds of causes, adherents of psychodynamic, behavioural, and humanistic-existential theory have clear ideas as to what it the most important kind of cause, and they will choose assessment methods that allow them to explore that kind of cause.

The Psychodynamic Approach to Assessment

As we have seen in Chapter 2, two basic assumptions of psychodynamic theory, as derived from Freud, are

(1) That people's behaviour is primarily determined not by their will or by 4 their Current environment but by their inborn drives and their psychosexualhistory, and

(2) that these latter factors operate unconsciously in motivating their behaviour. Proceeding on these two assumptions, psychodynamic assessment procedures attempt to Filter out all situational influences and to provide the subject with the free and loose atmosphere so that the "core" personality of unconscious memories, drives, and conflicts will reveal itself in its purity.

This assessment strategy involves two basic techniques :

(a) The First is the depth interview, in which subjects are encouraged to talk about their past, and particularly their childhood histories, as freely and as candidly as possible. Of special interest to the examiner is the subject's handling of sexual and aggressive impulses during the pregenital psychosexual stages, along with any possible traumas that occurred during these presumably crucial stages. Hence the examiner may prompt the subject to talk about these matters.

(b) The second major psychodynamic assessment tool is the projective test. This technique, as we have been, gives the subject some stimulus to respond to, bat at the same time keeps the stimulus vague enough so that it will not restrict the subject's verbalizations to a specific context and thereby allow his or her defenses to remain intact. The hoped for result is that, faced with this ambiguous stimulus, the subject will be forced to fall back on imagination and thus to project onto the image whatever is lurking in the unconscious.

These psychodynamic assessment techniques may be said to have the same virtues and vices as psychodynamic theory itself. On the one hand, they represent one method of tapping the inner reaches of the personality, levels that " lie below the individual's surface behaviours. On the other hand, they tend to accord the status of fact to assumptions that cannot be empirically validated assumptions regarding the primacy of sexual and aggressive drives, the ineradicable influence of psychosexual development, the importance of Oedipal conflicts, and so forth. Furthermore, psychodynamic theory assumes, as we have seen, that any verbalization is interpretable in terms of unconscious motivation. But if a person who is asked to use imagination in interpreting an inkblot sees in that inkblot two staring eyes, does this really mean that the person is paranoid ?

Essentially, what all these criticisms come down to is a serious concern regarding the faith that psychodynamic assessment places in the clinician's subjective judgment. Numerous studies have been conducted on the predictive validity of clinical interpretations (Goldberg, 1959; Holtzman and Sells, 1954; Meehl, 1954), on the reliability and validity of such interpretations when aided by projective tests and self-report inventories (Golden, 1964; Kastlan, 1954; Little and Shneidman, 1959-, Sinnes, 1959), and on the validity of interpretations made by trained clinicians as opposed to those made by lay persons (Goidman, 1959; Soskin, 1959). Summarizing this vast literature on the accuracy of clinical judgment, Mischel and Mischel conclude :

The results have been surprisingly disappointing. Oft the whole, clinical inferences (e.g. about the meaning of projective test answers) have not been shown to have impressive validity. Experienced clinicians tend to be no better judges than inexperienced non professionals such as secretaries. Equally ' upsetting for clinicians, training does not seem to increase the accuracy of inferences about dispositions. In fact, predictions may get worse when the judge goes beyond common stereotypes. Such negative conclusions have been found regardless of the kind and quantity of information on which judges base their interpretations. Thus, while clinical judgments are often better than purely random guesses, they usually predict less well than docs information from cheaper, simpler sources like biographical facts and social case history (1977, p.358).

The problem of clinical judgment is one that plagues mental health workers of all persuasions. But of all the psychological perspectives, the psychodynamic is the one that relies most heavily on inference and interpretation, and therefore, this problem is particularly to psychodynamic approaches to assessment.

The Behavioural Approach to Assessment

Unlike psychodynamic theorists, who see behaviour as controlled by intrapsychic forces, the behaviourists, as we have seen in chapter 2, regard behaviour as issuing primarily from the individual's interaction with the environment. Thus, when people report that their actions or feelings are distressing to them, the behaviourists, in assessing the problem, will concentrate on determining with the greatest possible accuracy what it is in the environment that is reinforcing the maladaptive response (Kanfer and Phillips, 1970).

Because they sec behaviour as variable in relation to the environment, behaviourists place little faith in such stable trait oriented assessment methods as the projective tests and the MMPI. Indeed, behaviourists are generally not interested in interpreting human actions as signs of anything else-underlying traits, interapsychic conflicts, or whatever. Rather, they view behaviours as samples, specimens of how a particular person responds in a particular situation. For example, in diagnosing a patient who complains of shyness and anxiety in social situations, a behavioural clinician would not care greatly whether such behaviour was a sign that the trait "introversion" was particularly pronounced in this person. The behaviourist would simply regard the patient's social behaviour as a sample of a particular response pattern and would concentrate on finding out what concrete stimuli - and, in keeping with the new cognitive behaviourism, what thoughts - were eliciting and maintaining that response pattern. The main tools for obtaining such information are interviews, self-monitoring diaries, and direct observation.

An interview conducted by a behaviourist bears little relation to the depth interview favoured by psychodynamic clinicians. Generally, a behavioural assessment interview takes the form of a functional analysis. What this involves is a systematic dissection of the person's complaint: what precisely the problem behaviour is, how it developed, what the person has done to try to combat it, and most important of all what specific thoughts and situations tend to provoke the maladaptive response. In addition, the interviewer will try to get some idea of the person's strengths and preferences, since these are important in formulating a treatment program. In such an interchange, unlike the psychoanalytic depth interview, the subject's remarks are assumed to be fairly frank statements of the problem rather than veiled clues to underlying dynamics.

To supplement information gathered in the interview, many behavioural examiners will ask subjects to keep a self-monitoring diary of their problem behaviours.

For example, a woman who is afflicted with vague anxieties would be asked to note down when her anxiety occurs and the circumstances surrounding these episodes. If the diary should reveal that one situation in which her anxiety regularly occurs is when she is taking the bus home from work, then his correlation will provide a starting point for determining the stimuli that are maintaining the anxiety.

Finally, a widely used behavioural assessment method is direct observation of the problem behaviour. As described earlier, the subject may be observed in the school, work, or home environment in order to identify the discriminative stimuli that trigger the maladaptive responses. Or the behaviour sampling may take place in the clinical situation itself.

In evaluating the behavioural approach to assessment, it should be noted first of all that this approach generally fulfills very well its stated objective that is, the detailed and concrete analysis of the problem behaviour and the environmental conditions that support the behaviour. On the negative side, behavioural assessment is subject to the same objections that have been leveled at behavioural theory in general : that it treats human beings as if they were on a par with experimental pigeons and white rats, and that it attends only to the symptoms and ignores what are presumed to be the underlying causes, rooted in the total personality structure or in organic functioning. In answer to these criticisms, behavioural clinicians point out that a technique that works for human beings should not be discarded because it also works for white rats and that if problems can be solved by dealing with environmental contingencies, then there is no need for speculation as to unverifiable "underlying" causes.

The Humanistic-Existential Approach to Assessment

The behavioural assessment procedures tend to avoid diagnostic labeling because behaviourists feel that such labels obscure the actual problem. Humanists and existentialists also avoid labelling in the assessment process, mainly because they consider diagnostic labels an affront to the patient's individuality. The central focus of humanistic-existential psychology, is precisely this matter of Individuality the uniqueness of each human being and the validity of his or her unique perceptions. And the central aim of humanistic-existential therapy is to restore to patients their power as individuals the power to be true to themselves, to choose their own goals, and to take responsibility for their actions.

In accordance with this orientation, humanistic-existential assessment procedures are aimed at helping both the therapist and the patient become more fully aware of precisely what the patient's unique self really is. The experienced humanistic therapist is adept at using the interview to extract information about the individuals and their ways of perceiving themselves and their world. In addition, some humanists may employ a device such as the Q-sort. This test, described above, has been used extensively by Carl Rogers, and other humanists in measuring patients' self-concepts.

Relying on the interview or on a test such as the Q-sort procedures in which there are no "right" answers, only revealing ones - has a distinct advantage. First, such an approach focuses on obtaining a clear picture of the individual in all his or her idiosyncratic reality rather than on forcing the personality into theoretical molds. Second, of all the assessment procedures that we have discussed, these techniques are probably the least contaminated by the pathological bias that we discussed earlier in this chapter. The major weakness of this phenomenological approach to assessment is that it must assume that what the individual says in interviews or in a Q-sort is true, at least for himself or herself. Hence no account is taken of the possibility of intentional or semi-intentional distortion, which could seriously interfere with the therapist's effort to participate sympathetically in the patient's internal world.

(B) ASSESSMENT OF GROUPS

In group assessment, the focus is on the group as a social system instead of on particular individuals within the group. Here, too, interviewing, testing, observing, and other psychosocial assessment procedures may be used, but the primary concern is with determining social roles, communication patterns, task performance, and other aspects of the group's structure and functioning.

Unfortunately, there are few research findings or guidelines on the assessment of group systems.

In the assessment of groups a wide variety of assessment techniques have been used, including videotaping of interactional patterns to permit more precise analysis, drawing on data from epidemiological studies, and observing "high-risk" groups, over a period of time to delineate conditions that may be causing problems.

The reliability and validity of these instruments needs to be checked.

(C) MEDICAL EVALUATION OR ASSESSMENT

For the medical evaluation, data are collected relevant to the individual's general physical state and any physical pathology that may have a bearing on his maladaptive behaviour. Medical data may also be collected concerning adverse physical conditions-such as malnutrition - in given groups or entire societies.

On an individual level, the medical evaluation commonly includes the following:

(i) **General physical examination:** The physical examination consists of the kinds of procedures most of us have experienced in getting a "medical checkup". Typically, a medical history is obtained and the major systems of the body are examined.

(ii) **Neurological examination:** Since brain pathology is involved in some mental disorders, a specialized neurological examination is commonly given in addition to the general medical examination. This may involve the use of electroencephalography to check on brain-wave patterns.

(iii) **Special diagnostic techniques:** where EEG's reveal dysrphythmias-abnormal brain-wave patterns or where other data indicate the possibility of brain pathology, a variety of specialized techniques may be used in an attempt to arrive at a precise diagnosis of the nature and extent of the problem.

Medicine and allied sciences are contributing many new procedures of value in assessing conditions that can affect brain functioning. Radioactive isotopes can help locate brain lesions and other types of nervous system disturbances techniques have been developed for the detection of rare metabolic disorders; and new methods have made it a simple matter to detect the use of heroin and other drugs of dependence. And as we have seen, new techniques have made it increasingly easy to identify genetic and chromosomal abnormalities These techniques not only make it possible to diagnose conditions such as Down's syndrome in mental retardation, but also permit preventive assessment For example, potential parents may be examined to see if they carry particular genetic aberrations that may adversely affect their offspring.

(D) CLINICAL INTERVIEW AS A PSYCHOLOGICAL ASSESSMENT TECHNIQUE

Clinical Interview also called as interview or clinical case history is a very useful technique of assessment which majority of the clinicians follow.

The standardized tests of personality, cognitive abilities, and neurological functioning basically involve a subject's responding to some type of impersonal questions or tasks. By contrast, in the interview, the subject is face to face with an interviewer who asks for information that is necessary for understanding the interviewee's personality. Because information flows only in one direction, interviewing differs from everyday conversation and calls for a great deal of skill to put clients at ease, build feelings of trust, and obtain relevant information. There arc many who see interviewing as the most important way that clinicians collect information about their clients (Stevenson, 1971).

The style of the interviewer and the contents of an interview may vary according to the interviewer's theoretical-background. Psychodynamically oriented interviewers are likely to focus on past life experiences, while behaviourists are more likely to focus on current life circumstances. Most clinicians, regardless of theoretical background, will try to obtain as much information as possible.

Areas explored in a clinical interview usually include the individual's current life setting, specific problem behaviours; a chronology of problem development; description of past and present treatment; and on assessment of the individual's physical characteristics, emotional state, self description, and intellectual functioning. The interviewer wants to find out as much as possible about social factors such as group membership, family structure and relationships, education, type of work and community involvement. In addition, the clinician is interested in possible precipitating factors such as the individual's perception of levels of stress, and any recent life changes such as losses, physical illness, and marriage.

In other words, in the clinical interview, one wants to find as much information as possible about the individual which is relevant to the problem behaviour. In practice, interviewers often depart from such a format as the need arises.

Interviews can be unstructured or structured. In an unstructured verbal interaction, interviewers usually are free to cover as wide a range of topics as they desire. There are typically few constraints on what may be asked during such broad-ranging interviews. However, part of the price for this flexibility is a loss of standardization and reliability that may make the data from structured interviews inapplicable in systematic research. On the other hand, like the Rorschach inkblots, unstructured interviews can sometimes yield information that can lead to fruitful hypotheses about the basis for people's problems.

While unstructured interviewers usually are free to cover as wide a range of topics as they desire and in any order, structured interviewers are required to ask the same questions in the same manner to all interviewees. The structured interview is frequently used in research projects when the data from interviews *need* to be compared. In clinical settings probably the most common *use* of the highly structured interview is the mental status exam.

"The purpose of the Mental Status Examination is to evaluate a person suspected of neurological or emotional problems in terms of variables known to be related to those problems" (Kaplan & Sacuzzo, 1982, p. 213.) In the mental status interview, the interviewer attempts to assess a person's appearance, attitudes and general behaviour. By asking a structured set of questions, the interviewer attempts to evaluate such characteristics of disordered behaviour as disturbed thought processes or inappropriate emotions. Mental status examiners can assess intelligence by using brief sets of questions that require memory, judgement, and abstracting abilities to answer. Finally, the examiner wishes to see if the person can direct and focus attention onto relevant tasks. An inability to attend properly or disturbed perception usually are associated with more severe psychopathology.

The mental status exam is an integral part of the assessment process. When properly used, it can provide essential information necessary for accurate diagnosis and effective treatment.

Like with the unstructured interview the benefits of the structured interview come at a cost. The standardization of the interview interaction may result in a more rigid and artificial communication process that some clients may perceive as cold, unfeeling, and nontherapeutic.

The psychometric merit of interviews as assessment tools probably varies with their degree of structure (Anastasi, 1982). The more structured the interview, generally the easier it is to establish reliability. However, the unstructured interview approximates normal conversation and may facilitate freer expression of feeling. Regardless of the degree of structure, however, in the diagnostic process information gained through interviewing is usually combined with information from other assessment procedures to make decisions.

Behavioural Interviewing: Assessments of specific behaviour often occur in a behavioural interview. In this procedure, the interview focuses on specific problem behaviours and "their frequency (such as anxiety attacks). Like A" a typical clinical interview, a behavioural interview attempts to clarify the development of the disorder, but the focus is on behaviour and the learning process which led to it. Thus, the behavioural interview centers on the environment in which the behaviour occurred, the reinforces in the environment, the persons who might be involved in reinforcement, and possible modifications of the environment which can be made to change the reinforcement contingencies (Hersen & Bellack, 1976).

(E) INNOVATIVE APPROACHES TO ASSESSMENT

Perhaps the most dramatic innovation in clinical assessment during.

The last decade has been the increasing sophistication and use of computers in individual assessment. In addition, there has been an increasing reliance on the use of specialized tests to obtain more accurate individual assessment data, as well as a trend toward using model soften with computer assistance in the assessment of social systems.

(i) **Use of Computers**-Computers arc used primarily in three ways in assessment: (a) to gather information directly from the subject; (b) to put together all of the information that has been gathered previously through interviews, tests, and other assessment measures and (c) to stimulate and predict the functioning of social systems. Here we shall deal with the use of computers in individual' assessment.

By comparing the incoming information with data previously stored in its memory banks, the computer can perform a wide range of assessment functions. It can supply a diagnosis, evaluate the risk of certain kinds of behaviour, suggest the most appropriate form of treatment, predict the outcome, and print out a summary report concerning the subject.

Over time, the computer builds an increasingly large data base covering many 'cases, which enables continual refinement of its probability statements. Interestingly enough, the computer is superior to individual clinicians in many of these functions. Goldberg (1970) demonstrated that a computer, programmed with the assessment strategies utilized by 29 clinical psychologists, was more proficient than the individual clinicians in differentiating between neurotic and psychotic individuals on the basis of MMPI profiles. Similarly, Mirabile, Houck, and Glueck (1970) demonstrated that a computer could out perform clinicians in selecting from among three chemotherapy programs for psychotic subjects. In predicting the risk of suicidal or assaultive behaviour, the computer appears to be far superior to individual clinicians (Greist et al. 1973 Sletten, Altman, & Ulett, 1971). Computers can also be used to compare a patient's adjustment in the community prior to and after treatment, and to show whether the outcome of treatment was better or worse than the state wise average for a particular disorder (Evenson, Sletten, Hedlund, & Faintich, 1974).

In making predictions for an individual, the computer uses an actuarial procedure much like that used by life-insurance companies in predicting risks. It conclusions are only statements of probability, based on what has happened to a large number of other, supposedly similar, people. For such an approach to work successfully, two conditions are of critical importance : (a) there must be consistent and objective criteria for interpreting test responses and other data; and (b) these criteria must have an adequate statistical base: that is, they must have been derived from information gathered on a large sample of subjects similar to the one being assessed. Both these conditions, in turn, imply a stable world, one that does not change in relevant particulars. To the extent that there has been change in the "real world" since the computer was programmed, its conclusions are subject to possible error.

(ii) Use of specialized tests: A number of psychologists have suggested that so-called "all-purpose" tests designed to measure a variety of factors within the same scale or test instrument be discarded. It does not seem productive to attempt to obtain a verity of assessment data or to answer all assessment questions by means of a particular tests instrument. In fact, it would seem unrealistic to expect a given Jests or even a small battery of tests to supply all relevant psychosocial assessment data for particular patient or subject. Thus, as Walker (1974) has pointed out, "an increasing number of well-researched, highly sophisticated, and intensive batteries of tests designed for specific purposes are being developed," (P.12). By means of these scales, specific questions relevant to the assessment of a given individual can be answered with a high degree of assurance.

(iii) Improved assessment of social systems: Since one major trend in modern science is toward increased emphasis on social system-marital dyads, families, communities, organizations, and even societies-a good deal of research attention is being focused on ways of analyzing such systems. Some of the forms this attention has taken are for e.g. studying social roles, communication patterns, task performance, and other characteristics of marital, family, and larger, groups. These techniques arc ways of assessing interpersonal interactions as a basis for making improvements in the functioning of the system.

Another innovative technique that appears to offer great future promise involves the construction of computer models of social systems. Computers then stimulate the actual functioning of the system. This not only permits detailed analysis of the system in operation, but also makes it possible to study the effects different changes would have on the overall operation of the system. Simulations of complex social systems arc handicapped today by our inadequate knowledge of many of the key variables that affect their functioning. As these variables are better understood, however, computer simulation can become an increasingly accurate replica of "real-world" social processes.

2

Disorders of Psychophysiology

Psychophysiology disorders are an important group of disorders which are also known as psychosomatic disorders. These disorders have been of concern to mental health professionals since a long time. Freud and his followers clearly demonstrated how psychological factors can lead to the development of physical disorders. Freud most convincingly demonstrated the role of psychological factors in the causation of physical disorders. Similarly Walter Cannon, the famous physiologist also demonstrated that how various emotions affected the physiological processes and brought about physiological disorders on the basis of his work, it became possible to understand how interrelationship among people, could result in psychosomatic disorders.

clearly demonstrated how psychological factors can lead to the development of physical disorders. Freud most convincingly demonstrated the role of psychological factors in the causation of physical disorders. Similarly Walter Cannon, the famous physiologist also demonstrated that how various emotions affected the physiological processes and brought about physiological disorders on the basis of his work, it became possible to understand how interrelationship among people, could result in psychosomatic disorders.

DSM-II for the first time labeled psychometric ailments as psychophysiological disorders. In these disorders, there is an emotionally caused physical symptom involving a single organ system usually innervated by the autonomic nervous system. The physiological changes found in these disorders are the same as those associated with certain emotional states except that they are more intense and longer lasting.

In this chapter we would first define what are psychophysiological disorders and discuss the various types of psychophysiological disorders.

Following this we would discuss in detail the common psychophysiological disorders. Some of these common psychophysiological disorders are peptic ucler, asthama, migrain and tension headaches, essential hypertension and coronary heart diseases.

We would then discuss the General theories of causation of psychophysiological disorder. Some of these general theories include the organ system approach, psychological theories, behavioural theories and the medical approaches.

Psychophysiological Disorders

Psychophysiological disorders were once called as psychosomatic disorders. They refer to a group of disorders, in which physical conditions are disturbed presumably due to emotional stress caused by psychological factors.

Thus, psychophysiological disorders refer to those disorders which are thought to be due to emotional factors and which are also scientifically traceable to a clear organic cause. The term 'psychophysiological disorder' is not used in DSM-IB.

The term "Psychosomatic" has become familiar not only in medical and psychological literature but also in popular speech. Much publicity has been given to such "psychosomatic illnesses" as peptic ucler, high blood pressure (essential hypertension), coronary heart disease, rheumatoid arthritis, and bronchial asthama. The term was originally applied to those physical disorders in which emotional stresses have led to identifiable organic pathology.

The concept of psychosomatic illness is an old one, dating from some of the earliest recorded writings. Even the term psychosomatic is not very new, having been proposed at least as early as 1818. Nevertheless, the psychosomatic movement in medicine and the widespread recognition of psychogenic factors in physical disorders are of relatively recent origin. The publication in 1935 of Dunbar's book on "Emotions and Bodily Changes", which survyed relevant world literature of both experimental and clinical nature, did much to lunch the movement. The first journal and the first association devoted to the study of psychosomatic problems were established within the next few years. The high incidence of psychosomatic disorders among military personnel and among civilians exposed to wartime stresses during World War II also contributed to the growing concern with these problems.

Several antecedent developments in psychology, physiology, and psychiatry contributed to the rise of the modern psychosomatic movement. A major contribution stems from research on the effects of psychological factors on physiological functions, as studied in both humans and animals. The pioneer animal experiments of Pavlov (1928) on the conditioned salivary reflex and of Cannon (1932) on physiological effects of intense emotional stimuli are outstanding examples of this research. The investigations of Selye (1946, 1973) on the "general adaptation syndrome" following prolonged exposure lo any kind of stress shed further light on the role of certain hormones in mediating physiological responses to stress. More limited experimental studies on human subjects, as well as clinical observations on patients, provided additional data on changes in blood pressure, respiration, gastric motility, glandular secretions, and other physiological reactions resulting from emotional stress. Such research established that temporary ana preversible physiological changes accompany anxiety and other emotional states and lead *io* development of certain disorders.

These disorders were called psychosomatic disorders by such early investigators as Helen Flanders Dunbar (1943) and Franz Alexander (1950). Unfortunately, this term came to be used incorrectly by most people to suggest that the symptoms or problems were "all in the head" and "not really a physical illness". This belief was particularly common in regard to disorders whose symptoms are not obviously physical, such as headaches, stomachaches, and muscular pain such as backaches. To avoid the negative meaning of "psychosomatic", the term "psychophysiological" was introduced DSM-II. This term is quite popular among health care professional, since more and more of them now believe that all physical illness has psychological components. Emotional and psychological factors appear to have pervasive effects on our general physical well-being.

In the past few decades, however, there has been mounting evidence that this distinction between psychgophysiological and purely physiological disorders is a false one, and that almost any physical complaint may be affected by psychological processes. Consequently DSM-III has dropped the term "psychophysiological disorders" from its nomenclature. Instead, DSM-III explicitly acknowledges that psychological factors may affect any physical condition, and provides the diagnostician with the opportunity to rate the likelihood that psychological factors are involved in physical disorder.

Psychophysiological disorders should be distinguished from somatoform disorders because both are concerning bodily processes. The following are some important distinctions between them:

(i) One important difference between psychophysiological disorder and somatoform disorders is that psychophysiological disorders do cause physical damage whereas somatoform patterns typically do not.

(ii) Psychophysiological disorders usually involve internal organs like the lungs, viscera, heart, etc. but somatoform disorders generally involve those bodily organs which are external like hand, eyes, voice etc.

(iii) Patients suffering from psychophysiological disorders typically are quite concerned with and anxious about their symptoms and feelings. On the other hand individuals having somatoform disorders are attention seeking but hardly concerned or anxious about their symptoms. They show no feelings. Some researchers have described this in terms of "Labelle indifference" i.e. they are indifferent to their symptoms and feelings.

TYPES OF PSYCHOPHYSIOLOGICAL DISORDERS OR CLASSIFICATIONS OF PSYCHOPHYSIOLOGICAL DISORDERS

Psychophysiological disorders have been classified in a wide variety of ways by different researchers. The most useful classification system of psychophysiological disorder has been one given by DSM-INDIVIDUALS. According to it Psychophysiological disorders are characterized by physical symptoms in nine specific organ systems. The nine major organ systems are identified below, with examples of Psychophysiological disorders:

1. Skin disorders: Disorders such as neurodermatosis (inflammation), hyperhydrosis (dry skin), and eczema (severe flaking, scaling, and itching).

2. Musculo/skeletal disorders: Tension headaches, backaches, cramps, muscle spasms, and rheumatoid arthritis.

3. Respiratory disorders: Bronchial asthma, sighing, hiccoughs, hyperventilation, sneezing, and coughing.

4. Cardiovascular disorders: Tachycardia (rapid heart rate), hypertension (high blood pressure), migraine headaches, fainting, vagal depression of the heart rate.

5. Hemic and Lymphatic disorders: Disturbance in the blood or lymph system. Recent speculation suggest that leukemia, for example, may have a psychophysiological component.

6. Gastrointestinal disorder: Peptic ucler, chronic gastritis, ulcerative or

mucous colitis, constipation, diarrhoea, "heartburn", and hyperacidity.

7. Genito-urinary disorders: Problems in menstruation (such as "cramps") or urination.

8. Endocrine disorders: Malfunctions of the endocrine glands resulting in disorders such as hyperthyroidism and diabetes.

9. Disorders of Special sense organs: Glaucoma (increase in pressure within the eye) and disorders of the inner ear's semicircular canal, (leading to problems in balance) are thought to be examples.

It should be very clearly remembered that while these disorders may be psychologically influenced in .some or even a majority of individuals, it is possible that for others, psychological factors have only a small or non-existent role in the genesis and development of the disorder. In some individuals, the cause of one of these diseases may be almost completely physical.

Besides the above DSM-II classification system, some researchers have emphasized some paychophysiological disorders more than the others. For e.g. Mehr (1983) discusses the following five psychophysiological disorders and considers them to be very common. These are :

(i) Ulcers, (ii) Asthama, (iii) Tensio and Migrane headaches, *(iv)* Essential hypertension, and *(v)* coronary heart *disease.*

Whereas Bootzin and Acocella (1980), besides the above mentioned disorders, include in the list of common' psychophysiological disorders the following (i) obesity (ii) eczema, and (iii) insomnia.

CLINICAL SYMPTOMS RESPONSIBLE IN THE DEVELOPMENT OF PSYCHOPHYSIOLOGICAL DISORDERS

(a) Peptic Ulcer is one of the most common psythopysiological disorders found among executives and those staying in urban areas. It is genera characterized by the presence of a crater like holes or lesions in the lining stomach or deodenum due to excess of HCL and pepsin in gastric juice. The hole is produced by the excessive secretion of hydrochloric acid and pepsinogen which is present in the gastric juice. Usually the inner value of the digestive track protected from the various gastric acids by the layer of mucus. During stress, lack of normal blood supply to the mucus and excessive secretion or gastric juice erode the mucus and results in crater like wound in the intestinal value which is referred to as ulcer. Thus, an ulcer can be described as an open sore, varying from the size of a pinhead to the size of a quarter, in the wall of any part of th digestive system. However, ulcers usually develop either in the stomach, i which case they are called gastric ulcers, or in the duodenum (the area lyir between the stomach and small intestines, in which case they are referred to as duodenal ulcers).

Some common symptoms of ulcer include the abdominal pain which is of uniform quality, disappears at times and tends to be chronic. Ulcers are usually physic in character and flare up during the time of stress and ebbs off when the stress is reduced. It has been found that usually 10% of the people suffers from the ulcer at some or other time during their life. The relative occurrence of ulcer in male and female have varied over the past few decades. Gorove Tudor have reported that 80 years ago 12 women had ulcers for every ulcered male. Today men with ulcer outnumber woman by approximately 3:1. However, the extent of ulcer among women is again on the rise since last two decades.

Recently, Cheren and Krappa (1980) suggested that gastric and duodenal ulcers may have different etiologies. Compared with gastric ulcers which tend to appear in the age group of 60s, duodenal ulcers occur most frequently when the people are in their 40s and 50s. Duodenal ulcers not only occur early in life but are more frequently found in lower social classes and more in women than men.

Causes of ulcer: A wide variety of factors have been implicate in the development of ulcer. Usually the researchers have found that physical predisposition along with frustration and stress of everyday life leads to the development of ulcer. Researchers have suggested that individuals who develop peptic ulcer arc likely to meet the following 3 criteria :

(i) Biological predisposition.

(ii) Specific stress resulting from life events.

(iii) Psychological and Intrapsychic factors.

We would now discuss the above three causes in detail

(i) There is a biological predisposition towards high level of pepsinogen secretion which is usually inherited.

The predisposing biological condition for an ulcer is thought to be acquired genetically. For e.g. it has been found, that compared with normal controls people with certain types of ulcers have longer hyper secreting stomachs and produce more acids and pepsins. It appears, then that the biological conditions necessary for the creation of an ulcer may be present long before the ulcer actually forms. This partly explains Why, when no people experience the same degree of stress, only one may develop an ulcer.

Thus, from the discussion we see that Individual physiological predispositions arc clearly important.

Mirsky (1958) has demonstrated that marked individual differences in pepsingogen levels exist even at birth (pepsinogen breaks down into the digestive enzyme pepsin). The importance of this Finding is reinforced by a study of 2073 Army draftees (Weiner *et al,* 1957), which identified 63 men with the highest levels of pepsinogen and 57 with the lowest levels. All 2073 men had been given a complete physical, including intenstinal X-rays, and were administered a series of projective personality tests. Four of the high-level pepsinogen men had ulcers at the start of the study, and by the end of Army basic training, 5 more men in this group were found to have developed ulcers. None of the low level secreters had ulcers at the beginning of the study, and none developed them during basic training. The data suggest that a biological predisposition towards high pepsinogen levels is an important factor in the development of ulcers under stress.

(ii) Specific stress resulting from life events: Those who develop ulcer usually have stressful life events. Stressors like immobilization or conflict or feelings of helplessness to control the situation etc. Lead to development or ulcer. Wiess (1970) has demonstrated that those individuals who experienced more stress which was severe and of longer duration developed ulcer as compared to control group in whom such stress were absent.

There have been several interesting animal studies aimed at determining what specific kinds of stress are most likely to cause ulcers. Perhaps the best known is a series of experiments with monkeys by Brady and his colleagues (1958). Brady bad two monkeys sit next to each other in restraining chairs. Both monkeys received electric shock, but only one, called the executive monkey, could prevent the shock from occurring to both monkeys by pressing a lever. The other monkey also had a lever, but it had no effect on whether the shock occurred. Both monkeys received the same number of shocks.-After 23 days of such experience, the executive monkey died. An autopsy revealed that he had developed a severe ulcer. A subsequent autopsy of his partner monkey showed him, to be ulcer-free. The results of Brady's experiment were quoted in the popular press, for it was easy for the layperson to sec the similarity between the stress placed on the so-called executive monkey and the stress experienced by the human business executive. Seligman (1975), however, criticized Brady's results on methodological grounds.

Another type of stress that may lead development of ulcer is separation from loved one, especially parents. Proponents of psychoanalytic theory have suggested that separation from parents might create the kinds of stress that translate into peptic ulcers. To investigate this possibility, Ackerman et. al. (1981) used information from hospital records, tape recorded admission interviews and follow up questionnaires to assess whether adolescents who were separated from their parents were more prone to develop peptic ulcers. In support of this relationship more adolescent-aged peptic ulcer patients were round to have experienced separation from parents in the year prior to admission as compared with appendicitis patients.

(iii) **Psychological and Intrepsychic factors:** A wide variety of psychological and intrapsychic factors have been implicated in the development ulcers, for e.g. Franz Alexander, a psychoanalyst has suggested that unmet dependency needs and anger oriented reaction, persistent, conflict and repressed hostility leads to development of ulcer.

(b) **Asthama** is a common disorder of the respiratory system which is characterized by wheezing, excessive coughing, suffocation, etc. Incidence of asthama is 2 to 5% in general population at a given period of time. In India also about 3% of the population has been reported to be suffering from asthania. Males suffer more from it as compared to females and about approximately 60% of the asthmatics are below 17 years of age. Some common symptoms of asthama includes shortness of breath, excessive coughing and wheezing caused by narrowing the airways of the lungs, swelling of the air walls and secretion of excessive mucus. The asthma attack usually appears any time and may last for an hour to several hours and on rare occasion days. Asthma attack is associated with panic and severe reactions. There is also fatigue and exhaustion, irritability and anxiety.

There are atleast two main forms of the disease, (i) Extrinsic (caused by external factors like allergies or bacteria) and/ (H) the intrinsic (caused by internal psychological factors). Rees (1980) estimates that about 40 percent of all cases are caused by extrinsic, allergic factors. While extrinsic asthama tends to develop before the age of 40, intrinsic asthama more often occurs in those people over the age of 40 who have no hereditary or allergic components in their etiological history.

The Casual factors in asthama: A wide variety of biological and psychological factors are responsible for the causation of asthma.

Biological Factors: (1) Majority of the reported cases of asthama is due to infection or allergy. Reese indicated that in 30% of the cases, psychological factors are not important. He suggested that physiological predisposition is a major cause of asthama. Infection of the respiratory system is one of the precipitating factors which makes the respiratory system weak and increases the chances of asthma. Researchers have found that allergic reactions to specific irritants such as pollen, molds and animal dander lead to development of asthama. It has also been found that infectious conditions such as whooping cough, tonsillitis and premonia lead to asthamatic attack.

(2) Some researchers have suggested that malfunctioning of the immunological system of the body is the cause of asthama. According to some researchers, strong emotions may act to block the sympathetic nervous system, ultimately leading to the release of biochemical substance known as Histamines which constrict the lung passage and Finally leads to asthama.

(3) Some individuals have inherited hypersensitivity of the respiratory mucoso which is one of the chief cause of asthama. Some people are so sensitive to harmless substances that they react to it by developing asthama.

Psychological Factors: Many researchers have suggested that psychological factors may also an important role in the causation of asthama. Three main psychological factors are as follows :

(i) Asthama is a learned behaviour.

(ii) Family interaction, and

(iii) Disturbed parent child relationship.

Some psychologists have suggested that expectations about the attack by the patient seems to be one of the primary psychological factors responsible for the-development of asthama. Phillips (1970) demonstrated that when asthamatic Patients were given neutral solution and believed that they would cause breathing defects, they, manifested asthamatic response. However, when they believed they were inhaling neutral solution (infect, airway spasm inducing drugs), they reacted with less intensity than they would ordinarily do. The effect of suggestion and expectation in the development of asthama has already been confirmed in a study carried out by Luparello *et. al.* In which 19 of the 40 asthama patients responded to a placebo (neutral) mist when they Were told that it contained air pollutants, 19 of the 40 patients showed significant symptoms of asthama.

Asthamatic response can also be learned through classical conditioning. Recent work with bio-feed back equipment suggest that autonomic reaction to stimuli can be generalized and so some people might learn to respond to certain 'stimuli with asthamatic attack. However, some studies have indicated that learning is secondary factor in the causation of asthama. Lachman has demonstrated that how asthama can be classically conditioned to rose and then generalized to an artificial rose.

Parent child relationship and family interaction is also another cause of asthama. This factor contributes not only towards the development of astbama but also in maintenance of asthama, in many cases, particularly among the children. Purcell has demonstrated that asthama is due to family interaction. Stressful family environment and disturbed parent child relationship makes the child emotionally upset and either results in asthama or increases the intensity of attack. It has also been found that whenever the child receives unanticipated and subtle rewards for behaviour asthamatically, asthamatic attack develops.

With respect to parent child relationship researchers have observed that parental over protection, over rejection and perfectionism have been associated with asthamatic patients (Cheren & Knapp, 1980). Similarly Lipscomb and Parker (1979) found that parents of asthmatic children were perceived as being more overprotective of these "sick children" than they were of their siblings. Notably, Lipscomb and Parker implied that it was over protectiveness in the father and not the mother that was associated with asthamatic symptoms.

Sick-role model has also been used to explain the development of asthamatic reaction in children. The recognition that the sick-role can be reinforcing for a child (as well as an adult) has led to the common treatment recommendation that asthamatic children be treated no different at home than the healthy sibling.

(c) **Tension and Migrane Headaches:** Tension and migraine headaches are two common psychophysiological disorder. 90% of the headache has been found to have emotional cause. Though these two disorders are lumped together they are primarily disorders of two different organ system. Tension headache is disorder of musculoskeletal organ system while migraine is a disorder of the cardiovascular system, which is composed of the heart, arteries and veins.

There are roughly about 20 million migraine suffers and 100 million tension headache suffers in the United States. However, the figure for India is not yet known. But it is estimated to be roughly within the same proportion.

Tension Headache: Tension headache is commonly described as a feeling that one's head is being compressed by circular vise. The duration of this disorder varies from few circular vise. The düration of this disorder varies from few hours to few months. The common tension headache is characterized by intense pain usually encircling the head although some suffers report it to be localized on one side. Martin (1972), along with many other researchers have described the tension headache as a muscle contraction headache.

This type of headache usually develop due to periodic intense contraction of face, scalp, neck and shoulder muscles. Thus, tension headache is due to vaso construction caused by the contraction of the muscle serving the skull. This develops due to the reduction in blood supply to arteries and veins in the skull. Tension headache patients, even when they are free of pain, are more vaso constricted. People suffering from this disorder usually do not take any treatment except for some pain killers like aspirin or any analgesic. Formal treatment consists of giving some muscle relaxant drug or pain reducing sedative. Bio-feedback and relaxation exercise have been of valuable help and serve as muscle relaxant in many number of cases.

Migraine Headache: Migraine headache is also called as one side headache, which lasts for few minutes to few hours. It has intense pain which is localized and associated with nausea, and giddiness. Migraine headache is a disorder of cardiovascular system. There are 3 types of migraine, headaches.

(i) Classic Migraine: Which include 'aura' which precedes actual pain by few minutes to hour. The 'aura' is usually accompanied by visual disturbance tingling feeling or numbness.

(ii) Common migraine is a term used to refer to migraine headache which is not accompanied by an 'aura'.

(iii) Cluster migraine: The term cluster migraine is used to refer to migraine headache which is accompanied by sharp, stabbing pain which occur in multiple episodes.

Symptoms that arc experienced during cluster migraine includes dizziness, fever, mood changes, blurring of vision, exhaustion and vomiting.

Migraine typically has the following symptom pattern :

(i) Recurrent throbbing pain, usually on one side of the head at onset.

(ii) Nausea, vomiting, and irritability at the sight of the headache attack.

(iii) Temporary visual disorders preceding the headache.

(iv) A history of migraine headaches in the immediate family.

(v) Dizziness, sweating and other vasomotor disorders.

(vi) Positive response to administration of the drug, ergotamine tartrate, if given early m attack..

(vii) Variable duration, but usually 2 to 8 hours.

Causes of migraine headache :

(1) Biological causes: Migraine headache usually appears to be primarily due to changes in the vascular system. More particularly in the coronary arteries. Some researchers have suggested an inherited genetic pre-disposition in the causation of migraine headache.

A great deal of research evidence has suggested that when individuals are unable to cope with personal frustration, and conflict they develop temporary increased intracranial pressure which may produce vasoconstriction leading to migraine.

The vascular explanation of migraine headaches states that pain-sensitive extra cranial arteries dilate and cause intense discomfort. However, there is other work suggesting that it is the constriction of these same arteries, especially the carotid artery, that causes the pain of the migraine. In any case, the flow of blood through the cranial arteries seems to be implicated as the major cause of the pain experienced by the migraine suffer. These vessels constrict or dilate in response to the release of biochemical substances such as serotonic and histamine.

2. **Psychosocial causes:** With respect to psychosocial causes, a great deal of research evidence has suggested that when individuals are unable to cope with personal function and conflict they develop temporary increased interacranial pressure, which may produce vasoconstriction leading to migraine.

Kolb (1963) described a typical migraine-headache victim as a tense, driving obsessional perfectionist with an inflexible personality maintaining a store of .bottled up resentments that can neither be expressed nor resolved.

Consistent with the description, when asked to report the circumstances preceding their migraine attacks, many victims state that they were in an emotionally stressful situation and felt tremendous amount of rage.

Similarly, Harrison's (1974) review of studies of migraine headaches also concluded that unexpressed anger was involved in the disorder. In an attempt to find empirical support for a psychosocial explanation of migraine headaches, Henryk Gutt and Rees (1973) compared office workers who had migraine headaches with those who did not. They found that migraine suffers "subjectively" experienced more symptoms of emotional distress than controls.

(d) Essential hypertension: Essential Hypertension is also chronic high blood pressure. About 10 to 15% of the population generally suffer from this disorder. Urban population and those of certain occupations suffer more from this disorder as compared to others. When a prolonged condition exist in which there is intermittent and chronically elevated blood pressure which is not normally due to any other disorder (like kidney disorder, renal artery disorder, obesity etc.) or due to the use of drugs, then it is called essential hypertension. This disorder is not noticed as the symptoms are not obvious. However, some symptoms which are apparent include feelings of dizziness, fatigue etc. There may also, be palpitation, insomnia and headache. This condition if it is not treated properly or if untreated, may lead to coronary heart disease or death. There are many causal factors in the development of hypertension.

(i) Physiological pre-disposition is a chief cause. In some individuals the sympathetic nervous system is hyperactive and may lead to greater vascular reactivity which increases blood pressure.

(ii) Some emotional factors, especially emotional arousal leads to increased stress which results in vasoconstriction resulting in hypertension. Cobb and Rose found that Air traffic controllers had six time more incidence of hypertension than the controlled group, because they experienced more stress.

(iii) Franz Alexander has suggested the co-relationship between certain personality traits and hypertension.

Alexander concluded on the basis of his research that "inhibited hostile tendencies play an important role in this phenomenon". Similarly Walter Cannon on the basis of his experimental work on animals demonstrated that chronic feelings of hostility are implicated in essential hypertension. Clinical and empirical studies focusing on the relationship between aggression and hypertension show that the two phenomenon are related.

(iv) David Mcdelland have found that hypertension is due to inhibited power motivation. He suggested that those who have strong desire to have power but inhibit its expression are likely to develop hypertension.

McClelland suggested that inhibited power motivation would be related to the development of high blood pressure. In three samples of men varying in age and baseline level of blood pressure, it was found that the inhibited power motive syndrome was associated with significantly high blood pressure.

(e) **Coronary Heart Disease** Coronary heart disease is one of the major cause of death not only in the United States, but also in India. In India, coronary heart disease sufferer is young adult from urban area facing a lot of stress. The two forms of coronary heart disease are as follows :

(i) Myocardial Infarcation and

(ii) Angina pectoris.

(i) **Myocardial Infarcation:** In common vocabulary is referred to as heart attack. These attacks usually are caused by an obstruction of one of the heart arteries which can lead to the destruction of portions of the heart muscle. If the destroyed heart muscle was responsible for maintaining heart functioning, then the heart attack will probably be fatal. The experience of myocardial infarcation is uniquely frightening and can generate a great, deal of anxiety.

(ii) **Angina Pectoris** is a less serious but still very painful form of coronary heart disease. In this disease people experience intense pain in chest, especially in the area behind the breast bone, and from the shoulder radiating down the left arm. These symptoms typically are caused by fatty deposits that block the arteries leading to the heart resulting in a decrease of oxygen to the organ itself. While the reduced blood flow creates pain, it is rarely fatal. Either emotional or physical exertion may trigger an attack of angina pectoris.

Causes of Coronary Heart Diseases: A combination of biological, psychological and socio cultural factors has been associated with the development of coronary heart diseases.

(i) **Personality Pattern and Coronary Heart Diseases:** Clinicians and researchers have found that certain individuals are more prone for the development of this type of disorders due to the situational challenges they face and due to their personality make-up. These individuals are called as type 'A' individuals. The concept of type 'A' was introduced by Friedman and Roseman in 1958. "They found that type 'A' individuals are twice as much likely to develop heart disease as type 'B' individuals. Type 'A' people are emotional, achievement oriented, competitive, time conscious, perfectionist and are always functioning above their physiological baseline. This leads to the development of coronary heart disease.

Research evidence has led some support to Fredman and Roseman's thinking. For e.g. Suinn (1978) found that type 'A' males in the 39 to 49 year old age group had six times as many heart attacks as type 'B' males. In an extensive study Roseman et. al. (1975) followed more than 3000,391059 year old men over an 8 year old period. Results showed that type A individuals were more than twice as prone to develop coronary heart disease as type B people. Further, in those men who already had evidence of coronary heart disease, type A men were 5 times as likely to have a second heart attack. Also the higher frequency of coronary Heart Disease in the Type A men was independent of such extraneous factors as education, health care and exercise levels.

(ii) **Combination of Biological and psychosocial factors** have also been identified in the causation of coronary heart diseases. Lipowski (1980) has identified six major factors that appear to be related to the development of coronary heart disease.

(a) **Dietary Factors:** Diets that are habitually filled with high levels of saturated fats, cholesterol and calories.

(b) **Blood chemistry:** Elevated levels of various innate chemicals such as cholesterol.

(c) **Organ disease or dysfunction:** Disorder like Kidney disease or diabetes Mellitus.

(d) **Living habits:** A deadly trio of smoking, overeating and physical inactivity.

(e) **Environmental factors:** Chronic dissatisfaction with life and work.

(f) **Familial factors:** A family history of coronary heart disease and related disorders.

THEORIES OF DEVELOPMENT OF PSYCHOPHYSIOLOGICAL DISORDERS

Different theories have been put forward to explain the etiology of psychophysiological disorder. According to some researchers psychophysiological disorders area result of poor organ system, whereas, according to psychoanalytic writers psychophysiological disorders are a result of unconscious conflict and frustration. Behavioural theorists have also explained the development of psychophysiological disorders on the basis of learning principles. Some have explained the development of this disorder according to Diasthesis Stress Theory.

1. **Organ System Weakness:** Weakness of a specific organ system is largely a result of genetic influences or may be a result of prior damage of a given system. Organ system specificity may also be related to the concept of general adaptation Syndrome in the development of psychophysiological disorder for e.g. Hans Selye has demonstrated that general adaptation syndrome along with damage to body's immunological system may lead to development of psychophysiological disorder.

Thus, from the above we see that some individuals have a poor organ system and is more vulnerable to stress of life. By the concept of organ system we mean that some organs are weaker and more susceptible to the development of certain disorders. For example, a person may be otherwise healthy but may have a poor respiratory system which is more vulnerable to infection and allergy. Such individual is more likely to suffer from asthama than from coronary heart disease or from ulcer. However, one of the major difficulties is to demonstrate that a given disorder is how much due to psychological factors and how much is due to physiological factors.

2. **Psychoanalytic viewpoint:** Psychodynamic viewpoint is explained in the work of Alexander and Dunbar. According to psychoanalytic approach, psychophysiological disorders are symbols of unsolved unconscious conflict and frustration. For example, Alexander has pointed out that frustration of unsolved dependency need during the oral stage lead to the development of fear. Similarly Mactell has demonstrated that hypertension is usually associated with high need for power. Graham and Grace have suggested that specific attitude are co-related with the development of psychophysiological disorders. For example, Asthama is associated with individuals who want to go away from the situation. A duodenal ulcer is commonly seen in individuals with repressed hostility. Hypertension develops due to anticipated threat. However, psycho-

dynamic theory is one of the most controversial, requiring further research.

3. **Behavioural Theories:** 'Lechman has pointed out that psychophysiological disorder is a learned disorder. According to him the autonomic nervous system response can be learned through learning. He has proposed 5 methods which lead to the development of a specific symptomatolgy.

These five learning processes are

(a) the role of stimulus-substitution learning,

(b) the role of emotional integration,

(c) the role of stimulus generalization,

(d) the role of symbolic stimuli,

(e) the role of ideation.

(a) **The role of stimulus-substitution learning:** According to this theory, classical conditioning leads to the development of psychophysiological disorder. If the neutral stimuli is associated with one action producing stimuli,

soon the person learn to respond to neutral stimuli. For example, while it is raining, a child is frightened not by raining but by lightening and thunder outside. However, on subsequent occasion, even a slight raining may lead to fear reaction in the absence of thunder and lightening.

(b) **The role of emotional reintegration:** A single component in the stimulus-situation earlier associated with a complex pattern of emotional reactions (i.e., physiological responses) may itself be effective in producing the

total complex pattern of emotional reactions. A boy, while fishing on a bridge (fell) 30 feet into the ice cold water, was swept down a rocky track, and almost was drowned. Now the sight of that bridge or river or of people fishing or of the rocky track serves to revive vividly all of the complex stimulus situation and emotional reactions associated with the earlier event.

(c) **The role of stimulus generalization:** An internal response that has been associated with a particular stimulus may come to be elicited by a variety of somewhat similar stimuli, that is, stimuli somewhat like the originally learned stimulus but varying along one continuum or another. Such stimuli become capable of eliciting an internal response an emotional reaction or aspect there of they did not elicit prior to learning. (Swimming may evoke the emotional reaction that the boy felt after falling in the icy water, as mentioned above).

(d) **The role of symbolic stimuli**: Stimuli that in the personal history of the individual represent effective emotion-provoking stimuli, may themselves become emotion-provoking. At the human level, such symbolic stimuli (or stimulus symbols) are frequently but not always language stimuli. (The Word "rape" may provoke strong emotional reactions in a woman who has been sexually assaulted).

(e) **The role of ideation:** Organismic effects of stimuli, probably largely in terms of central nervous system manifestations, may persist in the form of "central percepts", thoughts", or "ideas" (i.e., neural images or cognitive symbols) that can be revived in the absence of the originally relevant external stimulus situation, to produce a characteristic implicit emotional-reaction constellation. (An individual may think about an emotional event (being criticized by an employer) and may feel the associated emotion (anxiety).

According to Lachman, any one or more of the above processes may give rise to autonomic nervous system arousal leading to the development of psychophysiological disorder.

4. **Diathesis stress theory**: The term 'diathesis' means physiological or psychological pre-disposition. Diathesis when it is accompanied by stress is likely to develop a psychophysiological disorder, in an individual.

VARIOUS APPROACHES FOR TREATMENT OF PSYCHOPHYSIOLOGJCAL DISORDERS

A wide variety of treatment approaches have been adopted to tackle various psychophysiological disorders. We would discuss how the various approaches have been used to treat different psychophysiological disorders.

1. **Psychodynamic approaches in the treatment of psycho-physiological disorders:** Psychotherapy based on psychoanalytic theory gives mix results. It is effective with some people and with some disorders. It is suggested by Karasu that effectiveness of this therapy depends on patient's preparedness for the therapy. According to him first step of this preparation is health alliance where the therapist builds trust in the patient by being supportive. At the second life alliance stage the therapist becomes more reliable and trustworthy. At this stage the actual therapy may begin. However, this entire process can be very time-consuming as it may involve a period of 6-7 years.

A noteworthy study in the area of psychodynamic approach is that of Kellner (1975). Kellner (1975), in a survey of controlled studies concluded that psychotherapeutic approaches are effective for some patients with some disorder. For e. g. peptic ulcer, asthama, and migraine appear to be more amenable to such treatment than to hypertension and uncertain colitis. However, he points out that few of these studies have been replicated and the evidence remains tentative.

Hypnotism-Techniques can also be used to treat the patient. But success of this technique depends on the individual rather than the disease i.e. If the person has high hypnotic ability, hypnosis can be effective, but not otherwise. Bowers and Kelley (1979) have examined some disorders and the impact of hypnotic treatment on them. A major point which they have is that the characteristics of the person, rather than the type of disease, are important in determining the usefulness of the techniques. They indicate that high hypnotic ability in the subject is predictive of successful use of hypnosis in the treatment of psychophysiological disorder, while low hypnotic ability is not. Are view of the application of hypnosis to the treatment of skin disorder, headache, and asthma, however, indicates that the evidence that hypnosis can directly influence autonomic nervous system .functioning, even in people who can be deeply hypnotized, remains equivocal.

Another significant work with respect to psychoanalytic treatment of psychophysiological disorder is that a Malan (1973) who assessed the various therapy effectiveness survey review studies from the perspective of dynamic psychotherapy, found that the traditional psychotherapy approach is effective with psychophysiological disorders. One type of psychophysiological disorder that has been found to be especially responsive to this form of therapy is ulcerative colitis (ulceration and inflammation of the colon often accompanied by disturbances in normal bowel functions). On the basis of research at the psychoanalytic clinic for training and research at Columbia University's college of Physicians and Surgeons, it has been shown that clotis patients can be effectively treated with psychoanalytically-oriented psychotherapy (Kanish et. al, 1969 and O'Connor et. al 1964). This research also demonstrated that ulcerative colitis patients who are characterized as being overly dependent and symbiotic in their interpersonal relationships (i.e. who sec themselves as helpless victims of others, with a tendency to blame others for their frustration and faults) are most responsive to insight oriented psychotherapy. Weinstock (1962) has reported similar findings. Thus, there is evidence for the effectiveness of traditional psychotherapeutic techniques in the treatment of psychosomatic disorders.

2. **Behavioural Approaches to Treatment:** Since the early 1960s behaviour therapy has frequently been applied to psychophysiological disorders. In a survey of treatment approaches. Price (1974) reports that a wide variety of specific behaviour which influences the course of psychophysiological disorders. The techniques have been used to modify the environmental contingencies which seem to maintain symptoms, to directly inhibit a supposedly pathological automic nervous system, and to modify behaviours that increase the risk of illness (e.g., smoking cigarettes). The successful application of behavioral

techniques to physical illness has led to the development of a new specialty called behavioral medicine.

In the operant behavioral technique reinforcement like special attention or overprotection is totally withdrawn. In addition improved behaviour is reinforced by giving some rewards. This technique does not take into account physiological aspect.

Biofeedback is a technique which is becoming more and more popular. In biofeedback some instruments are used which will inform the individual about the psychophysiological processes, of which we are not usually aware. And then he is taught to bring them under voluntary control. With the help of biofeedback technique the individual can control blood pressure, skin temperature, muscle tension etc. According to some psychologists biofeedback is a very promising technique.

Table 4.1 briefly summarizes the psychosomatic disorders found to be responsive to the various behaviour therapy techniques and lists some of the relevant studies.

Table 4.1

Disorder	**Treatment**	**Investigators**
Asthama	Systematic desensitization	Moore (1965)
	Respiratory resistance biofeedback	Feldam (1976)
Dysmentinheo	Systematic desensitization.	Mullen (1971).
Essential hypertension.	Blood pressure biofeedback.	Benson, Shapiro, Tursky & Schwartz (1971) Eldere, Ruiz, Deobler, & Dillenkoffer (1973).
Migraine headache	Systematic desensitization, assertive training.	Mitchell & Mitchell (1971)
	Vasomotor biofeedback.	Friar & Beatty (1976)
	Temperature biofeedback, autogenic training*	Sargent, Green, & Walters (1973)
Muscle contraction headache	EMG biofeedback**	Budzynski, Stoyvo, Adler, & Mullaney (1973)
	EMG biofeedback, relaxation training.	Chesney & Shelton (1976); Haynes, Griffin, Mooney, & Parise (1975)
Neurodermatitis	Relaxation training	Ratliff & Stein (1968)

* Autogenic training is a relaxation techniques that uses simple imagery. It was developed by Schulz and Luthe (1959) for the treatment of a wide variety of psychological and somatic disorders.

** EMG biofeedback is a procedure that provides auditory and/or visual display of muscular activity EMG means electromyography.

If various emotional reactions result in psychophysiological disorders, then, systematic desensitization can reduce these emotional reactions. It has been found out that desensitization is effective in reducing asthamatic attacks.

Besides these techniques, relaxation training meditation can also be helpful to control psychophysiological disorders.

3. Medical Approaches: Medical approaches are used to great extent because people find difficult to accept that their disorder has psychological factors involved. Not only the patients, but many physicians also do not believe in psychological causes. They emphasize pharmacological treatment or surgical techniques and advise the patient rest or change of climate, e.g. for ulcer the physician may advise rest, balanced died, involving milk, multivitamin capsules and some medication or for asthama drugs like ephedrine and epinephrine a given.

4. Application of Treatment approaches to some specific psycho physiological disorders:

(a) Asthama can be treated best by medical approach. The exact treatment depends upon the type of symptoms. In emotional factors psychotherapy or hypnosis is used. Recently biofeedback is becoming popular. Alexander (1972) found that asthamatics with low somatic predisposition respond better to relaxation training than do those with high somatic predisposition.

(b) Migraine: Treatment of Migraine is a joint effort of biological as well as psychological approaches. Some of the more successful, but primarily symptomatic, biological treatments for migraine are tranquilizers, antidepressant drugs, histamine desensitization surgery and special diets. However, the most effective biological treatment for migraine headache has been the administration of ergotamine tartrate and its derivates. Administration of ergotamine tartrate early in the migraine headache attack usually restores the dilated vessels to their original state and reduces the severity of the headache.

Of all the biological approaches, variants of biofeedback procedures also seem to hold much promise. Holroyd ct. al. (1980) compared EMG biofeedback training with psychotherapy or a symptom monitoring control group. Only the biofeedback procedure effectively reduced headache symptoms. The efficacy of biofeedback procedures was further established by Andrasi and Holroyd (1980), Cram (1980), and Anderson et. al. (1981) who used a variety of techniques to lesson the pain brought about by migraine headaches. These results reinforce the conclusions of Addams et. al. (1980) that "a biofeedback approach directed at modifying the peripheral pain mechanism in migraine appears to be a promising treatment technique for this disorder".

From the psychosocial perspective, behaviour modification has been advocated by some as a treatment for headaches (Philips & Hunter, 1981). Behavioural techniques are based on the assumption that, if a person could relax in response to the cues that a migraine headache was developing, this might lesson the response of the endocrine and autonomic neurons. Using a population of 17 migraine-headache suffers, Mitchell and Mitchell (1973) found that pitting relaxation against the tension of migraine-headache cues was successful in reducing the number and duration of migraine episodes. In fact, after reviewing a large number of studies, Adams et. al. (1980) concluded that "hypnotic intervention relaxation training, various behaviour therapy techniques, and thermal and blood volume pulse biofeedback appear to significantly after migraine activity.

(c) **Essential Hypertension:** As Physiological predisposition is one of the major factors in essential hypertension, drugs reducing B.P. are given in medical treatment. But the drugs may have dangerous side-effects, so must be prescribed with caution.

Like migraine, biofeedback and relaxation training are very effective in hypertension. The subjects can be trained to lower their B.P. However, these approaches do not have enough empirical evidence.

Recent research on biofeedback and relaxation therapy has indicated promise for the treatment of hypertension. (Price, 1974). Both approaches can be used to train subjects to significantly lower their blood pressure. Patel and North (1975) have demonstrated that the combined use of Yoga meditation and biofeedback led to a significant average reeducation of 26.1 points in bloods pressure for hypertensive patients. Simply providing direct feedback of blood pressure levels without training in meditation also can lead to a 10-15 percent reduction in pressure (Kristt & Engel, 1975) But studies of the clinical application of these techniques are not completely positive. Although Agras, Taylor, Kraemer, Allen, and Schneider (1980) found that relaxation treatment significantly reduced hypertensives' blood pressure, Tylor et.al. (1977) found that relaxation therapy had no greater when evaluated one year after the treatment period. In this study, the immediate positive effects of relaxation therapy were lost due to the absence of what authors concluded was an essential requirement periodic maintenance training in the relaxation techniques. Surwit, Shapiro, and Good (1978) found that relaxation, treatment muscle tension reduction, and cardiovascular feedback were of little value with borderline hypertensives, and suggested that these approaches are useful when the initial values of the clients blood pressures are very high. The current status of biofeedback and relaxation approaches warrants further study and clinical trials. They do not have enough support to justify calling them established treatments (Engel, 1979).

(d) **Colitis:** Treatment methods for colitis derive primarily from the psychosocial and biological paradigms include psychoanalytic psychotherapy and drugs. Drug treatment, however, is primarily directed at reducing symptoms and not at remediating the underlying cause. In psychoanalytic therapy on the other hand, the therapist seeks to become the "key" person in the colitis patient's life and through this relationship to help the patient learn new, more effective ways of relating to people, thereby changing the course of the colitis.

In a through study of the effects of psychotherapy of ulcerative colitis patients, Karush and his colleagues conducted a 30 year follow-up of people who had received various combinations of treatment involving psychotherapy and medical and surgical procedures (Karush et.al. 1977). They found that patients who had received psychotherapy were more improved than others the large intestine) or a colostomy (removal of all or part of the colon or large intestine leading to the rectum). Surgery is suggested only if there is intractable diarrhoea or the threat of further disease such as cancer.

(c) Ulcer can best be treated with a wide variety of approaches. Good diet, regular food intake, milk etc. is very useful. Antacids can also be very useful in controlling the development of ulcer.

Pchological approaches like controlling one's negative emotions and managing anxiety can also prevent the development of ulcers.

In one study (Brown & Richards, 1980) patients with duodenal ulcers were taught to manage anxiety and to express negative emotions appropriately. Eleven of the 22 male patients who had confirmed X-ray diagnosis of duodenal ulcers completed this training in eight 75-minute session over a 2-week period. The other II patients received an attention placebo treatment. Those patients who had received training consumed less antacid, reported fewer days of symptomatic pain, and experienced less severe symptoms over the entire follow-up period. In fact, after 3 *Vi* years, the treatment group did show a significantly lower rate of ulcers.

Although psychotherapy may be effective in helping people handle stress more adequately, it probably doesn't directly change underlying inherited physiological predisposition that is, on a genetic basis, people who tend to hypersecrete stomach acids probably will be most vulnerable to developing ulcers when stressed. In light of this, people who develop ulcers should be made aware of the possibility that proneness to ulcers doesn't necessarily reflect a psychosocial defect or weakness it may simply be the result of chronic gastric hyperactivity over which they have no control.

(A) TYPE A PERSONALITY AND CARDIOVASCULAR DISORDERS

The concept of type A behaviour pattern was for the first time discussed by Friedman and Rosenmann (1959) in the contest of medical setup. According to them certain people, because of their personality characteristic and life style have a particular pattern of functioning which makes them more vulnerable to the development of cardiovascular disorders.

Individuals who have type A personality pattern display the following characteristic of behaviour.

1. They are highly achievement oriented, ambitious and competitive.

2. Type A individuals tend to become irritable and impatient.

3. The high need for success, in most of them, leads to a preference for working alone when under pressure, and to become angry when anything or anyone gets in the way.

4. Type A individuals do not believe in avoiding problems or responsibilities, and they want to do things perfectly. These various pressure lead to problems with sleeping.

5. Time is all important to them. They tend to arrive early for appointments and gets irritated if anyone is delayed or if anyone keeps them waiting.

6. In social situations. Type a fee] uncomfortable and have a sense of insecurity.

7. Type A individual tend to focus attention on the task at hand and to ignore any distractions that could interfere with getting the job done.

8. Type A's complain less about the hard work. They work as hard as is necessary to get the main task done, even when the demands and interruptions increase.

9. Though type A respond well to a challenge, the price they pay is an accompanying increase in cardiovascular activity.

10. Type A individuals fear failure more often than others.

11. In interpersonal relationship Type A's need to control the situation and to do better than opponents. The result is a belief that they know a great deal about other people and that they can predict what others will do.

12. Type A have poor family relationship, experience more interpersonal

conflicts, have less intimate interpersonal relationship and are perceived to be selfish and narcissistic.

13. Type A orientation is associated with masculinity among both, males and females.

14. Type A individuals have internal locus of control are more confident arid extrovert.

(B) GENERAL ADAPTATION SYNDROME

The concept of General Adaptation Syndrome was introduced by Hans Selye. This syndrome consists of a sequence of 3 successive physiological stages which are called as (1) the alarm reaction, (2) the stage of resistance and (3) the stage of exhaustion

(1) **The alarm reaction** Consists of two phases, a shock phase in which there is an enlargement of adrenal cortex, a withering away of the thalamus gland and the appearance of gastrointestinal ulcers, and a counter shock phase in which body temporarily recovered from these symptoms. Most of the effects of the body during the alarm reaction particularly in the shock phase, are degenerative in nature but Selye noted that the changes of the adrenal cortex actually do flourish on stress.

If the stress was prolonged, (2) a stage of resistance set in and most of the symptoms of the alarm reaction begin to subside. The adrenals returned to normal size. The glucose and chloride levels of the blood were restored and the thalamus began to recover its normal appearance. In this stage, the physiological adjustment to the stress seemed optimal and the state of the body was not as it appeared. However, there was a serious weakness in the animal's adjustment Their resistance was strictly limited to the particular stress to which they had been exposed, the introduction of other stressors lead to further degeneration and even death. It is as though the protective defenses, of the animals were limited in amount. When they were given over entirely to handling one stressful situation, there were few or no reserves to use against other stressors.

Moreover, the stage of resistance did not persist indefinitely. (3) If stress continued the animals eventually weakened, and the stage of exhaustion began. In this final stage, serious physical changes occurred particularly in the brain. These included hemorrages. Cerebral arteriosclerosis, and epileptic seizures which brought death.

(C) ROLE OF AUTONOMIC NERVOUS SYSTEM IN EMOTIONAL AROUSAL

Autonomic nervous system is a part of peripheral nervous system which consists of peripheral motor fibres running to a variety of organs. Autonomic nervous system causes many of the emotional and motivated activities initiated by the old fore-brain and in particular by the hypothalamus. Autonomic nervous system is divided into 2 parts, one part is sympathetic nervous system, which is composed of fibres leaving the brain and sacral regions of the spinal cord. The sympathetic system consisting of fibres leaving the central portion of the spinal cord. Autonomic nervous system plays a very important role in emotion. Typical changes occur in the physiology of the body. Walter Cannon, a physiologist regarded these changes as adaptive, since they are frequently seen in pre-emergency when the organism is threatened with injury or it is actually injured. The autonomic nervous system changes prepares the body for emergency action. This is called as "fight or flight" response.

The sympathetic and parasympathetic system tend to act in opposing ways. The sympathetic system prepares the body for action. The parasympathetic system usually function when the body is at rest. When the sympathetic system is active, heart beat increases to pump more blood. Blood is shunted away from the Viscera to the muscles, providing extra oxygen and nutrients where they are most needed during activity. Breathing becomes deeper and more rapid, which ensures a plentiful supply of oxygen. The pupils of the eyes dilate to allow for better vision. The liver releases sugar for energy. All these action mobilizes the body's resources.

The parasympathetic system helps the body's organs to protect and conserve their resources. The heart beat slows down, blood is shunted from the muscles to the viscera, the pupils of the eyes contract, breathing is more relaxed and shallower. Because of the nature of the physiological process that. They initiate the two system tend to be associated with emotional states. Sympathetic arousal is interpreted as nervous tension, anxiety, fear and excitement, parasympathetic arousal as calmness.

(D) STRESS LIFE EVENTS AND PHYSICAL ILLNESS

Researchers and clinicians have observed that there is a significant relationship between physical illness and certain life events. Many individuals who have undergone certain stressful life events show definite psycho-physiological disorders.

Many tests have been developed to scale certain life events which lead tc stress and subsequent physical illness.

One of the best known life event scale was developed by Holmes and Rahe in 1967.

They constructed a list of various life-changing events. Then asked large number of subjects to assign value to each of the events according to the intensity of stress and period required for adjustment. Thus, marriage is given value of 50 . and accordingly various other events like death of spouse, divorce, fired at work, pregnancy, beginning or ending of school, etc, spouse has highest score of 100 in terms of stressfulness and lowest value of II is assigned for minor violation of the law.

In number of studies it was found that there is definite relationship between stressful events and illness. In one study of 2500 U.S. Navy officers, it was found that those officers who had more risky jobs suffered 90% more illness than the officers with less risky jobs (Rahe, Maten and Arthur). Similarly in one other study by Cobb and Rose (1973), it was found that air traffic controller suffered from hypertension nearly six times more than the group of second class airman who were licensed to fly airplanes.

The impressive evidence for the relationships between stress and disease has not gone unchallenged. Correlations between stressful events and disease in random populations are usually quite moderate, sometimes as low as 0.10 (Bowers&Kelly,1979).

This moderate or low correlationship between stress and life event scale can be explained by the fact that some individuals are better equipped than others to handle such stressful life events. They have what is called as psychosocial support system which helps them to adjust better with stress and these life events, and this raises their immunity against the development of physical illness due to these life events.

3

Stress Related Disorders

Stress is a common phenomenon of everyday life. All of us experience Stress to some degree in one or another from throughout lives. However, some forms of stress are pathological and lead to development of wide variety of symptoms and disorders. Prolonged exposure to stress leads to wide variety of physiological changes that may effect our health and functioning.

A wide Variety of changes in our social system, technological developments and scientific revolution has brought about sweeping and radical changes in our value system, and have placed higher demands on human beings for effective -functioning. This very often creates stress. Modem Man is also not free from wars and natural catastrophes. The history bear witness to the fact that many historical wars like World War I & II, Korean War, Vietnam War etc, have created stress not only among soldiers and their family members but also among the general public. The consequences of these wars in terms of psychological casualties is well documented and needs to be studied in detail.

Natural disasters like flood, famines, illnesses, accidents also bring severe stress in many individuals. The effects of these stress is long tasting and difficult to overcome.

In this chapter we will first define stress and discuss the important characteristics of stress. We would also distinguish between stress and stressor and discuss the characteristics and consequences of major stressors and their consequences.

Following this we would discuss the nature and characteristics of stress associated with combact or war. Such stress is also called as chronic intense stress. We would discuss the various disturbances that develop as a result of stress experiences due to combact or war.

Besides the destructive aspect of War, one type of stress experienced by individuals, during War, which is very traumatic, is the experience of being a prisoner of war or experience of concentration camp. We would discuss the nature of this particular type of stress also.

Stress is not limited to War. It occurs in our daily life also. We would discuss the nature of civilian catastrophe or typical crisis situation in our daily life. Such stress is also harmful and can disrupt our functioning and adjustment by affecting us physically as well as psychologically.

We would then discuss the various techniques of coping with stress. We would end .this chapter with a few short notes.

DEFINITION OF STRESS

Stress can be defined as a demand placed on our psychological and physical functioning that threatens an individual's adaptation to a given situation.

The tern stress is generally used in two sense: (1) It is used to refer to the negative feeling and emotions that are generated in us. (2) The term is also used to refer to the presence of various stressor, that is, various situations that give rise to stress. The type of the stress experienced depends not only on the situation and events which give rise to it, but also on the individual's perspective, constitutional make-up and the strategies that he has-developed to cope with the stress. Bowers and Kelly (1979) has pointed out four important characteristics of stressful events:

(1) People feel a sense of loss of control of the events in their lives. They feel helpless to change what is going on and to successfully intervene in the process.

(2) There is an anticipation or occurrence of physical or psychological pain. For example, the individual fears being injured or killed (as in a disaster) or is threatened with a loss of self-esteem (as in a divorce).

(3) There is a loss of social or emotional support. In a disaster, friends and

relatives may be missing or killed. Less drastic events such as divorce, job loss or marriage may separate individuals from family members and old friends.

(4) The event or some aspect of it is perceived as unpleasant or aversive and the individual tries to actively avoid it.

STRESSORS AND ITS TYPES

Any event or a situation that give rise to stress is called as a Stressor. Different stressors differ in a number of ways. For example, some stressors like illness, robbery have short term effect, whereas, others like death of loved one, poverty etc., have long-term effects. Some stressors, like death of loved one, criminal victimization etc. effect only a few individuals, whereas other stressors, like hurricane, earthquake etc. effect large number of people. Terrorism is a severe stressor, the irritating habit of-a hostel room mate are inconsequential. Obviously, these differences offer several bases for classifying stressors. According to Lazarus and Cohen (1977) stressors can be classified into following three types:

(1) Background stressors

(2) Personal stressors, and

(3) Cataclysmic events.

(1) **Background Stressors** are the hassles of everyday life. They are the persistent, nagging, irritations at home, school and work that effect us all. Some of the examples of background stressor include:

(a) Early in the morning when you have for the college the bus conductor asks you to give a change which you don't have. Arguments result which according to you creates unpleasant situation.

(b) At work your boss or a particular colleague bit of irritating you.

(c) While you are sleep the phone bell constantly rings and its repeatedly a wrong number.

(d) Your house maid is very irregular and causes you discomfort due to this habit of hers.

(e) Working in the night shift or working under some pressure is also one type of background stressor.

By themselves these background stressors are not harmful. However, the effects of stress accumulate. A brief exposure to any one of them would have little or no effect on any one. Prolonged exposure to them, however, can leave the individual to stress disorders. The cumulative effect of background stressors are harmful. Background stressors interestingly, also include positive events like election to an office, promotion at work, vacations, marriage, dating etc.

(2) **Personal Stressors** are inevitable in the lives of all of us. We will experience different types of personal stressors in varying degrees during the course of our life. However, in some individuals many personal stressors may occur one after the other and cause considerable stresses whereas in others personal stressors may occur after long periods of time giving them an opportunity to overcome them gradually. Some of the common personal stressors are as follows:

(a) Separation.

(b) Transition stress.

(c) Unemployment.

(d) Divorce.

(e) Bereavement (i.e. death of a loved one)

(f) Criminal Victimization and

(g) Conflict.

We will now discuss these in brief.

(a) Separation occurs at each and every period of our life. The first type of separation that a young child experiences is during that weaning period. It is a period when child is no longer breast fed. He has, to eat and drink on his own. He has to walk and move without support. Weaning period, often, is a source of stress.

Going to school especially the first day at school, is also a source of stress in many children. It is during this period that the child has to remain away from his home into a school or a nursery which is a new environment for the child. The class teacher as well as other children may not give the child the same attention and care that he gets at home. A child may also experience many unpleasant experience which may create stress in him/her.

During puberty and adolescent the child experiences different types of stress. At puberty girls are told to come home early, not to talk to boys or strangers etc., whereas, an adolescent male would realise that he is no longer a child and neither an adult.

Some other types of separation that might lead to stress arc job transfer, marriage, change of residence. Divorce and death also lead to separation.

Separation is a stressful experience because it- leads to loss of companionship, comfort and emotional support. Separation can bring anxiety, require newer coping skills and may-create fear or threat in an individual; regarding his adjustment. Hence, it creates stress.

(b) **Transition Stress** In the course of developing from infant to child to adolescent to adult, the individual experiences a series of new stressors connected with the transition from one stage of development to another. During these transitions individuals are likely to feel a discrepancy between the new demands placed on them and their assessment of their abilities to meet these demands. A transition stress can occur at an early age, as the results of a recent study by Jerome Kagan (1983) very clearly indicate.

The experimental situation devised by Kagan reveals the existence of transition stress in very young children. Similar stress occurs at later ages when the life of an individual changes in important ways; going off to school, experiencing the puberial changes of adolescence, leaving home for work or college, marrying and beginning a family, retiring. In the case of retirement, people often experience a reverse from of stressful discrepancy. The individual's abilities are greater than the demands of retirement.

(c) **Unemployment** is another major source of personal stressor because unemployed people in our society are looked down upon. Besides, unemployed individuals, especially youth, may have low buying power. Many of their needs may not be met leading to frustration and conflict in them. Unemployed people may also have interpersonal problems, poor self esteem and experience helplessness and dependency.

Based on his analysis of thirty years of data, M. Harvey Brenner (1972, 1981 and 1982), the Johns Hopkins University expert on the long-term effects of stress on the nation's health, has projected the following unhealthy consequences of every one percentage point of increase in the unemployment rate; suicide, up 4.1 percent, homicides, up 5.7 percent, deaths from heart disease, stress-related disorders, and cirrhosis of the liver, up 1.9 percent, admission to state mental hospitals, men up 4.3 percent, women up 2.3 percent.

Various clinical accounts of the stressfulness of unemployment is reinforced by a study of the physiological consequences of joblessness (Kasl and Cobb, 1970). The participants in this study were married, stably employed men who lost their jobs when their plant was permanently shut down. Over a span of twenty-six months, their stress reactions were studied by means of their blood pressure. During these months their jobs ended, some men were unemployed for a prolonged period, some took temporary work, and some found another job. The blood pressure of a group of men who kept their jobs during the same period were also studied, the major results were these:

(i) Individuals who continued to be employed showed no important changes in blood pressure. Psychologically they remained reasonably well satisfied with their situations.

(ii) When workers were advised that they would probably lose their jobs, their blood pressure began to rise as they were forced to deal with the discrepancy between their earlier expectations and their new uncertain situations.

(iii) With unemployment blood pressure rose further and remained high, even when men took temporary work. The men also reported a greater awareness that they were under stress.

(iv) When the men went back to work, their blood pressure began to decline, and their outlook on life became more positive. Extensive data obtained more recently support these findings (Kasl and Cobb 1980, 1982).

(d) **Divorce**: Divorce is now a major source of stress, especially in the case of children. And the rate of divorce is on the increase. Divorce is more stressful for women as well as children especially in our society.

Divorce places strains on children in three principal ways :

(i) The First is by removing one of the children's parents from the home.

(ii) The second is by decline in the economic status of their mothers, with whom they usually remain.

(iii) The third source of pressure is from the heightened stress on the divorced mother herself.

In a national survey (Champbell et. al., 1976) divorced women gave more affirmative responses, even than widows, to questionnaire items such as the following: feel life is hard, feel tied down, always feel rushed, worry about bills, feel frightened worry about nervous breakdown.

Divorced men like women, of course, also suffer. By comparison with non-divorced people, they arc over represented in the statistics for motor vehicle accidents and fatalities, they are more frequently psychiatric patients they visit physicians more often every year because of higher rates of illness, disability, and alcoholism. They arc more frequent victims of homicide, and they more often take their own lives.

(e) **Bereavement: D**eath of a spouse is the most powerful stressor on the life stress scales. This tragedy is particularly stressful since it must be endured alone. The death of a spouse brings in its wake the loss of companionship, sex, comfort, often a home, and the most important source of economic and social support. Friends are unable to understand or accept the grief and mourning of the widow or widower as it becomes prolonged, and they gradually drift away. Bereavement is a particularly common problem among the women in our older population. Because of the greater longevity of women, the ratio of widows to widowers is four to one.

The stress of bereavement is sometimes fatal. For men and women who become widows and widowers, the mortality rate increases abruptly, especially during the first six months after the death of a spouse. These mortality statistics prove that people do die of broken hearts, literally as well as figuratively (Lunch, 1977). Cardiac disorders take the lives of many widows and widowers, even of those who are under thirty five years of age.

Other data indicates that widows younger than sixty-five consult physicians at thrice the expected rate for their ages (Greenblatt, 1978; Parkes, 1972). These widows also spend more time than other women of their ages sick in bed at home or in the hospital. They use sedatives at seven times the normal rate, they drink too much alcohol, and they use medication excessively. All these practices are ones that hasten dying. Suicides are an additional testimonial to the grief of bereavement. During the first year of widowhood, the suicide rate is 2.5 times that of other women of their age, from the second through the fourth year, the rate is 1.5 times greater for widows than for other women of their age.

(f) **Criminal victimization** is another important source of stress. Many a times we may become victims of criminal acts which may lead to considerable degree of stress in each one of us depending upon the severity of crime committed on us. Rape is the most severe form of crime, as compared to molestation. Robbery, housebreaking, chain snatching are less severe as compared to kidnapping and threat to murder. In certain geographic locations such types of stress are more common. For example, terrorism and its resulting consequences are more experienced by people of Punjab than that of West Bengal. Similarly communal riots are more commonly feared in places like Meerut, Moradabad and Aligarh than at places like Gujarat or Madras. There are also sex differences in this type of stress. For example, women are more likely to experience stress with respect to the fear of being molested or raped as compared to men.

(g) **Conflict:** Conflicting motives are a final important source of personal stress. States of conflict and the stress that accompanies them are familiar to all of us. We experience conflict in many ways. One of our common conflict is deciding to forego one goal to attain another, for example, giving up to night's social evening to work on a term paper that it due tomorrow. In terms of emotions, conflict is a state in which opposing feeling tug at one another. We are irritated at the sight of another student's cheating and consider reporting the incident, but the feeling that we are not the sort of person who tells on another, restrains us. The more important the opposed values in conflicts of this type, the greater the conflict. The wartime conflict between patriotic and religious values is one of the most difficult of these. Patriotism may require as soldier to slay an enemy; God's commandment insists that "Thou shalt not kill".

Some of the earliest theoretical analysis of conflict were by experimental psychologists who applied the basic principles of learning and motivation to the subject. They treated conflict in terms of positive tendencies to approach certain goals and negative tendencies to avoid others. They identified four major ways in which these tendencies could oppose one another and thus defined four major types of conflict : (i) approach-approach, (ii) avoidance-avoidance, (iii) approach-avoidance, and (iv) double approach-avoidance, or Multiple approach avoidance conflict.

(i) **Approach-Approach:** In this type of conflict a person is faced with two attractive alternatives, only one of which can be selected. There are two courses that you want to take, but they are scheduled for the same time. As this example suggests, approach-approach conflicts are usually easy to resolve; you choose one course and decide to take the other next semester. Approach-approach conflicts becomes serious only if the choice of one alternative means the loss of an extremely attractive alternative.

(ii) **Avoidance-Avoidance Conflict:** A second type of conflict, avoidance-avoidance, involves two negative goals and is a fairly common experience. A boy must do his arithmetic homework or get spanking. A student must spend the next 2 days studying for an examination or face the possibility of failure. A woman must work at a job she intensely dislikes or take the chance of losing her income. Such conflicts are capsuled in the saying, "caught between the devil and the deep blue sea." We can all think of things we do not want to but must do or face even less desirable alternatives.

(iii) **Approach-Avoidance Conflict**-The third type of conflict, approach-avoidance, is often the most difficult to resolve because, in this type of conflict, a person is both, attracted and repelled by the same goal object. Because of the positive valence of the goal, the person approaches it but as it is approached, the negative valence becomes stronger. If, at some point during the approach to the goal, its repellent aspects become stronger than its positive aspects, the person will stop before reaching the goal. Because the goal is not reached, the individual is frustrated.

As with avoidance-avoidance conflicts, vacillation is common in approach-avoidance conflicts; people in these conflicts approach the goal until the negative valence becomes too strong, and then they back away from it. Often, however, the negative valence is not repellent enough to stop the approach behaviour. In such cases, people reach the goal, but much more slowly and hesitatingly than they would have without the negative valence; and until the goal is reached, there is frustration. Even after the goal is reached, an individual may feel uneasy because of the negative valence attached to it. Whether a person is frustrated by reaching a goal slowly or by not reaching it at all, emotional reactions such as fear, anger and resentment commonly accompany approach-avoidance conflicts.

(iv) **Double Approach-Avoidance or Multiple Approach-Avoidance Conflicts** Many of life's major decisions involve multiple approach-avoidance conflicts, meaning that several goals with positive and negative valences are involved. Suppose a woman is engaged to be married; suppose, further that the goal of marriage has a positive valence for her because of the stability and security, it will provide and because she loves the man she will be marrying. Suppose, on the other hand, that marriage is repellent to her because it will mean giving up an attractive offer of a job in another city. With respect to her career, the woman is attracted to the new job, but also repelled by the problems it will create for her marriage.

3. **Cataclysmic Event** is a momentous, violent, sudden happening, affecting many people such as natural disasters and combat. It is a powerful stressor.

History has many elaborate descriptions of the cataclysmic events especially in this century where wars, famines, floods etc. have increased beyond Human expectation. The recent years, we have seen cataclysmic events like terrorist acts, wars and natural disasters like Bhopal Gas Tragedy, train accidents etc. The two broad categories of cataclysmic events which we would discuss here areas follows:

(a) Reaction to disaster, and

(b) War and Combat.

(a) **Reaction to Disaster:** Tornadoes, hurricanes, floods, droughts, earthquakes and volcanic eruptions, all these disasters strike in unpredictable pattern and often permit neither preparation nor escape. More detailed observations of persons living through such catastrophes indicate that they suffer from a disaster syndrome that is reminiscent of the general adaptation syndrome. It consists of three stages:

(i) The first of which is a shock reaction. In this stage come 10 to 20 percent of the people remain calm, and another 20 percent go into a state of panic but most individuals are confused, stunned and paralyzed by the magnitude of disaster. This reaction may serve a 'useful purpose, for, like those in the silent exodus from Hiroshima; it isolates the victims from an overwhelming reality, at least for the time.

(ii) In the second state **a recall reaction,** people become aware of the disaster and begin to face reality. Depression and hostility are common part of the reaction.

(iii) In the third stage, the stage **of recall,** depression and hostility give

Way to tenseness and restlessness. People may relieve the events of the disaster, or they may repress these traumatic experiences. Only later does the process of renewal and rehabilitation begin to take place. Usually, the victims do not require hospitalization. But high levels of anxiety and distress may continue to have debilitating effects on the individual. As we saw in Selye's work and shall see again in connection with the stress of combat, the individual who has suffered trauma often remains susceptible and breakdown when faced with other stress later on.

(b) **War and Combat:** Nature's catastrophes comes in an unexpected fashion, there is relatively little anticipation of the threat. By contrast, war usually comes upon a people with some degree of warning, bringing with it the expectation of hunger, separation, bereavement and terror. Actual combat *adds* an additional element of fearful expectancy and thus heightens the stress of men going to battle. Neuropsychiatry casualties are inevitable in wart' .Tie, but time has brought changes to the most common types of breakdown, the conditions that produce them and the forms of therapy available.

Before World War I breakdown in combat was viewed as cowardice. During the First World War, the perception of breakdown changed. At first dazed and confused soldiers were considered the victims of "Shell Shock" which was taught to be due to brain damage caused by the impact of nearby explosions. But as the war progressed "Shell Shock" came to be recognised as a psychological reaction to stress, and the casual factors were thought to be personal. The victims were seen as individuals whose vulnerability to stress had been an aspect of their basic personality even before their war time service.

In the World War, too stress reactions to combat were called combat exhaustion, a designation that put the blame once again on the stressful conditions of battle. The principle symptoms were extreme fatigue, sleeplessness, terror, tremors, strong startle reaction to the slightest sounds, mutism and either stupor or agitated excitement.

One type of stress disorder related to war is called as post traumatic stress disorder. It is an anxiety disorder following in the aftermath of a traumatic event outside the range of usual human experience, the individual has intrusive recollections and recurrent dreams of the event, feels estranged from others and has lost interest in ongoing activities, is easily startled and has trouble concentrating and sleeping.

REACTIONS TO COMBAT OR STRESS IN COMBAT

Situational stress especially during combat situation has received a great deal of attention from psychologists and other mental health experts. The word "shell shock" was used to define severe reactions to stress during World War 1. However, during World War II many new terms developed to describe individual reactions to combat situation. It is a chronic intense stress situation. These terms are called as "combat exhaustion", "combat fatigue" and a "post-traumatic stress disorder".

In the Korean War the frequency of these disorders was less, but ranged from approximately 4 to 5 per cent. In Vietnam war the incidence of acute stress reaction was 1.5 per cent. The symptoms of a combat reaction developed sequentially from initial irritability to hypersensitivity, jumpiness and startle reactions. Sleeplessness then develops followed by fatigue.

Individuals during combat reaction shows acute emotional turmoil instability and insecurity.

Goodwin (1980) has pointed out that the following disturbances are commonly seen in Vietnam veterans with chronic stress reactions :

(1) **Depression:** The veteran who experienced the death of a comrade is likely to develop depression. The depression is often associated with a feeling of helplessness over the futility of war not supported at home.

(2) **Isolation:** Veterans often feel isolated from non-veteran peers, friends and family. They feel that only another Vietnam veteran can understand what they have been through. They sometimes experience hostility of civilians who opposed the war which is unlike the reaction to veterans of previous wars, who are hailed as "heroes".

(3) **Rage:** Many Vietnam veterans feel anger, even rage at "the system" and people who put then in an intolerable no-win situation. Most do not act out the rage, but are frightened that it will "break through" into their behaviour.

(4) **Surivival Guilt:** Many veterans feel survival guilt because they survived and friends or comrades died. They feel that if they had behaved differently the others might have lived.

(5) **Anxiety:** Many settings can evoke anxiety in these veterans people walking behind them on the street, standing in an exposed place, a loud noise. Though these men know their anxiety is irrational, they respond to these stimuli as if they were still in combat.

(6) **Sleep Disturbances**: The period before sleep is often filled with anxiety-provoking memories of Vietnam. During sleep, many have nightmares about combat experiences.

(7) **Intrusive thoughts:** Daytime events often trigger unpleasant thoughts (and associated emotions). A helicopter flying overhead, for example, may trigger intrusive thoughts or memories of a violent firelight and feelings of panic or rage.

(8) **Avoidance of feelings:** Many veterans describe themselves as emotionally dead. They feel no love, no caring, no joy. They seem to have pushed away all feeling in order to avoid feeling pain.

Some other common symptoms including ejections, weariness, hypersensitivity and tremors and emotional turmoil.

WAR AND CONCENTRATION CAMPS

War is a very stressful experience. During a war certain individuals are captured. These individuals are called as Prisoners of War. Sometimes civilians can also be held captives, one such experience, experienced was during the World War II, where Jews were captured and put together under torturous experiences that came to be called as concentration camp.

A common symptom experienced by prisoner of war is what has come to be known as "DDD" syndrome, a term, which was first used in the Korean Conflict which has been described by Farber, Harlow and West. "DDD" stands for debility, dependency and dread. It included debility due to semistarvation, fatigue and disease; dependency on captors due to separation from comrades; and dread due *feat* of death, pain from being captured and endless imprisonment. For many prisoners of war, anxiety and depression were constant campanions, others became emotionally isolated to avoid such feelings and some simply gave up and died.

Recent Research (Hall and Malone 1976; Hunter 1978) indicates that most returned prisoners of war have difficulties in mental functions including time distortions and confusion, depressive symptoms, fears and anxieties nightmares, flask backs (re-experiencing past perceptions and emotions), and mood swings.

Marital adjustment problems were quite prevalent, with the divorce rate for prisoners of war at 26.9 per cent two years after their return.

Some studies indicate that some prisoners of war feel that they have changed for the better during the prisoners of war experience. Schein, Cooley and Singer (1960) found that 21 percent of American prisoners of war in the Korean conflict felt they benefited from learning to deal with the experience. More recently. Sledge, Boydstein and Rabe (1980) found that over 61 per cent of a large sample of American prisoners of war released from Vietnam camps felt in retrospect that they bad grown from coping with such adversity. The prisoners of war felt that the harshness of their experience changed their personal values, so that they could communicate better with others, had greater self understanding and more patience with others.

Concentration Camp experience: Few experiences are more chronically stressful than existence in a prisoner of war camp. However, the nazi concentration camps of World War II seem to have been even more stressful than the prisoner of war. Over 6 million people (mainly Jews) were systematically tortured and killed in these camps.

Within the camps, reactions of apathy withdrawal and emotional repression were common (Chodoff) 1970). Many inmates refused to believe that friends and relatives who suddenly disappeared had been gassed and cremated; they denied that the smoke they saw was from the cremation. Bruno Bettelheim (1943, 1960) has described many disturbed inmate behaviours such as extreme regression, stealing, hoarding and identification with the aggressors. A few inmates became "capos" and worked for the Nazis to gain favoured status. The hopelessness and the helplessness of the situation appears to have led many to give up or at the other extreme, to almost complete psychological denial (Dimsdale, 1974).

Among survivours, long-term emotional disability is common. Nappe (1971) found that of 190 survivors of camps and other types of Nazi persecution, 70 per cent had a chronic depressive reaction, 23 percent showed combined depression and aggression and 2 percent had developed a schizophrenic reaction during the persecution. Mattusk ((1971) found that many survivors displayed chronic adjustment reactions, long after release from the camps. His Findings suggest that survivors have their symptoms, even when they do not report them. Berger (1977) had found additional symptoms of chronic guilt and 'self loathing, inability to cope with anger, chronic depression, impoverished relations with others and continued apathy all of which may appear years later. He calls this the survivor syndrome.

Dor- shav (1978) extensively studied 42 camps survivors and 20 controls in Isreal. She found that they were more limited in imagination, less creative, not open with others aloof, had poorer emotional control, were more conservative and took fewer risks than the matched controls. In addition, they were depended on others for a sense of safety and security, but were less able to emotionally "connect" with others.

POST TRAUMATIC STRESS DISORDERS

Post Traumatic Stress disorders are acute psychological reactions to intensely traumatic events-events much more disturbing than most ordinary human troubles. These include assault, rape, natural disaster such as earthquakes and floods, accidents such as air planes, crashes and fires and wartime traumas such as torture and bombing. Predictably most of our knowledge of post-traumatic stress disorders comes from war survivors, people who lived through Nazi concentration camps. The bombing of Hiroshima, or simply the day to day agonies of combact in World War II and the Korean and Vietnam war.

Post-traumatic stress disorder is a new category in DSM-III, because post-traumatic stress disorder is *normally* characterized by anxiety, DSM-III classifies this syndrome under the 'anxiety' disorders they differ from other anxiety disorders, however, in that the source of stress is an external event of an overwhelming painful nature, so that the person's reaction, through it may resemble other anxiety disorders seems to some degree justified and "normal".

Following are its important features:

(i) Post-traumatic stress observed can be extremely debilitating. Victims may go on for days, weeks and months re-experiencing the traumatic event, either in pained reaction or in nightmares.

(ii) Victims of post-traumatic stress disorders show a diminished responsiveness to their present surroundings a sort of "emotional anesthesia" they may find it difficult, for e.g., to respond to affection or to interest themselves in things that they cared for before the trauma.

(iii) Some typical symptoms of post-traumatic stress disorder include physical symptoms like insomnia, decreased sex drive and hightened sensitivity to sound. Psychologically, they suffer from depression, anxiety and intense irritability, exploding over the slightest frustration.

(iv) Post-traumatic stress disorder also leads to memory disturbances. Long and short-term memory is affected. Survivors forgot the phone numbers of relatives or of the family pet.

(v) Another common reaction seen in post-traumatic stress disorder is what is called as "survivor guilt", or "why should I have survived when so many others did not?"

Symptoms of post-traumatic stress disorder generally appear shortly after the trauma. In some cases, however, there is an" incubation period" for days or even months after the event the person is symptom free, and then, inexplicably, the traumatic reaction begins to surface. In the usual case, symptoms clear up by themselves within about six months, some however, may linger for years for e.g. in a survey of Vietnam war veterans who had been discharged for atleast five years, one-half of the veterans still reported nightmares and episodes of "hot headed" behaviour while one-third reported difficulties with emotional intimacy.

There are individual differences with respect to how effectively individuals cope with stress. Some individuals can cope with stress very effectively whereas, others breakdown during stress situations. At times, we can cope with one stressful situation very effectively but breakdown while coping with another different stressful situation. The manner in which stress effects us depends to a large part, on the interaction between the stressfulness of precipitating events and the predispositions of individuals to react inadequately

to stress. Individuals' personality factors also contributes to how effectively we cope with stress.

COPING DEFINED

Coping is facing and finding effective means of overcoming problems and difficulties. People vary in the means they have of coping with stress. Frances Cohen and Richard Lazarus (1979) have suggested that the behaviour of peoples who cope effectively with stress have five primary characteristics which arc as follows:

1. **Information Seeking**: They seek information about how to deal with the problem and what their alternatives are. They ask, to themselves questions like what is the problem? What do I need to know to deal with it What are my alternatives? etc.

2. **Direct Action**: They are prone to take direct action in trying to reduce stressor's impact. They ask themselves questions like what can I do that will help solve the problem?

3. **Inhibition of Action**: They avoid impulsive, ill timed actions that make

the problem worse. One such type of impulsive action that needs to be avoided is not panic or become emotional, not to become aggressive etc.

4. **Intrapsychic Processes:** Various intrapsychic processes also help in coping with stress. Such intrapsychic processes include the use of cognitive, or thinking mechanisms, such as reappraisal of the situation. Another intrapshychic process is the use of defense mechanism that people use when they feel endangered, anxious, insecure and threatened. For example, they may deny that the situation exists. Or they may try for an intellectualized detachment. They may block the emotions aroused by their distress from conscious awareness, becoming calm and detached in the stressful situation. There is no hierarchy of adaptiveness in these processes. Even denial which has been considered the hallmark of immaturity may be a healthy choice in Overwhelming situations. Denial may buy us the time needed before we move against an intolerable situation.

5. **Flexibility**: Those who cope effectively with stress arc flexible in their approach. Flexibility is the hallmark of adaptive behaviour.

VARIOUS TECHNIQUES OF COPING WITH STRESS

Some of the strategies that helps us to cope with stress are as follows

:

1. **Social Supports:** Coping does not occur in a vacuum. For every one effective mode of coping will be more successful in some situations than others. Coping is more successful if certain types of social support are available. Besides individuals differ in their personality characteristics which in turn determine the extent of support that an individual will generate not only for himself/ herself but also for others. The two most important types of social support areas follows:

(a) **Family**: One important source of social support is the family. A family marked by discord can have a powerful negative effect on a child's development of effective coping strategies, Families that are integrative and responsive to the needs of all their members can increase the likelihood that the child Will grow up to become a competent adult. And members of family can, of course, be the best, most dependable and closest source of comfort and aid for the person in trouble.

(b) **Agencies of Community and Government** is the another source of social support. These can be informal, such as the friends and neighbours who come to the aid of the people in distress, or they may be formal. For example, Women's Welfare Organisation, Handicapped Children's Society etc. Support Groups such as AL-Anon, can be a source of strength to families facing the problem of alcoholism in one of their members. The process whereby such support systems facilitate adaptation to stress is not entirely clear, but their effectiveness is evident.

2. **Transcendental meditation programme** also called as TM in short, was developed by Maharishi Mahesh Yogi and his followers. This technique has been found to be of considerable use in helping us to overcome stress, thereby increasing our ability to cope with it. This technique has evolved from the philosophy of eastern religions, especially from the practice of Yoga. The person learning the TM technique is given a special sound to repeat while sitting in a relaxed position. An instructor helps the student learn to repeat the sound mentally without concentration or effort, so the thinking process can become more and more deeply settled and quiet. About ten hours of instruction, spread out over a week or so, are all that are needed to earn the technique.

The physiological measurements reported to accompany the TM state are consistent with relaxation and lowered stress, and this relaxation seems to persist in experienced meditators even when they arc not meditating. During meditation, the heart rate slows down a little, the breathing rate goes down and, in well practiced mediators, may even ease for periods of up to 30 seconds, with no deeper breathing needed, afterwards to make up for it; the consumption of oxygen, decreases, muscle tension is reduced, blood levels of lactare and cortisol, which respectively, are associated with anxiety and stress decreases, the resistance of the skin to the passage of a weak electric current, i.e. the galvanic skin response, or GSR rises (this is also a sign of relaxation) and several changes in the electroencephalogram, or EEG indicative of relaxation occurs. Thus many stress-opposing bodily changes are characteristic of the TM state.

TM meditators report that they feel more relaxed and less anxious, are more efficient in their daily activities, get along better with other people and are more creative and selfactualising than they were before the training. They also say that they have a "heightened sense of awareness". All this help to cope with stress.

3. **Herbert Benson's Relaxation-Response Training:** In addition to TM technique, stress reduction has been achieved by the use of techniques such as systematic desensitization, a technique developed by Joseph Wolpe. Hypnosis and the relaxation-response technique of Herbeit Benson and his colleagues. In the Benson technique, the person sits for 20 minutes or so in a comfortable relaxed position, progressively relaxes the muscles from feet to head concentrates on breathing and saying "one" after each cycle of breathing in and out and suppresses unwanted distracting thoughts by thinking, "Oh. Well" when they occur.

While the Benson method results ill many of the same physiological responses as the TM technique, there may be a difference in the overall pattern of response, especially in the EEG and skin resistance changes. Controversy exists around the relative merits of Benson and TM technique. However, the fact is that they both help to cope with stressful situations. Both seem to be good ways of achieving some relaxation and stress reduction.

4. **Crisis Intervention** is one of the therapeutic techniques of dealing with the crisis situation such as divorce, job loss, death of a loved one or retirement. The primary objective of crisis intervention is to help the individual to cope with the crisis situation through counselling. Crisis intervention is based on the assumption that if the individual facing the crisis situation is provided with a supportive, encouraging and motivating environment, then the individual learns the ways of dealing with stress. The crisis counsellor provides a supportive environment to the individual in which the client can express his feelings, emotion, discuss the problem and evaluate the various ways of dealing with stress. The counsellor also provides feedback and effective strategies for dealing with stress. The counsellor, not only provides emotional support but also directs and assists the client to learn new techniques of dealing with stress.

5. **Stress inoculation** training is a therapeutic technique developed by Donald Meichenbaum (1975). According to him our self defeating thoughts make adjustment during stress difficult. According to him in stress inoculation training individuals are taught to engage in cognitions (thoughts), which enhance their ability to deal with stress. In this approach the individuals is trained to think positively about "stress". The counsellor provides strategies for successful coping while practicing the self-instructional coping statements. The client also learns physical relation exercises which reduce many of the subjective experiences of anxiety. Stress inoculation training has been demonstrated to be an effective cognitive behaviour modification technique, *and is* commonly used to enhance individual's ability to cope with' many types of stressful situations.

4

TheAnxiety, Somatoform and Dissociative Disorders

Anxiety, Somatoform and dissociative disorders were once called by a general term called as neurotic disorders. This term was used to refer to a group of disorders which showed intense anxiety, in which there was touch with reality and exaggerated use of defence mechanisms. Neurotic disorder was considered to be a less severe disorder as compared to psychnotic disorder in which there was loss of reality presence of hallucination and delusion and deterioration from previous level of functioning. However, DSM-UI has omitted the use of the term neurotic as it reflects a psychoanalytic bias.

In the anxiety disorders the anxiety is more easily seen and recognized than in the somatoform and dissociative disorders where it may be thought of as having been converted into physical like symptoms or memory difficulties. However, all three types tend to substitute maladaptive (self-defeating) and selfdeceptive maneuvers and strategies for conscious, reality-based responses to problems. Such strategies help to avoid anxiety but at cost of continual or episodic signs of fatigue, tension, and unhappiness. Because of their symptoms, neurotic people may be kept from realistically coming to grips with the causes of their anxiety, and their behaviour patterns may become stabilized and self-perpetuating. In this chapter we would first discuss the nature and symptoms of anxiety disorder, its types and its etiology or causes.

Following this we would discuss what are phobic disorders, its clinical picture and etiology. Phobia refers to intense, irrational, pathological fear. This fear is of interest because a person totally avoids the feared objector situation.

We would then discuss the nature, symptomatology and etiology of obsessive compulsive disorder.

Following this we would discuss- the somatoform and dissociative disorders. There is ample literature available With respect to this disorders; most of the literature is psychoanalytic in nature. These disorders have received a great deal of attention in literature and mass media. Somatoform and dissociative disorders may take a wide variety of forms. We would discuss these various types of somatoform & dissociative disorders along with its clinical picture and etiology.

Anxiety is a common experience of modern society. It is so common hat the present age is called as the age of anxiety. More or less everyone experiences anxiety but it is not considered as abnormal unless and until it disrupts functioning to such an extent that the individual becomes incapacitated. The experience of anxiety is considered as abnormal when

(a) The anxiety is so unpleasant that it interferes with human relationships, (b) with life goals (such as study or work) (c) or is extremely painful and disruptive. Anxiety disorders differ from normal anxiety primarily because if the intensity & frequency.

According to Marks and Lader (1973) anxiety disorders are estimated to occur in 2.5 percent of the population, at a given period of time.

Individuals with the anxiety disorder were in the past called as neurotic. Traditionally the disorders associated with anxiety have directly or indirectly included free floating forms of anxiety, an experience of generalized irrational hear not attached to specific object or situation. Phobias or unrealistic fears of specific objects or situation and various other types of neurotic disorders.

The experience of anxiety is central to many disorders some of which include panic disorder, generalized anxiety disorder and phobic disorder.

CLINICAL PICTURE IN ANXIETY DISORDERS

The clinical picture associated with anxiety disorder has three aspects which are as follows :

(a) Physiological aspect

(b) Behavioural aspect and

(c) Subjective experience

(a) **Physiological aspect of** anxiety- When an individual experiences anxiety many physiological changes take place. Autonomic nervous system is activated and many autonomic nervous system changes take place. The autonomic nervous system arousal associated with anxiety is called as "flight or light response" as these changes prepare the individual either to go away from the danger or to fight the danger.

People experiencing anxiety, typically feel that their heart is pounding. In anxiety provoking situation heart rate increases. In addition, depth and rate of respiration escalate, palms tend to respire generalized increase in tension of the voluntary musculature occurs. These events are relatively available to the subject's awareness.

Also possible are other physiological changes that the subject is less likely to be aware of, such changes include changes in stomach activity glandular secretions etc. (Katkin 1975). People are likely lo be completely unaware of some of these changes unless assisted by special equipment.

These changes include

(i) Increased electrical resistance of the skin due to prespiration (Katkin 975, **Khrer** 1977)

(ii) Increased blood pressure (Lader & Mathews, 1970) and

(iii) Increased diameters of the pupils of the eyes. (Janiste 1976)

(b) **Behavioural aspects of anxiety:** Anxiety is also associated with some behavioural changes which show that the person is anxious, e. g. there may be changes in the pitch of voice, some people may start biting nails under anxiety, some may tremble and some may try to avoid the situation. However, these behavioural changes may also be seen under some other emotions, e.g. people may avoid some stimuli because it is boring, or people may tremble in anger. So to be sure about the reasons of behavioural changes, we must always consider the verbal report of the individual. Only the explanation given by the individual can tell us objectively whether the behavioural changes are due to anxiety or some other emotion.

(c) **Subjective experience or aspect of anxiety:** Anxiety by nature is a subjective experience. A same situation will elicit different degrees of anxiety in different individuals. The subjective experience of anxiety is often, but not always correlated with physiological events described above when someone is threatened, physiological changes occur and subject's assessment of these changes may result in the subjective awareness of anxiety for e.g. if on your way to take an exam you feel your stomach churning and your heart pounding, you might report that you are anxious. However, if you bad this same physiological experience just after being rudely insulted your subjective report might be one of anger. The subjective experience may very with situational factors, even when the behavioural or physiological signs or symptoms are the same or similar.

The subjective experience of anxiety is best measured through the self report of the individual.

The self-reports can be either very formal and structured, or they can be very informal. So, if the person simply puts in words his experience, it becomes informal report, but if he answers to some questionnaire or inventory it becomes a structured or formal report.

PANIC DISORDERAND GENERALIZED ANXIETY DISORDER

Both these disorders are primarily manifestations of severe anxiety. Common symptoms of both these disorders include (a) apprehension; (b) a sense of impending doom, worry and fear of losing control; (c) more tension such as shakiness, twitches, trembling and jerky movements; (d) autonomic manifestations such as sweating, pounding heart, hot and cold spells, flushing and rapid breathing; (e) there is also increased breathing and the individual have;.(f) Insomnia and (g) depression.

The primary differentiation between panic disorder and generalized anxiety disorder is in intensity and duration.

In panic disorder there is sudden and inexplicable attack of the anxiety symptoms. These attacks arc very acute and disabling. They last for relatively short time like few minutes. Very rarely they last for an hour or so. Usually, they are not associated with any specific stimuli or object and so they are unpredictable. The individual never knows in advance when the attack is going to occur.

In generalized anxiety disorder, the anxiety is chronic and long lasting. The individual is consistently anxious in many life-situations, so it is also referred as “free-floating anxiety”. The ANS of the person suffering from generalized anxiety disorder seems to be hyperactive. The symptoms associated with anxiety are not as intense as in panic disorder, but the person always ‘on edge’, can be easily discouraged, is extremely sensitive to criticism and is often midly, depressed. They experience relatively constant mood of anxiety.

ETIOLOGY OF ANXIETY DISORDERS

The three common theories of the development of anxiety disorder are as follows:

(1) Biophysiological issues; (2) Anxiety as a learned behaviour disorder (3) Psychoanalytic explanation of anxiety disorders.

(1) **Biophysiological issues:** Physiological or constitutional make up of an individual largely determines whether an individual will develop anxiety disorder or not.

There is a great deal of research evidence that indivates that innate differences exist in the case with which individuals are aroused and in the magnitude of people's autonomic reactivity. Some individuals have and autonomic reactivity. Some individuals have an autonomic nervous system which is very labile i.e. easily aroused. Such individuals are more likely to develop anxiety disorder. People with easily aroused nervous system are more likely to experience a subjective sense of extreme anxiety.

Slater and Shields (1969) suggested through research that there is a genetic influence in the predisposition to develop anxiety disorders. They studied II identical and 28 fraternal same sex twins to find out whether differences in automatic reactivity has an inherited base they found that 41% of the identical cotwins had anxiety disorders but only 4% of the fraternal cotwins. Such differences suggest a genetic influence in the predisposition to develop anxiety disorder. However, Eysenck opposed these findings, after evaluating the available evidence he concluded that the concept of genetic transmission in this broad range of disorders has not yet been adequately supported.

2. **Anxiety as a learned behaviour disorder:** Learning theorists have made interesting contributions to the conceptualization of anxiety. Most theorists view the basic physiological response as being innate and present at birth in the form of the startle response. This startle response through the process of conditioning takes the form of anxiety disorder.

According to Skinner anxiety response is learned because it is reinforced. Some social learning theorists like Albert Bandura and Walter Mischel have suggested that anxiety disorder can be modeled behaviour.

Children learn to be anxious by modeling such behaviours from their parents who themselves are anxious. Some social learning theorists have also focused on the process of internal mediated responses in the causation of anxiety. The behavioural approaches suggest that individual differences in anxiety may partly be due to combination of (1) Innate factors that influence autonomic arousal (2) Conditioned learning and (3) Learned cognitive beliefs.

According to cognitive learning theorist anxiety disorder is a result of certain cognitive factors. Some clinicians believe that the influence of the learned irrational beliefs or expectations of anxiety is important for e. g. a person who believes that "I always make a fool of myself" might become anxious in a public setting because of the perceived danger that foolish behaviour might occur. Ellis and Beck have pointed out that people with anxiety disorders tend to have irrational beliefs about how people should behave and about their own likelihood of experiencing "catastrophic events". Thus according to Beck and other cognitive therapists irrational beliefs and thoughts give rise to anxiety disorders.

(3) **Psychoanalytic explanation of anxiety disorders:** According to psychoanalytic view anxiety is at the base of almost all neurotic disorder.

Freud conceptualized anxiety as based on the flooding of excitation during the birth trauma and subsequently as a signal of a threatened over stimulation by id impulses. Wachtel has described anxiety as a fear of our deep seated desires. The function of anxiety is to signal the need for repression and/ or the activation of the defence mechanism, such as projection or regression.

Later psychodynamic theorists have proposed alternative notions about anxiety. Alfred Adier saw anxiety as being due to a sense of inferiority. Karen Homey introduced the concept of basic anxiety which she felt develops as a result of lack of security in a potentially harmful world. She proposed that "basic anxiety" leads to feelings of isolation and helplessness and the individual develops "strategics" to cope with these feelings by developing certain neurotic needs. Harry Stack Sullivan, a neofreudian, like Homey conceptualised anxiety as a response to frustration of the need of security.

PHOBIC DISORDERS

Phobia is an intense irrational fear of some object or situation. It is a pathological, morbid and intense fear. Phobic behaviour is an avoidance behaviour associated with anxiety.

Many types of phobias have been identified according to the object or situation feared. Three broad category of phobias include

(1) Agoraphobia (2) Social phobia & (3) Simple phobia or object phobia.

(1) **Agoraphobia** is most commonly seen in clinical practice the individual with agoraphobia has a significant fear of either being alone or being in public places. An individual fears being in public places as a result of anticipation tha

if something happens to the individual, either no one will be available to help or those who will be available will be strangers and may not help.

Agoraphobia frequently develops after a series of panic attacks and the individual often feels that the anxiety attack is the threatened event which may occur when alone or in crowds. As with other anxiety disorders, agoraphobics are often midly depressed and manifest mild obsessive compulsive 'behaviour, perhaps in an attempt to deal with anxiety. Agraphobics tend to be passive, shy and dependent, anxious and are often female than male.

In extreme cases of agoraphobia individual remains in the house only and docs not go out.

(2) The social phobia involves an irrational fear and avoidance of situations in which one must interact with others. The fear usually involves the possibility of humiliation or embarrassment by others. A common example is disabling anxiety over public speaking.

(3) Simple phobia is a phobia of any object or event other than the one listed above. Simple phobia includes many objects. The most common phobia is of animals, fire, blood etc.

Following table lists some common factors of object phobia.

Some Common Forms of Object phobias

Name	**Object (s) feared**
Acrophobia	High places
Agoraphobia	Open place
Ailurophobe	Cats
Anglophobia	Pain
Anthrop phobia	Men
Aqua phobia	water
Astraphobia	Storms, thunder, and lighting
Claustrophobia	Closed places
Cynophobia	Dogs
Hematophobia	Blood
Monophobia	Contamination
Nysophobia	Contamination
Ocholophobia	Crowds

Pathophobia	Disease
Pyrophobia	Pire
Syphilophobia	Syphilis
Thanatophobia	Death
Xenophobia	Strangers
Zoophobia	Animals or a single animal

ETIOLOGY OF PHOBIA DISORDER

(1) **Psychoanalytic explanation:** (a) The psychoanalytic perceptive conceptualizes phobic behaviour as a defence against the recognition of threatening sexual or aggressive impulses. Anxiety, which is experienced when the impulses threaten to break through into consciousness, is displaced on to the phobic object. By avoiding the phobic object or situation, the individual avoids recognition of the impulses and reduces the danger that will break through, (b) Another psychodynamic concept of phobia is the displacement of anxiety to defend the self concept, (c) More recently, Ariti (1979) proposed another psychoanalytic theory of phobia. According to him, phobia is a result of particular interpersonal problem of childhood. When children are afraid that other adults particularly parents, are not reliable, they consciously transform this fear of others into fear of some impersonal object or situation. This fear surfaces in adult- hood, when they undergo major stress. However, as psychoanalytic theories stress on unconscious process, it becomes difficult to prove or disprove the theory.

(2) **Behaviour Explanations** (a) The most common explanation of the development of phobic disorder is that of behaviours. The conditioned fear hypothesis of phobia has been a classic one since Watson and Rayner's experiment on little Albert (1924). The conditioned fear also generalized to other objects similar to furry rat such as rabbit, a furcoat and a Santa Claus mask. (b) Preparedness theory was given by seligman. According to this theory human beings have a predisposition to be easily conditioned to some stimuli but not to others. Individual can be easily conditioned to some stimuli than others, (c) Social learning theorists like Bandura think that phobic responses may also be learned through modeling or by imitating the reaction of others. Learning of phobic responses through modeling is also called vicarious conditioning. Thus, a child may learn to be anxious or afraid by observing its parents. Besides, vicarious learning may also take place through verbal instruction or communication.

(3) **Multiple Causation View**: Phobia seems to be due to multiple factors. Weeks (1978) approaches phobias as a problem of multiple causation.

She has found that persons with phobia, particularly agoraphobia first experience heightened autonomic arousal. Then they have a panic experience during the time of major stress and are indecisive about coping procedures. In her formulation, deep rooted psychodynamic conflicts may well be operative in the development of phobic behaviour.

OBSESSIVE-COMPULSIVE DISORDERS

Obsessive compulsive disorder is one of the common forms of neurotic disorder obsessions arc un welcomed thoughts. They are thoughts that intrude repeatedly into awareness and are experienced as irrational unwanted and difficult to control.

Compulsion is an irresistible impulse to repeat some action or activity again and again e.g. washing bands, counting staircase or some other acts.

Obsessions and compulsion usually occur together, though they can also exist separately. These behaviours actually have no functional end but may be momentarily tension reducing.

Adhter ct. al (1975) studied a group of 82 obsessive compulsive subjects and found several categories of obsessions and compulsions, which are as follows:

(1) **Obsessive doubts**: Recurrent thoughts that a previously completed ask had not been appropriately finished were found in 75% of the subjects.

(2) **Obsessive Thinking:** Interminable chains of thoughts about future events that might affect them were experienced by 34% of the subjects.

(3) **Obsessive Fears**: Fears about loss of self-control and doing something embarrassing plagued 26% of the subjects.

(4) **Obsessive Impulses**: Of these interviewed, 17% had strong impulses to engage in behaviours ranging from silly acts, such as drinking ink, to assaultive behaviour.

(5) **Obsessive Images**: A small proportion (7 percent) were bothered by cognitive images of imagined events or by images of events recently seen. These images were most often unpleasant for example, a woman imagined her infant being flushed down a toilet.

COMPULSIONS

(1) **Yielding Compulsions**: Of the subjects, 61 percent yielded to an obsessive urge and were compelled to engage in the act.

(2) **Controlling Compulsions:** Of the subjects 6% were able to avoid acting on an obsession by repetitively engaging in an alternative behaviour. In effect, the alternative ritual gave control over the threatened urge for example, counting to 10 to avoid an obsessive sexual impulse.

The compulsions and obsessions are characteristically ago alien, that is foreign to an individuals perception of themeselves and thus distressing.

Causal factors in the development of obsessive compulsive Disorder or Etiology in their development of obsessive compulsive behaviour: The following arc the factors involved in the development of these disorders.

(1) **Physiological factors**: Researchers like Rachman & Hodgson (1980) have suggested that over reactivity of Autonomic Nervous system predisposes. The individual for such disorders.

(2) **Habituation of Arousal response**: Habituation of autonomic arousal response is another area related with obsessive compulsive disorder. Habituation is common in most individuals i.e. when individual is repeatedly exposed to a specific stimuli, the degree of autonomic arousal decreases. In simple terms, the individual becomes used to or habituated to the stimuli. But it is assumed that, obsessive-compulsive patients do not get habituated, and so every time they arc exposed to the stimuli they are aroused to the extent of first exposure. Only engaging in compulsive act reduces the arousal. This is the reason why obsession-compulsion lasts for years. However, further studies are necessary to prove this.

(3) **Learning and obsessive-compulsive disorder:**

Ability to Control Aversive Stimuli: Individual's ability to control the compulsives are in a situation that is undesirable or harmful, they overestimate the likelihood that the harmful outcome will occur. So they have "If anything can go wrong, it will" view of life. This cognitive set Or way of thinking necessitates avoiding the source of threat and that increases chances of obsessive-compulsive behaviour.

(4) **Modelling and Reinforcement:** This cognitive set can be learned in family. As social learoing theory suggests that in family, through modelling such behaviour is learned. The families of obsessive-compulsives are very formal in their relations, lack warmth and the parents fail to model humour, spontaneity, and may also punish the child for such trait. These are clear do's and dont's rule of thought and conduct, concepts about good, bad, right and wrong children are constantly reinforced, positively or negatively, for their behaviour. The child which deviates from rules experiences anxiety and this anxiety is reduced by engaging in compulsive behaviour. As Meyerand Chesser (1970)

suggest this reduction of anxiety and fear reinforces compulsive behaviour. However, the studies have also indicated that children of obsessive-compulsive parents, arc not likely to have obsessive-compulsive disorder. But the obsessive parental behaviour makes the child anxious, which can later develop compulsive disorder.

(5) **Superstitions Behaviour:** More direct operant reinforcement may also play some role in obsessive-compulsive disorder. Skinner demonstrated that pigeon can learn superstitious behaviour (i.e. Purposeless ritualistic behaviour) by shaping and reinforcement. So, the child in family where compulsiveness is important may experience shame and guilt when it is engaged in wrong thoughts. This shame, guilt and anxiety can be reduced by engaging in some compulsive behaviour.

Thus, the individual who has predisposition to overactive ANS, through modelling learns rules of conduct, feels highly anxious with bad thoughts, finds that compulsive behaviour reduces anxiety, learns compulsive behaviour easily as it is reinforced.

(6) **Psychoanalytic explanation:** Psychoanalytic writers view obsessive and compulsive acts as resulting from instinctual forces, primarily aggressive in nature which arc not under control. Obsessive compulsive acts are defence reaction to keep in check these instinctual forces and impulses and are due to rigid and harsh toilet training which results in fixation at anal stage. The obsessive compulsive behaviour represents the struggle between id and ego defenses or defense mechanisms. When id is dominated in the struggle, result is obsessive thought and when defense mechanism are dominated, the result is some-ritualized behaviour i.e. compulsion.

(7) **Inferiority Complex:** According to Dr. Aflred Adler, obsessive compulsive behaviour results due to inferiority complex. According to Adler many obsessive compulsive acts, are due to impulses which arc unacceptable to the individual and due to the fear of punishment. So individuals avoid the thought and anxiety by becoming ritualistic in certain behaviour. According to Adler if parents arc dominating, the child does not become enough competent to face the world. Thus he adopts a compulsive ritual to make the world orderly and exert control over the world, which makes him feel comfortable.

SOMATOFORM DISORDERS

Unlike the anxiety disorders and stress disorders, where anxiety is clearly observable, in somatoform types of disorders, anxiety is less obvious because it appears to be expressed in physical symptoms. The DSM-III divides the somatoform disorders into two main groups. In the first group are patterns involving physical symptoms similar to those seen in actual physical diseases: somatization disorder, psychogenic pain, and hypochondrias is. Often the psychologically based symptoms in this group are so "real" that they are quite difficult to discriminate from physically based problems. The second group of somatoform patterns are the conversion disorders in which the symptoms are more easily discernable from actual physical disorders. Overall these disorders affect about 0.25% of the population (Robins ct. al. 1984).

TYPES OF SOMATOPORM DISORDERS

There are 4 different types of somatofonn disorders, these are as follows

1. Somatization disorder, 2. Hypochondriasis, 3. Psychogenic pain disorder, 4. Conversion disorder

We would discuss these disorders in brief:

1. **Somatization disorder** is also called as Briquet's Syndrome who was a French physician and who in 1859 described this disorder. In this disorder there are repeated and multiple vague somatic complaints 'for which there is no physiological cause. The common complaints are pseudoneurological i.e. neurological disorder without organic neurological causes like double vision, or headache, allergies, nausea, stomach problem, menstrual and sexual difficulties. Such people experience pain and sickness in exaggerated manner and they keep on having medical treatment. This disorder usually occurs before the age of 30.

2. **Hypochondriasis:** In hypochondriasis, the person is pre-occupied with his or her state of health and feels that he or she is suffering from some severe disorder of bodily organ. There is unrealistic interpretation of relatively common physical complaints. The complaints are not restricted to any logical symptoms and they have trouble in giving precise description of their symptoms. They read a lot on medical topics and feel certain that they are suffering from every new disease they read or hear about. They are sure that they are seriously ill and cannot recover. As there are no physical causes, no treatment is possible, so they keep on changing their physician, until the physician treats the disorder which is not existing at all. Usually, they are treated with placebos i.e. such substances which have no physical effect on body.

These patients are so preoccupied with their health, that many of them keep detailed information about diet, functioning of body, etc. Besides they also keep themselves well informed about the latest medical treatment by reading popular newspaper and magazines. Usually this disorder occurs after age of thirty. Hypochondriacal people may be characterized as fitting snugly into the role of a sick person. Their apparent sickness can elicit sympathy and attention from others, as well provide an excuse for failure.

3. **Psyehogenie pain disorder:** In this, the individual experiences pain where there is no physical cause or they experience exaggerated pain for normal cause. This pain disturbs their routine and they keep moving from doctor to doctor.

Psychogpnic pains usually involve the back and neck and arc often precipitated by a significant change in relationships. Individuals in psychogenic pain, however, arc unaware of the connection between their "pain" and the emotional stressors that may be involved with precipitating it. On the contrary, they are likely to argue that emotional difficulties have nothing to do with their pain. As a consequence of their attitude, they are very difficult to treat psychologically.

(4) **Conversion Disorder:** Conversion disorder has a long history dating back to the earliest writings of abnormal psychology. Hippocrates called it hysteria and thought it was solely limited to women and was brought about by the - wandering of the uterus through the body. The term "conversion" was originally derived from Freud who thought that energy of a repressed instinct is diverted into sensory motor channels and blocks the functioning, leading to the development of physical symptoms. In DSM-II (1962), conversion disorder, as they are known today, was called as 'hysterical-neuroses conversion type and in DS-III it is listed as a somatoform disorder. In the earlier days of World War I, this was the most common disorder reported but now the frequency has come down to 5 to 20%.

Like Somatization disorder, conversion disorder too has physical symptoms in the absence of real physical or organic cause. The difference in these two disorders is that in somatization disorder various physical symptoms related to various parts of the body are present, but in conversion disorder it is restricted to one particular body organ. Some of the common symptoms in conversion disorder include

(i) Complaints of motor functioning which may involve (a) complete or partial paralysis (b) selective loss of function of specific organ (c) speech disturbances and convulsions.

(ii) Complaints of sensory functioning which includes (a) disturbances in vision like total or partial blindness, double vision etc. (b) disturbances in hearing and loss of sensitivity (anesthesia).

(iii) Other complaints. Some other complaints present in this dis order include lump in throat, coughing spells, false pregnancy or pseudopregnancy etc. Individuals with conversion disorder are highly suggestible, dramatic, attention seeking have shallow emotional relations and have a tendency to manipulate and exaggerate.

Diagnostically it is important to distinguish between conversion disorders and other disorders having a neurological base. The two important signs are as follows:

(i) **Selectivity of Symptoms:** The symptoms of conversion disorder are highly selective for e.g. during fits a person instead of falling may slide down so as not to hurt himself or herself or person suffering from conversion paralysis may not show consistent symptoms. So he or she may not be able to walk or stand but can move the legs in bed. This selectivity of symptoms is helpful in differential diagnosis.

(ii) **La Belle Indifference:** A second diagnostic problem with conversion disorder is differentiating them from 'malingering' i. e. intentional faking of illness, cither to gain something or avoid something. The true conversion disorder is out of conscious or voluntary control. As Theador and Mandelcom reported a case of a girl who was psychologically blind in her peripheral vision made more errors than the originally blind person in identifying the target. This difference in malingering and actual conversion disorder can be found out by what is called la belle indifference. La belle indifference is lack of concern about the symptoms. The conversion disorder patient is relatively indifferent about his or her illness, but is willing to talk and discuss endlessly and dramatically about it whereas malingers are more guarded and conscious about their illness. However not all conversion disorder patients show la balle indifference, for Stephen and Kamp found that only l/3rd of the conversion disorder patients showed la belle indifference.

ETIOLOGY OF SOMATOFORM DISORDERS

It is difficult to explain why one individual develops psychogenic pain whereas other develops hypocondriasis and some develop conversion disorder. We would discuss the etiology of conversion disorder. This to some extent will help us to generalize the causation to other somatoform disorder. In the following paragraphs we will discuss the etiology of conversion disorders.

(a) **Psychoanalytic Theory of conversion Disorder**: According to psychoanalytic theory, roots of conversion disorder in women are in unresolved Electra complex. The young female represses her sexual impulse towards the father, which produces pre-occupation with sex and an avoidance of it. In later life when the sexual impulse reawakens, these repressed impulses are transformed or converted into physical symptoms, which keep the impulses from being acted upon.

More recent modification of the psychoanalytic theory have tried to account for conversion disorder in both males and females, giving less importance to electra conflict arid oedipus conflict. In general these theories focus on strong emotions, such as sexual desire or aggression, which cannot be expressed because of the fear of the consequence. Consider the individual who experiences a range impulse against a loved one, and feels extremely guilty and fear for having this, "evil" feeling. The act may be defended against unconsciously by having one's arm become paralised so that the person cannot strike out or some who wishes to see a forbidden sexual act may become blind because such desires are "bad".

According to some psychoanalytic researchers induction of hypnotic behaviour may lead to conversion disorder. According to these researchers there seems to be a similarity between conversion disorder and hypnotic experience Many investigators have shown that hypnotic induction and suggestion can cans "normals" to develop conversion disorder that are hard to distinguish from "naturally" occurring cases. Perhaps the same mechanism arc operative in hot the cases.

(b) **Learning theory approach to conversion disorder**-According to learning theorists conversion disorder is a learned behaviour disorder. However as yet there is no convincing evidence that simple learning results in conversion disorders, although learning may well contribute to their development.

Interestingly many people who have a conversion disorder have had actually acquaintance with the symptoms. They manifest from a relative who "modelled" the behaviour (i. e. the relative was actually blind, deaf or paralyzed, (Mucha and Reinhardt) (1970). This type of learning need not be conscious or under voluntary control. Investigators such as Schwartz (1973) have convincingly demonstrated that humans can. learn to modify physiological activity previously thought to be outside voluntary control and awareness.

A very interesting model of somatoform behaviour has been proposed by Ullman and Krasner (1975). They suggest that these behaviours are a manifestation of a learned role enactment. In conversion disorder, they suggest the subject has not really lost any voluntary function but engages in behaviour that matches his or her concept of the social role which a person with the true physical disorder would enact.

Ullman and Krasner go on to suggest that once the person has adopted the role (e. g. being blind) and has acted in this manner, a return to healthy role is unlikely. The "Sick" role is maintained by the immediate benefit of avoidance of unpleasant situations and the positive secondary gains.

3. **Religions Background and development of conversion disorder-** The socio-cultural theories relate conversion disorder with religious. Background of the individual and with the norm of morals existing in the society. According to them when the standards or mores regarding sex, aggressions were too rigid proportion of conversion disorder was high. But when in 20th century, there was general relaxing of sexual norms, when society became more flexible, percentage of conversion disorder went down.

TYPE OF DISSOCIATIVE DISORDERS

The dissociative disorder refers to a group of related disorders which there is certalna ltered sate of consciousness.

The dissociative disorders are described in DSM-III (1980) as sudden temporary alterations in the normally integrative functions of consciousness, identity or motor behaviour. DSM-III includes(1) psychogenic amnesia; (2) psychogpnic fugue; (3) depersonalization disorder and (4) Multiple personality.

In the past, these above four types of dissociative disorders were considered to be a category of the hysterical neurosis, along with conversion disorder. Some of the personality characteristics of the above mentioned disorder include (a) poor self awareness (b) childlike emotionality (c) and a high degree of suggestibility and dependency.

The clinical picture of the various above mentioned disorders is as follows:

(1) **Psychogenic amnesia** occurs due to psychological causes. The amnesia has no physical cause. It refers to one's life.

Psychogenic amnesia occurs in the absence of physical cause. Faced with an unbearable situation or experience the individual use massive repression or avoidance learning to keep thoughts about the experience out of awareness, leading to amnesia.

The amnesia usually occurs in situations which the person cannot realistically escape.

The "forgetting" may involve a few hours or days or more rarely, a whole life-time of memories of places, people and one's own name and experience may be forgotten the person's basic behaviours and personality structure remain intact.

Somnambulism is another dissociative state which is not included in DSM-III under the category of dissociative disorder. In DSM-III it is classified as a sleep disturbance. Somnambulism commonly called as sleep walking, usually occurs in early hours of sleep. The individual moves with open eyes, is apparently able to sec obstacles, has a bland expression, and may engage in purposeless but complicated behaviours with varying degress of effectiveness. The sleeper is very difficult to awaken and usually return to bed, but sometimes lies down elsewhere and waken in the morning, wondering how he or she got there.

There is no memory of the events of the episode, although at times the walker may remember dream fragments.

Somnambulism seems to occur in some adults under stress from environmental or personal conflict. It remains a poorly understood disorder, with a few reports of successful treatment.

(2) **Psychogenic Fugue** is quite similar to amnesia, but has the notable difference. Individuals in a fugue state not only lose their memory but also travel away from their usual environment. They develop a new identity, which may range from vague memories of different past life to a complex identity with a complicated, vividly remembered, non existent past.

Psychogenic fugue is such a rare disorder that virtually no controlled 'research has been completed in it. It may simply be one type of amnesia.

The fugue can be of short duration or can be very long, when such patients .regain their memory, they totally forget what happened in the period of fugue. These people have the same personality characteristics as people with dissociative disorders i.e. they are immature, self centered, suggestive experience unbearable stress upon which there is no escape.

(3) **Depersonalization Disorder** is considered by Mehr to be the most frequent disorder found even among normal individuals.

Depersonalization involves a sense of things or experiences as being "unreal" and a feeling of estrangement from oneself or one's surroundings, both feelings have an unpleasant quality and are experienced as a distinct change from one's usual mode of functioning.

Depersonalization disorder involves feelings that are extremely unpleasant and result in anxiety and feeling of lack of control. This disturbs the normal functioning of the individual. The person may feel that he is out of his body and the body is distorted. Sometimes people also report that they were dead and floating above the body. They can see doctors trying to bring their bodies back to life and feel pulled back into the bodies when the doctors succeed. Few also report glimpses of hell and heaven.

This disorder is episodic by nature and lasts for few minutes or hours. This is the most frequent disorder of dissociative type, so it is thought that it must be mildest form of dissociation and must be more easily curable. It is assumed that depersonalization must be an attempt to escape from stressful situation. However, the data about the disorder is not very clear.

(4) **Multiple personality** is one of the most dramatic dissociative disorder that has received a large share of attention in the popular media. This disorder has been infrequently seen but the incidence of reports is now increasing.

Some authorities have suggested that typical multiple personalities appear in the set of threes, consisting of a moralistic character, a character who acts out behaviourally and a relatively well balanced character. Others have found that any variety of personalities *is* possible. Each personality has a relatively unique and stable identity with its own emotional structure and thought processes, but usually one appears to be the primary personality from which others have been dissociated.

The existence of truly different personalities' has received validating 'support from the work of Osgood, Luria, Jeans and Smith in their study of Evelyn.

The casual development of the multiple personality remains unclear, although many theories have been advanced. In general, theorists have focused on the existence in the individual of major conflicting desires, which are repressed, but are so strange that they break through. However, the desires are so unacceptable to the original personality that, in breaking through to behaviour a new personality is formed to allow their expression, because in such individuals the development of alternative personalities may be the only available coping mechanism.

CAUSAL FACTORS IN THE DEVELOPMENT OF DISSOCIATIVE DISORDERS OR ETIOLOGY OF DISSOCIATIVE DISORDERS

There are two theories regarding the development of dissociative disorders. These two theories are as follows:

1. Psychoanalytic conception of dissociative disorder and, 2. Learning

theory approaches to dissociative disorder.

According to psychoanalytic view, in dissociative disorder one part of the mind or consciousness splits off or becomes dissociated from another part to control an unacceptable impulse. The psychoanalytic concept suggests that some infantile sexual impulse of the oedipal stage are repressed. When there is some stressful event in later life, these repressed impulses are about to break through.

At this time to defend the self from anxiety, the dissociation occurs which is unconsciously expressed; in fugue state or new personality e.g. Nancy saw her mother engaging in sexual act with her boy friend. Nancy became very angry and wanted to kill her mother. But she had to repress her thought as it was unacceptable. So she dissociated into Kitty who in fantasy killed her mother. This case history of Nancy suggests how unacceptable feelings can be expressed by dissociation.

Some researchers, especially Ullmann and Krasner have explained the development of dissociative disorder on the basis of learning theory.

Under hypnosis, people can concentrate on the object and neglect all other stimuli around them. Similarly, it was seen that people can learn to block certain brain processing mechanism so that they don't become aware of the information brought in. This suggest that people can learn "to not to respond to" or "to not to think about" a specific stimuli. Blise has reported that people with multiple personalities can be hypnotized more easily. Thus, it is possible that people can enter in fugue by "not thinking about" their previous life or they can have amnesia about a traumatic event by not thinking about it. Thus, some theorists suggest that hypnotic suggestibility predisposes the individual to dissociative disorders.

According to social learning theorist, dissociation is extensive role enactments. Thus, in multiple personality, the persons act "as if" they have different personalities. Some theorists also suggest that multiple personality is unintentionally suggested by a therapist during the treatment of some other problem. The role enactment is also possible in fugue and in amnesia. Becoming another person is the most intense modelling or role enactment.

Thus, learning through modelling, role enactment and reinforcement is important in the development of these Dissociative disorders. Dissociation is assumed to be an escape from extremely unpleasant and anxiety-provoking stimuli.

VARIOUS APPROACHES FOR TREATMENT OF ANXIETY DISORDERS

A wide variety of treatment techniques arc available for anxiety disorders. Most of these treatment techniques are used in combination. Some of the most commonly used treatment techniques for anxiety disorders are as follows:

1. **Chemotherapy** means the use of a wide variety of medicines to alleviate symptoms of tension, anxiety and stress. These medicines also induces muscle relaxation, helps overcome insomnia and remove some physical symptoms. Antianxiety and antidepressant medicines are most commonly used.

The most commonly drug used is Benzodiazepine and mepiobamate. Among the most commonly used Benzodiazepine are the chloidiazepoxide, alprazolam, diazepam, flurazepam, Torazepam and nitiazepam. These medicines have hypnosedative, anxiolytic, muscle relaxant & anticonvulsant actions. These drugs are used in the treatment of anxiety and tension and muscular spasm.

The anti anxiety drugs are also called as minor tranquilizers and are used for reducing tension, fear & psychosomatic illness. The most common antianxiety drugs are Tranxene (Chlorazepate), liabrium (Chloidiazepoxide hydrochloride) or vallium (diazepam). These drugs are generally prescribed, besides psychiatrists, by the family physician for people who are not under psychiatric treatment but are undergoing through periods of stress and strain. These drugs produce many side effects, some of which include drowsiness, fatigue, impaired motor coordination, dryness of mouth etc. These drugs can be addictive and withdrawal symptoms can occur when the drugs are discontinued. These drugs should not be used by women in pregnancy, by children who are under six years of age, with depressed persons and with individuals who are engaged in hazardous occupations that requires alterness.

Another commonly drug used to treat anxiety disorder and associated affective disorder is the antidepressant drug also called as mood elevators. The discovery of improniazid led to the development of newer mood elevating drugs which have less side effects. One of the most important and useful antidepressant drugs is the MAO inhibitors (Monoaminc Oxidase Inhibitors). Among them the most widely used are the Phanelzinc (nardil),Is cocarboxazid (Marplan), Tranylcyprominc (Pamate) etc. Besides MAO inhibitors, the other antidepressant drugs are the tricycles derivatives (such as to franil and imipraminc) and the lithium. Antidepressant drugs, too, produce many side effects. These drugs can have adverse effects on the brain, the liver and the cardiovascular system. Lithum can also lead to toxic effects, convulsion, delirium, and in rare cases, death.

II Psychodynamic Therapy : In psychoanalytic therapy, unconscious, repressed impulses and sex instincts are emphasized. So the focus is on uncovering these issues. Techniques like free association or dream analysis is used to find out the source of anxiety.

The basic goal of psychodynamic therapy is to relieve this situation by exposing and neutralizing the material that the ego is spending its energy to repress. The assumption is that once the terrors of the unconscious are confronted, they will lose their power to terrify. Hence, if the patient can face and understand his or her repressed conflicts, the ego will be liberated from the all-consuming task of masking these conflicts and can devote itself to more useful and creative tasks.

Orthodox psychoanalysis uses two basic techniques to achieve this goal. The first is free association. Hence the patient lies back on a couch and simply says whatever comes to mind, without the censorship of reason, logic, or "decency". Unconscious material will eventually surface and will be interpreted by the therapist that is, the therapist will point how the patients remark indicate this or that unconscious preoccupation. The second technique is dream interpretation. whereby the patients reports his or dreams accurately as possible and the therapist explain the elements of the dreams as symbols of unconscious wishes and conflicts. In other forms of psychodynamic therapy *far* more common today than classical psychoanalysis-underlying conflicts are excavated in a more conventional manner, the patient sitting face to face with the therapist and simply discussing his or her problems as frankly as possible.

It is assumed that when the therapist begins touching sensitive parts of the patient's unconscious, the patient will begin to show resistance, arguing with the therapist, missing appointments and so forth. This too is interpreted to the patient. A final important component of the psychodynamic therapy is analysis of the transference. Presumably, patients transfer to their therapists the hostility and affection that as children they felt for their patients. These emotions, again, are interpreted to the patient, in the effort to clarify conflicts left over from the parent-child relationship. Through these means, the patient comes to reexperience and understand repressed events of the past and repressed impulses of the present, and as a result the ego is freed from the full-time job of maintaining defenses.

In treating patients with severe anxiety and post traumatic stress disorders, the therapist may also use hypnosis, under hypnosis the patient is encouraged to recall the traumatic experiences to which he or she has been subjected. This unleashing of the traumatic memory relieves some portion of the patients anxiety. Then the patient and the therapist work together to analyze the patient's defenses against this anxiety.

III. **Behaviour Therapy :** Behavioural treatment is the most successful treatment of anxiety disorders. As it assumes that anxiety is learned response, a specific or generalized stimuli, it emphasizes on modification of such learned responses.

Behavioural therapy is aimed directly at the removal of symptoms. Behaviorists are not interested in tapping the patient's unconscious, nor do they spend a great deal of time determining how the symptoms came about in the first place. Their concern is with the patient's current behavioural problems.

Behaviorists have a number of different techniques. One of the most popular of these is *systematic desalinization* (Wolpe, 1973). In this technique patients draw up a "hierarchy of fears" a list of increasingly anxiety-arousing culminating in the situation they most fear (e.g. holding a snake, being pressed against another person in a crowded elavator). Then they are taught to relax their muscles as completely as possible, and in this State of relaxation they imagine the situations in their hierarchy one by one, progressing from the least feared to the most feared over a number of therapy sessions. By the end of the treatment, if it is successful, they are able to imagine their most anxiety arousing stimulus and still remain relaxed a response that in most cases will generalize to the real life-situation.

A variation on this technique, called *in vivo desensitization,* involves leading patients through their hierarchies in the real-life situations themselves. For example, a dog-phobic person, usually in the company of the therapist, will first look at pictures of dogs, then listen to a dog barking in the next room, then enter a room where there is a caged dog, and so on, until at last he or she is able to remain relaxed in the presence of dogs.

IV. **Humanistic-Existential Therapy:** Although humanistic-existential therapies are quite individualistic, they all emphasize the fact that the responsibility for change lies with the individual. All the therapist can do is create an emotional environment n which change might take place.

One of the most popular humanistic treatment approaches is client-centered therapy, designed by Cart Rogers (1942-1951). In this approach, therapists make no value judgements about what the client says and offer no advice about possible courses. Instead, they become a "mirror of feeling" for the client. What this means is that the therapist responds to the client's remark by restating their important emotional components. This gives clients the sense that their feelings have validity, since they are understood by someone else. It also helps clients to expand their self-concept, incorporating into it all their feelings and experiences instead of sorting them into separate mental pigeonhole of "what I am" (bad, weak) and "what I should be" (good, strong) Rogers (1951) has shown that this mirroring process, along with the "unconditional regard" that the therapist gives the client, does in fact improves the self- concept.

A technique called paradoxical intention, originated by the existential theorist Viktor Frankl (1975), can sometimes be helpful in the treatment of anxiety disorders. This technique asks patients to go ahead and indulge in their symptoms, even to exaggerate them. A person with a checking compulsion, for example, might be encouraged to spend the entire day doing nothing but checking the doors to see if they are locked or whatever the problem behaviour is. In this way, the person comes to learn that the symptom can be controlled if the behaviour can be performed more frequently, it can also be performed less frequently.

V. **Cognitive Rehearsals & thought stopping:** Cognitive rehearsal can also help to reduce the anxiety of the individual. In cognitive rehearsal, the therapist reconstructs the thoughts of the clients. Usually the patient expects failure in anything he or she would be doing. The therapist revives these thoughts and asks the patients to rehearse or practice new set of thoughts or behaviour. This gives the patient more confidence and reduces anxiety.

Irrational beliefs and expectations result in obsession and compulsion. If these thoughts are stopped or changed, it will reduce anxiety. In thought-stopping process, some distracting or disturbing stimuli is presented to stop obsession or compulsion. When this is repeated over again and again the client himself says "stop" when obsessive thoughts occur.

Some therapists like Foa, Steketee, Milby used 'response prevention' to control compulsion. Thus, instead of controlling the obsessive thought, only compulsive thought is controlled. When a comparative study was done to Find out effectiveness of thought-stopping and response prevention, it was found that response-prevention was very effective technique of controlling compulsive behaviour. But it did not reduce subjective sense of anxiety, which was reduced in thought-stopping. Thus, we can say that combination of thought-stopping and response-prevention can be more effective.

SOMATOFORM AND DISSOCIATIVE DISORDERS

Treatment of Somatoform disorder has been extremely difficult although .psychotherapy has been used, it has been relatively ineffective. Behaviour therapy seems to hold some promise for treating Somatoform disorders.

Fordyce (1979) has used behaviour therapy successfully with pain disorders, and the modification of environmental contingencies has often been used with hypochondrical and Somatization disorders.

The use of fairly strict behavioural approaches with conversion disorder has not been frequently reported. However Hersen et. al. (1977) have reported an example which indicated that the operant approach may have some utility.

The treatment of conversion disorder has often centered on a psychodynamic psychotherapeutic approach using hypnotism, particularly when the disorder is suspected to originate from traumatic guilt experience.

The various somatoform disorders remain relatively resistant to treatment. Since it is often extremely difficult to convince their subjects that their problem is behavioural or psychological not organic. Most individual with Somatisation and hypochondrical disorders who are in treatment have usually looked for help for other problems, such as depression, rather than for the primary symptoms. Most people with somatoform disorders avoid entering psychological treatment for what they perceive to be a purely physical disorders.

Treatment of Dissociative Disorders: Dissociative Disorders have been most commonly treated by psychodynamic psychotherapy. Many therapist see dissociation as an avoidance of anxiety-provoking or very unpleasant stressful experience. Thus psychotherapy focuses on the development of skills which will assist the individual in dealing with the anxiety-provoking material or the traumatic stress in such a way that psychological retreat is not necessary.

Hypnosis as a psychothcrapeutic technique is often used to uncover the precipitating factors in dissociative disorder.

The application of psychodynamic psychotherapy to multiple personality has been the subject of popular books and films. These popularised versions of cases suggest that this approach is time consuming but effective when used by talented therapists.

Behaviour techniques have rarely been used with dissociative disorders probably in part because of the low frequency of manifestation of the classic dissociation of amnesia, fugue and multiple personalities. However, since these disorders seem to function to avoid stress, anxiety or emotional trauma, we can speculate that behavioural anxiety reduction techniques (such as systematic desensitization) or cognitive techniques (such as thought stopping or cognitive rehearsal) might well work once the stress had been uncovered. Treatment of the Somatoform and dissociative disorders remain an area in which little controlled research has been done. The disorders (especially conversion disorder and the dissociative disorders) are relatively low in incidence and have not been studied to the same extent. Much of the information that we have about treating these disorders is based on anecdotal case material.

5

Sexual Dysfunctions & Disorders

.Sex has been an interesting topic through out human history. It has been a topic of concern to almost all. There are many restrictions, taboos and cultural norms that regulate our sexual functioning and behaviour. In most societies sex has been an inhibited topic. Free and frank communication on sex is a taboo.

The nature of human sexual response and the topic of sexuality has only recently become a topic of academic and research interest Until the Kinsey studies in the last 1940s and early 1950s and the work of Masters and Johnson in the 1960sand 1970s human sexuality was a topic characterized more by myth than by reality.

Attitudes and values about sexuality have varied dramatically through the ages and from culture to culture. There has been notable changes during the 20th century in people's attitudes and values about sex and in their patterns of sexual behaviour. Such changes are most obvious generations. Though it is impossible to state with certainty the underlying reasons, it is clear that most of the western civilization has truly undergone a sexual revolution. Prohibitions have lessened, attitudes have become more flexible. Permissiveness in behaviour is seen. More couples live together before marriage in a consenting sexual relationship than in the past and both women and mer. seem more liberated, less constricted, about sexual behaviour. Variations in sexual behaviour is commonly found. Homosexuality today is no longer regarded as a mental health problem. Masturbation is no longer considered to be abnormal. Inspite of all these changes, a wide verity of sexual problems is still manifested in human relationships.

In this chapter we would first discuss what is a normal human sexual response and when does sexual behaviour becomes abnormal.

Following this we would discuss human sexual inadequacy or sexual dysfunction. We would first define sexual dysfunction and discuss the different type of sexual dysfunctions. We would then discuss the etiology of different sexual dysfunctions.

Another important group of disorders of interest to psychologists that considerably affects human behaviour and that leads to a wide variety of problems in interpersonal relationship, Personal distress and legal complication is what is -ailed as sexual deviations or paraphilias. We would discuss the different types of sexual deviations and its etology.

We would then discuss sexual behaviour of special significance; among them, three are most important. These include incest, rape and homosexuality. We would discuss these three, out of these three We would discuss homosexuality in detail. Following this we would discuss the various treatment techniques available for sexual dysfunctions.

We would also discuss the various treatment techniques available for sexual deviations.

We would end this chapter with a few short notes.

NORMAL SEXUAL BEHAVIOUR

What is appropriate or normal sexual behaviour has concerned societies for thousands of years. With respect to sexual behaviour, normality is a culturally relative concept. Cultural norm, societal values and development of science and technology in a given culture greatly determines what sexual practices or behaviours are to be considered normal and abnormal. For e.g. homosexuality is a normal behaviour in most European cultures but in our society, it is still considered abnormal. Premarital sex is tolerated in many sub-cultures but others do not approve of it. Some sexual behaviour such as Incest are universally condemned. Thus, we see that some behaviours are consistently viewed as abnormal or pathological,-such as sexual activity between adults and young children, other behaviours such as homosexuality remain the centre of controversy.

If we want to arrive at criteria for the fully functioning and sexually well-adjusted person we would have to include three things. (1) he or she should be able to reach sexual satisfaction i. e. orgasm, (2) The person should be free from irrational sexual fears; and finally and most important, (3) there should exist the ability to enjoy sexual intimacy and to share sexual pleasure with the person one loves. These criteria often bring together an objective knowledge about sex with healthy attitudes and appropriate behaviour.

In distinguishing normal or "healthy" from abnormal or "sick" sexual behaviour, the comments of several experts may be helpful (Manner et. al. 1977). Healthy normal sexual behaviour; 1. is motivated by feelings of affection and tenderness; 2. is not used to discharge anxiety, hostility, or guilt, nor does it lead to these feelings; 3. does not inflict pain or harm on oneself or one's partner; 4. is not performed using force on a no consenting person.

While experts disagree to some extent with each other, their opinions are more similar than different. They all raise the issues of motivation, the infliction of pain or exploitation, involvement of human partners rather than nonhuman objects, internal distress, and consent in their definitions of healthy sexuality. Sexual health or sexual sickness is not generally found in the specific behaviour, but in its effect on the participants.

With respect to sexual behaviour any activity is normal as long as two people engaging in it are happy, satisfied, do not experience fear, guilt or embarrassment and they do not create a public nuisance.

PHYSIOLOGY OF NOPMAI UIIIUI&N SFYIIAI RESPONSE

It is only in the recent years that what constitutes a normal human sexual response has been studied systematically in detail by Drs. William H. Masters & Virginia Johnson, who poineered the direct observational study of sexual behaviour in their clinic at Washington University, St. Louis, Missouri.

Masters and Johnson found that human physiological responses during intercourse (and during sexual excitement) could be divided into' four phases, parallel for the male and female. They called these the excitement phase, the plateau phase, the orgasmic phase, and the resolution phase. (See Table).

Table

Physiology of Human Sexual Intercourse

Phase	Male	Female
Excitement	Erection of penis. Thickening of the scrotal skin. The testicles begin to elevate.	Erection of nipples. Swelling of breasts. Sex flux.
Plateau	Increased heart rate and blood pressure. (Sometimes) a sex flush appears.	Expansion of outer third of vagins (contraction of inner two-thirds). Elevation of uterus. Increase in size of labia minor and heightened sensitivity reactions.
Orgasmic	Loss of most voluntary muscle control, with massive contractions in genital area. Ejaculation accompanied by contractions of prostrate, seminal vesicles seminal emission (ejaculation).	Immediately before orgasm intense increase of all the above reactions. Clitoris withdraws. Vagina fully lubricated and extended. Orgasm characterized by a long and then shorter muscle contractions.
	Penis returns to normal size. Tetes descent into the relaxed Scrotum.	Clitoris returns to normal size and position. Sex flush disappears. Muscle relaxation in vaginal walk.

(i) **During the excitement phase** There arc major physiological changes through the body, including an increase in muscular tension, heart-rate, and blood pressure. There is also an accumulation of blood in some of the vessels of the body, which is called vasocongestion. This vasocongestion is responsible for what Masters and Johnson call the "sex flush" in women a blush like change in skin colour from the breasts to the abdomen, indicating sexual arousal. The genitals of both sexes begin to prepare for intercourse the penis hardens and the vaginal wall expands and becomes lubricated.

(ii) **The Plateau phase** extends these excitement reactions and adds new changes. The genitals of both sexes prepare further for the possibility of intercourse, the vagina becomes fully lubricated and the bead (glans) of the penis becomes more firm for entry into the vagina. Blood rushes to the genitals, and the woman's clitoris withdraws under the hook (prepuce) while the male's scrotum wall becomes harder.

(iii) . **Organic Phase:** During the organic phase, the body goes through intense muscle contractions as the individual experiences heightened feelings of pleasure and release from the building tension. Immediately preceding the orgasm, all of the excitement and plateau reactions reach their most intense levels. Orgasm begins with involuntary muscle contractions and a loss of voluntary muscle contractions and a loss of voluntary muscle control. As the blood which has become engorged is now forced out by these violent contraction, the individual experiences the relieving pleasurable feelings of orgasm.

(iv) The body returns to its "normal" state during the resolution phase, where all these changes are reversed : the muscles relax, blood circulates normally, and Voluntary muscle control is regained.

It must be emphasized that the pleasure and the subjective experience of sexuality cannot be fully explained by this physiological reaction. Most of the pleasure of sex is in the mind in our attitudes and our feelings about what is happening inside our bodies. From the man's ability to maintain an erection and the female's ability to feel the throbbing excitement of her clitoris right up through the ability to have an orgasm it is our mind that clearly holds dominance over our body.

The above sexual response may not follow the same sequence. It may also create dissatisfaction, in such a case sexual dysfunction results.

SEXUAL DYSFUNCTION

Sexual dysfunction is also called as sexual inadequacy and refers to a range of difficulties that reflect an impairment or inability to obtain sexual gratification. Usually these difficulties are a result of emotional and psychosocial factors which makes completion of intercourse with orgasm a virtual impossibility.

According to Kaplan (1979) sexual dysfunctions refer to a class of psycho physiological disorders that prevent the individual from having or enjoying sex.

Regardless of other source sexual dysfunctions almost always affect others and can put great strains on relationships.

TYPES OR FORMS OF SEXUAL DYSFUNCTION

In the last decade there has been immense progress in the study and treatment of sexual dysfunction. Much of this progress is due to the work of three researchers: William Masters and Virginia Johnson at the reproductive Biology Research Foundation in St. Louis and Helen Singer Kaplan of the sex therapy and education programme at New York Hospital.

One important product of their research has been a new system of classifying the various forms of sexual dysfunction. This classification system is very important for understanding and treatment of sexual dysfunction because previously all sexual failure on the part of male was called as "Impotence" and ., that on the part of women was called as "frigidity". These two terms were a blanket label applied to any sexual problem faced my men and women respectively.

The new classifying system of sexual dysfunction Which we are going to discuss below was first devised by Kaplan (1974) and was incorporated with slight modification in DSM-III (1980). This classification system is precise and groups sexual dysfunctions according to the phase in the sexual response cycle in which they occur.

1. **Disorders of the Desire Phase:** The first phase of normal sexual response, celled the desire shape involves sexual fantasies and an interest in having sexual activity. Failure to experience such interest on the part of either a man or a woman is called hypoactive sexual desire.

2. **Disorders of the excutement phase:** In the excitement phase many normal physiological changes take place. Absence of these changes lead to what is called as erectile dysfunction (in men) and general sexual dysfunction (in women).

3. **Disorders of the orgasm phase**: This orgasm phase is the third phase in sexual response cycle. In this phase, there is peaking of sexual pleasure accompanied by rhythmic contractions of the muscles in the genital region and in men, a simultaneous ejaculation of semen from the penis. If a man is unable to exert voluntary control over this response, with the result that ejaculates very quickly, leaving his partner and/or himself disappointed, be is said to have premature ejaculation. If on the other hand ejaculation is greatly delayed or does not secure at all the condition is called as deferred ejaculation. A corresponding delay of orgasm in women is called as orgiastic (or organismic) dysfunction.

There are two more disorders that do not neatly fit into this three part typology. These two disorders are:

(a) Vagnismus which makes Intercourse painfully difficult or impossible.

(b) Dyspareunia i.e.: pain during intercourse.

For convenience sake, we can now divide the sexual dysfunction into following types and discuss it accordingly:

1. Arousal-dysfunction.
2. Erectile dysfunction.
3. Ejaculation dysfunction.
4. Dyspareunia.
5. Vaginismus.
6. Orgasmic dysfunction.
7. Excessive sexual drive which is called as satyriasis in maie and nymphomania in females.

1. **Arousal Dysfunction:** Some individuals experience an inhibition of desire or loss of sexual interest. For males, this may result from fatigue, stress or tension.

2. **Erectile Dysfunction:** Erectile dysfunction has in the past been called impotence. Masters and Johnson distinguishes between primary impotence or dysfunction in which the male has never been able to achieve an erection sufficient for intercourse (a relatively rare condition), and secondary impotence or dysfunction in which the inability to attain an erection sufficient for intercourse at present is present, but the individual has been potent at least once in the life. Serious long-standing erectile dysfunction may be due to physical causes such as diabetes or the use of certain medications, but most investigators agree that most frequent causes are psychological. Reports of erectile dysfunction arc increasing, most likely because of the increased acceptance of seeking help for sexual problems. However, some researches (e. g. , Ginsberg, Frosch, & Shapiro, 1972) suggest that the increase is due to males' perceived threat of having to live up to the sexual performance expectations of "liberated" women.

3. Ejaculatory **Dysfunction:** Even if erection is normal, ejaculatory disturbances can occur. Related to this there are three disorders(a) ejaculatory incompetence, (b) premature ejaculation and (c) retarded ejaculation.

(a) In ejaculatory incompetence, the male cannot ejaculate in the vagina, although erection and entry may not be a problem.

(b) **Premature** Ejaculation refers to the male's inability to delay ejaculation for a sufficient time to allow entry and satisfaction of an adequately functioning partner.

According to Masters and Johnson, in premature ejaculation, a male cannot control his ejaculation for a sufficient length of time during intercourse to satisfy his partner in at least 50 percent of their coital connections. Lipiccolo (1975) suggests that males should be able to experience at least 4 minutes of genital stimulation without ejaculation.

(c) **Retarded Ejaculation:** The opposite of premature ejaculation, retarded ejaculation, occurs less frequently and refers to an irritability to ejaculate during intercourse.

4. **Dyspareunia:** Dyspareunia means painful intercourse. It involves persistent and recurrent gential pain during intercourse. It is rare in females and even rare in males. Generally, it has physical causes like lesions, infections or some other structural abnormalities..

5. **Vaginismus**: This disorder is very rare. It involves involuntary contraction of the muscles in the lower third of vagina which interferes with sexual activity. Very rarely medical intervention becomes necessary. Usually this occurs because of anxiety, fear, tension or lack of experience.

6. **Orgasmic Dysfunction**: Orgasmic dysfunction is one in which women have difficulties in experiencing orgasm. They arc labelled as frigid, implying that they lack warmth, are antierotic and unresponsive to males.

Masters & Johnson identified two types of orgasmic dysfunction :

(a) **Primary orgasmic dysfunction:** In this women have never bad an orgasm by either masturbation or intercourse.

(b) **Situational orgasmic dysfunction**: Exists in women who have had at least one orgasm, but are non orgasmic in one or more specific situations. For e. g., someone might be nonorgasmic with one individual but not another, or nonorgasmic in intercourse but not in masturbation. According to Kaplan (1974) about I out of 10 women seems to have some degree of orgasmic deficiency.

7. **Excessive Sexual desire** is of two types (a) satyriasis and (b) Nymphomania.

Satyriasis: In this disorder of function, the male manifests an insatiable desire, which constantly drives him to pursue gratification. He is totally preoccupied with these matters that they interfere with all other activities.

Nymphomania: Nymphomania is the parallel of satyriasis and may also be considered a motivational deviation in that the nymphomania constantly seeks sexual gratification. The chances of being singled out and perhaps even ostracized by family and acquaintances arc greater for the nymphomaniac than for her female counterpart.

ETIOLOGY OF PSYCHOSEXUALDVSFUNCTION

Psychosexual dysfunction and sexual inadequacy can be due to various factors. Masters and Johnson have classified these causes in two broad categories (1) Historical factors, and (II) Maintenance factors.

I Historical Factors

The factors which are involved in the dysfunction before the onset of the disorder are called historical factors.

(1) **Sexual trauma**: Early traumatic or painful sexual experiences like rape, incest, punishment etc. can result in develoonment of psychosexual dysfunction. Some studies (Glenn, 1972) have also shown that anxiety associated with size of penis can also lead to male impotency.

(2) **Socio-cultural Factors**: Sexual behaviour is influenced by social and cultural values to a great extent. These values affect women to a great extent. Due to changed social and cultural values, women are also considered as "naturally sexual." As Masters and Johnson suggest" many less severe psychosexual dysfunctions develop due to "performance anxiety" i.e. anxiety about performing adequately to satisfy the partner. Thus, fear of not being able to perform adequately increases the likelihood of failure and each failure increases the anxiety. It has been observed that this performance anxiety results in several male sexual dysfunctions.

(3) **Religious or Moral restrictions**: The strong moral and religious beliefs that "sex is sinful" affect people even when sexual behaviour is rational and acceptable. The guilt feeling associated with sex results in psychosexual dysfunction.

(4) **Ignorance and Bad Advice**: Many people are extremely naive about the sexual functioning of the body, expecting perhaps that sexual behaviour will "Just happen", that it is instinctual, and that one will "naturally" do the right thing. Quite the opposite, effective sexual behaviour requires knowledge, prac-

tice, and feedback from one's partner. This pervasive ignorance is compounded by bad advice from both amateurs and professionals'. S. Kaplan, 1974, 1977). People with sexual problems may be told to "forget about it, and it will go away", or they may be advised to "sleep around and put some spice in your sex life". Such advice is unlikely to be followed, and if it is, is more likely to compound the problem than solve it.

(5) **Homosexuality**: Some individuals enter into heterosexual relationships knowing or suspecting that they are homosexual (Masters & Johnson, 1970). The homosexual who attempts such a relationship often finds it a difficult task, leading to sexual dysfunction. Bieber and Bieber (1975) raise the interesting problem of the heterosexual who has feeling homosexual ideas, fantasies, or attractions. Such thoughts may be quite anxiety provoking and lead to heterosexual dysfunction, which compounds the anxieties and may lead to more severe dysfunction. Masters and Johnson found underlying homosexuality to be a cause of heterosexual dysfunction in about 20 percent of their dysfunctional subjects. Current work, however, indicates that homosexuality is one of the less common historical factors in psychosexual dysfunction.

(6) **Physical Causes**: Some sexual dysfunctions are the result of physical trauma, illness, or abnormality. Scars, infections, or other physical problems may lead to sexual dysfunction, as many drugs used to treat certain physical illness. A major drug often implicated in male sexual dysfunction is alcohol.

II. Maintenance Factors.

(1) **Fears About Performance:** Once sexual dysfunction occurs, individuals usually react with anxiety and fears about future performances. These fears and anxieties may be present before the First sexual experience, or occur during a functional initial experience, growing as time passes until dysfunction occurs. In either event, as the likelihood of a sexual encounter nears, the fears and anxiety level probably .increase. Frequently, this over concern grows into what Masters and Johnson (1970, 1975) call the "spectator role".

(2) **Spectator Role Adoption**: The spectator role may be a defensive maneuver and a manifestation of anxiety. The individual distances him herself from the sexual act in progress. One becomes a spectator observing the performance looking for flaws which prevent adequate functioning. Spectator role adoption may also be due to interpersonal problems between the sexual partners.' As Lobitz and Lobitz (1978) have noted, interpersonal problems can lead to sexual behaviour loaded with insecurity or resentment. The adoption of the spectator role prevents the passive, uncritical acceptance of sexual stimulation necessary for adequate function. The individual is unable to "get into" sexual enjoyment.

The etiology of sexual dysfunction can also be explained on the basis of various perspectives. The three most important perspectives used to explain the etiology of sexual dysfunction arc as follows :

1. Psychodynamic perspective.
2. Behavioural perspective.
3. Biological perspective.

We would now discuss the above perspectives briefly.

1. **Psychodynamic Perspective**: Freud claimed that mature genital sexuality was the product of successful resolution of the oedipus complex. Accordingly, psychodynamic theorists tend to attribute sexual dysfunction to unresolved oedipal conflicts. For e.g. (a) According to Otto Fenichel, impotence is based on a persistence of an unconscious sexual attachment to the mother. Superficially no sexual attachment is completely attractive because the partner is never the mother. Hence impotence results.

(b) Psycho dynamic formulation so for gastic dysfunction tend to stress the role of continued penis envy, and

(c) Vaginismus, too, has been interpreted as the expression of an unconscious desire to reject or injure the male's envied penis.

Except for the selected anecdotal evidence from clinical practice there is little empirical support for these theories.

2. **Behavioural Perspective:** The work of Masters and Johnson and Kaplan represent the behavioural perspective. The historical and maintenance factors discussed above arc a part of behavioural perspective.

Among the behavioural perspective the views of Kaplan are worth noting. Kaplan argues that sexual dysfunction is probably due to a combination of:

(a) Immediate causes and

(b) emote causes.

Mediate Causes are such factors as performance anxiety, over concern about pleasing one's partner, poor technique, lack of communication between partners and marital conflict. These Kaplan claim, are potent stressors, but in most cases, they are not potent enough to undermine, sexual functioning unless they are combined with (or based on) remote causes of sexual dysfunction.

Remote Causes include Intrapsychic conflicts that predispose the individual to anxiety over sexual expression, childhood upbringing, early moral and religious influence, conditioning of certain behaviour practices and values etc.

3. **Biological Perspective**: Generally the biological perspective focuses on the presence of certain neurological disease or disorders of the genitourinary system that make intercourse painful. Dysfunctions can also be caused by certain tranquilizers and antidepressants whose side effects include suppression of the ability to ejaculate in males.

Thus, from the biological perspective we see that physiological, neurological and biochemical factors play an important role in causation of sexual dysfunction. Internal lacerations left over from child birth can easily cause dyspareunia in women, and long-term use of oral contraceptives can reduce female sex drive. Erectile dysfunction may be due to diabetes, heart disease, kidney disease or alcoholism. Furthermore various medical treatments like renal dialysis tranquilizers, medications etc can interfere with erection and lead to sexual dysfunction.

SEXUAL DEVIATION

Unlike the sexual dysfunction, in which there are difficulties in 'normal' mode of sexual gratification, paraphilias represent methods of sexual gratification that are contrary to the established rules and mores of society. Generally these deviant behaviours are assumed to be modes of sexual release that are used when normal modes of release aren't available. In most instances of true paraphilias, people cannot establish intimate, loved relationships with others. They are forced, therefore into the pursuit of alternative no intimate and impersonal channels of sexual expression.

Paraphilias were once called sexual deviations, a label that many still use. The term paraphilia was for the first time used in DSM-III (1980).

This label comes from the latin words para (meaning roughly "deviation") and **philia** ("attraction for"). The change is intended to avoid the loadec connotation of the terms "sexual deviation" and "sexual deviate".

The paraphilias are sexual behaviours that require unusual, bizarr imagery or acts for sexual excitement and satisfaction. The behaviours tend t have an "involuntary" character and involve either: 1. repetitive sexual activit with nonconsenting partners; 2. repetitive human sexual activity that include real or simulated suffering or humiliation; or 3. preference for the use of a socially unacceptable or nonhuman object for sexual arousal. Individuals who manifest a paraphilia rarely seek therapeutic help. They are often satisfied with their sexual behaviour, or they are ashamed to admit their acts. Treatment is often sought at the instance of a spouse or other relative; and frequently the treatment is court ordered, since some of these behaviours are illegal in most cases.

Various disorders included in paraphilias are as follows :

(1) Tranvestitcs.

(2) Fetishism.

(3) Exhibitionism

(4) Pedophilia.

(5) Voyeurism.

(6) Sexual sadism and masochism.

Some authors like Bootzin and Acocella (1980) have also included, within sexual deviations the following disorders.

1. Trans-sexualism.
2. Incest, and
3. Rape.

However, we would be discussing Trans-sexualism as a short note and the other two, i. e. Incest and Rape, we would be discussing under the title 'Sexual behaviour of special significance'.

We would now discuss some common types of paraphilias.

(1) **Transvestites:** It is also called as tansvestism. It is a term that was first used by German Sex Researcher Mangus Hirschfeld in 1910. Transvestites are those individuals who cross-dress for sexual excitement. This is an exclusively male disorder. The males either masturbate or engage in sexual act when they cross-dress. Transverstism is different from transsexuals, as transvestites enjoy cross-dressing maintaining their anatomical sexual identity. Similarly, transvestites are not homosexuals. Most of them arc married and have heterosexual relation. The incidence of transvestism is rare, because the cross- dressing behaviour usually takes place in private and only immediate family and intimates know about it. Many case-histories report parental support and reinforcement associated with cross-dressing in childhood.

DSM-III ; Lists four operational criteria for transvestism.

(i) Recurrent and persistent cross dressing by a male, with or without sexual arousal.

(ii) Interference with cross-dressing results in intense frustration.

(iii) Hetrosexual arousal pattern, homosexual acts may occur but are not the preferred pattern, and

(iv) Does not fulfill the criteria for transsexuals.

(2) **Fetishim:** This term was coined by Alfred Binet in 1880. Fetishism is exaggerated interest in a particular part of the partner's body or in some inanimate object for sexual stimulation and satisfaction. Fetishtic objects include a wide range of objects like females under clothing, boots, shoes, stockings etc. However, these fetish objects must be used and newly purchased objects have no effect whatsoever. Like transvestites, this disorder is also very much common in males than females. However, the fetishist may face problems with law and police as they may involve in robbery to gain the fetish objects.

Gebhard (1976) states that fetishisms can be divided into two categories (a) Fetish items that are inanimate, such as shoes, lingerie, or gloves and (b) Fetish items that are a part of the female body, such as legs or breasts.

Gebhard also suggests that fetishists can be placed on a 4 point-continum depending on how exclusively they employ the fetish item for sexual gratification. At the low end of the continum might be a man who has slight sexual arousal toward some particular object worn by a female, the next step is stronger arousal toward the object, but this man may still be able to perform sexually with a female partner. At the third point on this continum, no sexual activity or orgasm can occur without the fetish item, for e. g. this female partner may be required to wear high heeled shoes to bed. At the ultimate end of the continum, the exclusive fetishist substitutes the fetish item completed for his "living sexual partner".

Thus, we see that Fetishism is the process of attaching a sexual value to an inanimate object of to a part of the body (as opposed to the whole person). If a person is unusuallly attracted to boots and leather objects, or lace, then this person has a fetish for inanimate objects. Sometimes, however, a person may be ususually attracted to one part of the body at the expense of the others to breasts, or to hair. Such a person may relate only to part of the person, and not be able to relate to the person as a whole. This is a different type of fetish.

Fetishism his both cultuial snd psychological components. Typically, the objects chosen for fetishistic value are those that society directly or indirectly associates with sex or with gender. Men form fetishes to things that are traditionally femining or traditionally masculine but to things that are specifically

identified with one sex or the other. Moreover, certain fetishes arc reinforced by the media, where such things as a women's breasts are put on display as erotic elements even in non-sexual contexts, where, in other words, we are ought to "worship" them and to find them stimulating. This becomes particularly important in advertising, where our fetishistic fantasies arc created to.

Fetishism may vary greatly in degree. On the one hand, every person exhibits some fetishistic interest. This is only to say that there are certain parts of the body or items of clothes that we invest with more sexual interest than we do others. However, the healthy person, according to most psychiatrists, is able to make the appropriate transition between the fetishistic object and the whole person. That is, a healthy sense, serves as a preclude to the paired sexual relationship.

As a maladaptive sexual behaviour, fetishism cither excludes the whole person we are presumably involved with, or all other individuals, from our sexual world, or it may involve some kind of antisocial behaviour. The cum who runs around stealing women's underwear from, clothes-lines is clearly exhibiting fetishistic deviant behaviour. Generally, fetishism occurs in conjunction with some other forms of sexual perversion, such as exhibitionism, assault, or exclusive autoerotism.

(3) **Exhibitionism, Sexual exhibitionism** refers to the exposure of one's genitals to a nonconsenting individual, usually with the intent to achieve sexual self-stimulation or autocratic (masturbatory) satisfaction. Many exhibitionists masturbate soon after exposing themselves, and some during the exposure however, most male exhibitionists' penises are flaccid during the act of exposure. Sexual exhibitionism under conditions of sexual arousal is rare in women, and when seen, it is usually in very seriously disturbed psychotic women. Women who exhibit their body for money (strippers, nude models) are primarily motivated by financial gain and attention and their behaviour rarely results in their own sexual arousal.

Male sexual exhibitionism is one of the most frequently reported "sexual offences" (M.P. Feidman, 1977). Exhibitionists are almost never physically dangerous. Like Pedophiles, to be discussed later, exhibitionists arc usually psychologically immature men who have difficulty approaching adult females on a nature level. Many are married, but have inadequate sexual relationship with their wives, and grave doubts about their own sexual adequacy (Witzig, 1968). The frequently exhibit when under increased levels of stress. Macdonald (1973) has described them as inhibited puritanical, and fearful.

(4) **Pedophilia:** Pedophiles are adults who derive sexual gratification through physical or sexual contacts with prepubertal children. Mostly the pedophiles are male. The term First used by Krafft- Ebing in 1912 was 'pedophilia erotica' which indicated adults' sexual desire for children. The .pedophiles are also called "child molesters".

In most of the cases, the adult knows the child well, either he is a relative or a neighbour. The sexual activity is just looking, touching or funding. Most of the pedophiles are not dangerous and are quite harmless, but some can be dangerous.

M. Cohen, Seghom and Calms (1969) have identified three categories of pedophiles.

(a) **Fixated molesters** who are fixated psychologically at an earlier level of development. Because of this fixation, they cannot develop nature and adequate hetero or homosexual relations with adults. They are comfortable only with children.

(b) **Regressive pedophile** can develop adult hetero- or homosexual relations, but they are not very comfortable and they find themselves inadequate when under stress. So they turn to children for sexual and emotional satisfaction.

(c) Aggressive **pedophiles** are inadequate psychologically as well as in their psycho-sexual adjustment. So the hostility and rage is expressed through sexual acts on children who can't defend themselves. Aggressive pedophiles can be dangerous to children as they may harm or injure the child.

(5) **Voyeurism**: Voyeurism is the practice of becoming sexually aroused by watching either "Live" or through some medium (such as film, books, videotape, etc.) another person or persons, partially or completely nude, involved in some form of sexual activity. Part of the excitement is that the person, the veyour, is watching does not know that he or she is being observed. Most of us are, to some extent, voyeuristic, that is, we become aroused by cortically explicit stimuli (Steel and Walker, 1974). A healthy and normative version of this is to become excited as we watch our friend undress in front of us.

But voyeurism becomes sexually unacceptable and psychologically unhealthy when we spy on people without their knowing it. The "Peeping torn" who secretly wanders through backyards looking through windows is considered unhealthy and deviant. There is a middle ground, too. The person who enjoys attending sexually explicit films may or may not be - considered deviant, depending on the social standard that predominates in his or her environment. Psychologically, whether this is healthy or not depends on how this excitation is integrated into other activities. Is the person only capable of becoming aroused by pornography?

Although it has generally been assumed that men respond move to voyeuristic stimulation than do women (after all, we don't have any "peeping Janes"), some recent research seems to indicate that the differences are smaller than have been suggested, and that in general "the pattern and intensity of reactions to explicit sexual stimuli are in general the same for men and women" (Schmidt, 1975, p. 355). It may be that social pressures prevent the woman from recognizing and reporting the stimulation she feels, since her sexual excitement can generally be recorded biologically before it is recognized by her.

(6) **Sexual sadism and Sexual Masochism**: The inflation of pain on another person to obtain or enhance sexual gratification is called sexual sadism. The need to have pain inflicted upon oneself to enhance sexual pleasure or to attain gratification is called masochism. Each behaviour is named after a historical figure,. sadism after the Marquis de Sade (1740-1814), who wrote - extensively about the joy of his sexual gratification through the infliction of pain on others and masochism after the novelist Leopold Sacher-Masoch (1836-1895); whose protagonists usually experienced sexual pleasure from pain. In addition to the sadist and masochist, some sado-masochists experience pleasure from both giving and receiving pain. When psychological pain such as frustration and humiliation are the primary behaviours, we refer to sexual dominance- submission syndromes.

Sometimes, the individual may be a Sado-Masochist who achieves sexual satisfaction by giving and receiving pain. However, mere fantasizing pain is not enough in sadism as well as masochism, but the individual must act out these impulses. Partners can compliment each-other in sadistic and masochistic tendencies and the partners can be heterosexual or homosexual. The sadistic-masochistic tendencies may alternate in the person.

ETIOLOGY OF SEXUAL DEVIATION

The paraphilias involve a wide range of behaviours. What general factors could account for this diversity of sexual behaviours which most people consider in acceptable has been of great interest to mental health experts.

We would discuss the etiology of paraphilia or sexual deviation from different theoretical perspective.

Psychoanalytic theory Psychoanalytic theory explains paraphilia as a displacement of normal or natural sexual behaviour. As most paraphilias are observed in meb, Freud suggests that when the Oedipus complex is not resolved properly the man develops castration fear and associates adult women with mother who is not approachable. And thus, displaces the normal sexual behaviour to such objects or behaviour which is less threatening or with which he can be more comfortable. Thus, according to psycho-analytic theory.

(a) Transvestite is developed because it is considered as symbolic possession of mother, in the from of one's 'own body dressed in a woman's cloth.

(b) Fetishism is developed because fetish objects arc unconsciously associated with mother.

(c) As Exhibitionism does not involve direct sexual act, it reduces castration fear and proves the man to be a sexual creature.

(d) Similarly, pedophilia is developed as sexual behaviour with child does not involve castration fear.

(e) The voyeurism is symbolically "peeping" at mother or mother and father, as this secret act gives feeling of power over parents.

(f) Sadism involves "demonstration of power over mother".

(g) As sexual behaviour is perceived as immoral, the individual feels to be punished to reduce the guilt and this feeling takes the form of masochism.

Thus, psychoanalytic explanations for development of paraphilia concentrate around immorality of sexual act, and castration fear. However, there is no direct evidence to support these explanations.

Learning Theory : According to Learning theory paraphilias are a learned behaviour disorders which arc learned by the various principles of learning for example, a learning process has been suggested in the development of fetishistic behaviour. The frequent experience of sexual gratification in the presence of an object may lead to classical conditioning. Even in the absence of the object, the fetish could be learned through fantasy association.

Modelling has also been found to play a role in the development of certain paraphilia's. Most of these behaviours arc modelled through mass-media or films, however, is it difficult to explain the development of these paraphilias on the basis of simple principles of learning alone, however, important points to be noted are as follows:

(i) As a result of experiences in childhood and adolescence reinforcement of cross dressing or parental attitude towards privacy can lead to the development of exhibitionism, inadequate development of masculine role may also lead to the development of paraphilias later on in life.

(ii) Fantasies about unusual sexual practices may be self reinforcing and may lead to the development of paraphilias.

(iii) Many paraphilias may be learned in a complex process that involves cither (a) direct reinforcement of the behaviour or (b) fantasies associated with masturbation and later experiences and sexual gratification.

(iv) Some individuals are predisposed to alternative forms of sexual behaviour because of personal inadequacies in heterosexual behaviour. They are likely to find that unusual forms of sexual activity avoid the anxieties about these inadequacies and also that the behaviour is reinforcing because of sexual stimulation and gratification. These are neat explanations of how paraphilias might be learned and maintained.

INTEGRATED VIEW OF SEXUAL DEVIATION

According to Edwards (1983) and Storr (1964) sexual deviations may be seen as simple exaggerations of normal male sexual tendencies. For instance, normal males "exhibit" their masculinity in body building, athletics, sports, cars and the like, deviant males may "exhibit" their masculinity by exposing their genitals or being voyeurs. Similarly, while many normal males are easily aroused by the sight or touch of female undergarments, the fetishistic male achieves gratification "only" through such objects.

Persons with sexual deviations often have deep-seated feelings that they are less than adequately masculine or feminine. Although almost everyone has been distressed by such feelings of "sexual inferiority" atone time or another. They seem to have a particularly powerful influence on behaviour for the person with a sexual deviation. A male who sees himself as being inferior is likely to have problems relating normally to women and may settle on modes of sexual release which augment, or at least do -not threaten, his fragile sense of masculinity. In a fetishist, an object such as a bra can take on the power of the .female who wore it and substitute for her. The fetishist is guaranteed success in his interaction with the substitute and thereby increases his sense of masculinity. In pedophilia, the male is typically afraid of mature females and therefore, chooses a child as an object. The child's powerlessness emphasizes the deviant's strength and masculinity and assuages his inferiority feelings.

According to theorists such as Edwards and Storr, sexual deviations may be understood as exaggerated normal patterns that may be used to satisfy needs for a sense of masculinity without the requirements of intimate personal relationships. In our society the pressures on males to confirm to a highly idealized model of strength, competence and virility can be enormous. Thus, feelings of sexual inferiority are probably more strongly felt by males. This may be One reason why the sexual deviations are much more common in men than women.

There are three different types of sexual behaviours that are of special significance. These are (1) Incest, (2) Rape and (3) Homosexuality. Incest is an old problem which is receiving great deal of attention. It is a Penal offence in our country. Rape is another criminal offence which is occurring with relatively high frequency inspite of stringent punishment. Homosexuality is a sexual behaviour of significance because it has become highly controversial. Some societies tolerate it, others have given it legal sanction whereas in many countries, including ours, it is a criminal offence punishable as per provisions of Law. There is also a controversy, over homosexuality, among mental health experts whether it is abnormal, "sick" or deviant. We would discuss these three types of sexual behaviour of special significance.

1. **Incest** is a sexual relationship between a parent and a child or a grand parent and grand children or between siblings, of any age. Incest has been universally condemned, however, a few socio-cultural settings have condoned incest, the most notable being the pharashs of ancient Egypt.

Incest is usually a taboo because the progeny born out of such incestuous relationship are usually abnormal. However, despite the taboo incest is more common than would usually be assumed. Kinsey and his coworkers (1948) reported that 0.5 percent of the males interviewed in their study admitted to acts of incest. Adams and Neil in 1967 found that 7 of the 18 children born out of incestuous relationship could be considered normal. By the age of six months 5 of the 18 had died, 3 had borderline intelligence, 2 were severally mentally retarded and I had a cleft palate, whereas on the other hand in a control group out of the 18 infants only 2 were abnormal. This indicates that children of incestuous relationship have a substantial risk of genetic defect. Even when aft infant is not born from such a relationship, the effects of the experience can be quite damaging psychologically to the participants. Since the behaviour is far outside the bounds of what most people regard as acceptable. Recent studies have indicated that the frequency of incest and pedophilia is much higher than suspected.

By far the greatest percentage of reported incest occurs between mothers and sons (about 4 percent of reported cases; Maisch, 1972), the mothers appear to be even more psychologically disturbed prior to the initiation of the act than do incestuous fathers. When father daughter incest occurs the father often initiates the original act, while his judgement is impaired by alcoholic intoxication.

The behaviour often begins when these fathers are under a strain which threatens their masculinity, commonly when the wife is rejecting the husband's sexual interest towards her. The husband then turns to a sexually developing child for sexual and usually emotional gratification. In families where the prohibitions against incest break down, the family is often disorganized. Family members do not communicate and, in fact, tend to deny sexuality. The wife-mother frequently denies the possibility of the act, and fails to protect the daughter even when she hears the daughter complain about it. Instead, she often attacks the daughter as a "liar" or as a seductress (Bernstein, 1979). To outsiders, these families appear quite normal and respectable and come from all social classes.

Cavallin (1966) reported that the typical incestuous father confines his extramarital sexual contacts to his daughter alone, and sometimes to several daughters, starting with the eldest and going down the line as the years pass. Furthermore, far from being indiscriminately a moral, fathers who seduce their sexually mature daughters are likely to be highly moralistic and devoutly attached to fundamentalist religious doctrines.

Father daughter incest often occurs in connection with disturbed marital relationship and may even be tacitly encouraged by the mother as a means of escaping her husband's sexual advances. As might be imagined, the psychological impact of such a relationship on the daughter can be profound. Among the problems that psychotherapists have encountered in women who were molested by their fathers are depression, anxiety, alcoholism, drug abuse and difficulties in relating with men.

(2) **Rape**: Rape is a forcible sexual intercourse which is against the will and without the consent of the individual who is raped. In recent times we see that more and more cases of rape are being reported to the police, though the actual incidence that occur is very high. Rape usually occurs where man is the perpetrator and woman is the victim. Rape is a very traumatic incident in the life of a woman, specially the Indian woman.

Rape is not a diagnostic category in DSM-III, but it involves a disturbance in normal sexual functioning. Legally, rape is divided into statutory rape which involves the seduction of a minor and forcible rape in which victim is over 18 years. In the present section, we shall concentration forcible rape which is forced sexual intercourse with a nonconsenting partner beyond age of 18 years.

Generally, the rapist is a male and the victim is a female. But there are some rare instances in which male is the victim female is the rapist. But now-a-days in U. S. rape by man of other man is also becoming common, e.g. Growth and Burgess (1980) have studied 22 cases of male-male rapes. The reports of male-male rapes are uncommon because of victim's shame and humiliation.

Psychologists have tried to find out that when an individual indulges in a rape, is he indulging in a sexual act or no. Many authorities say "no", some say that sexual gratification is at most a secondary factor in rape, others claim that rape is a ritualist process for the subjugation of women and has little to do with sexual gratification. Psychologists have analysed the profile of a rapist. Most of them are young adult males and 50% of them are married and most of the rapist will indulge again and again in rape. Rapist usually have a very high need to express power, anger and sexuality. Rapist consider sexuality to be simple vehicle for the expression these motives. There arc many different Hypes of rapist

1. Power assertive rapist,
2. Power re-assurance rapist,
3. Anger retaliation rapist, and
4. Anger excitation rapist.

We would discuss these different types of rapists in brief.

(a) **Power-Assertive Rapist**: For him, rape is an expression of virility, mastery, and dominance. During the rape, his inadequacy as manifested in his identity and life effectiveness can be denied through an act of power over another person.

(b) **Power-Reassurance Rapist:** He commits the rape to reassure himself of his own sexual adequacy and masculinity. His need is to place women. in a helpless position to eliminate his doubts and bolster his weakened self-perception.

(c) **Anger-Retaliation Rapist**: Rape for him is an expression of anger and rage. The motive is revenge and his aim is degradation and humiliation. These men often have histories of abandonment or rejection by important female figures in their lives.

(d) **Anger-Excitation Rapist**: This rapist is a sexual sadist who is excited by and finds pleasure in the suffering of his victim. His aim is to punish, hurt, and torture the victim. These rapists aic likely to have histories of assaultive behaviours which in many instances are not associated with sexual activity. Fortunately, only 5 percent of rapists apparently fall into this category.

In all these four different categories of rapist we find that rape is cither a expression of dominance, sexual adequacy and masculinity or it is an expression of anger, rage and sexual sadism.

Psychologists have not given much attention to the rape victims, such rape victims suffer from physical and psychological trauma. Most often the victim is blamed for being seductive and provocative. Women cope with rape in a variety of ways. The four most common are:

(1) Cognitive strategies,

(2) Verbal strategies,

(3) Physical action, and

(4) Some become psychologically paralyzed and numb.

Burgess and Holmstrom report that during the physical attack, many victims mentally disengage and try to stay calm, others scream some try to reason with rapist some struggle and some experience involuntary gagging, choking, nausea, and even loss of consciousness. Once free of the rapist and safe, a series of reactions may occur (Notman & Nadelson, 1976). Victims are anxious and fearful, but often not immediately angry. Anger, when it appears, comes later. Guilt and shame are universal, and supported by the rejecting attitudes of friends, family, and strangers. Very commonly, the victims go through a period of lack of trust in men. Many women are so distraught they try to start life over, they find new places of residence, new jobs, new friends. The victims' reactions can be considered a posttraumatic stress disorder.

3. Homosexuality: Technically the term homosexuality (from Greek word homo,, meaning "same as") designates sexual activity directed towards one's own sex, whether male or female. However, in popular usage homosexuality usually means male homosexuality, while female homosexuality, which has received much less attention than its male counterpart, is given the separate name Lesbianism (the name is taken from the Greek island of Lesbos, home of the presumably Lesbian poet Sappho).

Homosexuality was included in the DSM-I under sociopathic personality disturbances, in DSM-II, it was included in a section on personality disorders. In 1974, six years before DSM-III was instituted, the American Psychiatric Association (APA) voted to stop considering homosexuality in and of itself a mental disorder. In place of the previous classification APA substituted category called sexual orientation disturbance. This category was intended for individuals whose sexual interests are directed primarily towards people of the same sex and who also are in some way uncomfortable with their sexual orientation. The spirit of this change in perspective was carried over to DSM-III. However, the term sexual orientation disturbance has been omitted and replaced by the classification e.g. dystonic homosexuality under larger category of psychosexual disorders. Accordingly to DSM-III, unless homosexual individuals experience persistent distress regarding their own sexual orientation and have a strong need and desire to change their behaviour, homosexuality is not a diagnosable disorder.

Contrary to common belief, incidence of homosexuality is very large. On the basis of interviews of 5,300 American men and 5940 women Kinsey et. al. found that about 5'4%-of men were exclusively homosexuals and about 37% had homosexual experience at least once and about 28% of women had atleast one homosexual experience.

There arc various misconceptions about homosexuals e.g. it is believed that homosexuals have a typical personality type or male homosexuals are feminine in appearance and mannerisms, or they are limp-wristed, or female homosexuals (i. e. Lesbians) are tough-looking, etc. Howevcr, all these beliefs are misconceptions, and homosexuals are not much different from heterosexuals. An intensive study of 979 homosexuals was conducted by Bell and Weinberg in 1978 and the reports were compared with 500 heterosexual control subjects. It was observed that there was no difference in occupational choice and less than 10% of homosexuals were in 'feminine' occupations. There was no significant difference in the level of psychological distress, between the two groups, and most homosexuals could not be differentiated from heterosexuals in terms of "pathological" thought processes. Contrary to common belief, only 25% of the homosexuals regretted their homosexuality. However, 28% of homosexual men and 16% of the homosexual women were cither isolated or had psychological problems which may be due to lack of acceptance by society. In addition 50% of the male homosexuals were promiscuous and reported to have 500 sexual pattern in their life. This promiscuity is considered as pathology by many like Bieber.

Homosexual life styles: Bell and Weinberg have conducted extensive studies of homosexuals. On the basis of their studies, they have given

Five types of homosexuals as follows:

(a) **Close-coupled** homosexuals who live with a partner in a quasi-marriage situation and are perfectly happy and satisfied.

(b) **Open-coupled** homosexuals are those who have special sexual partners, but are not entirely happy and many have many partners.

(c) **Functional** homosexuals organize **their life** around their sexual experience and have great number of partners. But they neither regret about their homosexuality, nor they are disturbed.

(d) **Dysfunctional homosexuals:** These are the disturbed homosexuals with lot of many problems and they regret about their homosexuality.

(e) **Asexual** homosexuals are those who are not involved in other, have very few sexual partners and are isolated from others.

Besides the above categorization, homosexual life-style has also been categorised into the following 5 types :

(1) **The situational homosexuals** are those who become homosexual because heterosexual partners are not available. They do not consider themselves to be homosexuals, but their behaviour is a matter of sexual necessity. This situation is common in prisons.

(2) **The hidden homosexuals (closet homosexuals)** are thrive homosexuals who hide their secret from others. Only very close friend or relative may know about their sexual preferences. Most of the homosexuals fall in this category.

(3) **The adjusted homosexuals** are those who have homosexual relations with one partner or many, but are well-adjusted in life and are linked with gay-community.

(4) **The behavioural obvious homosexuals** These are the homosexuals who can be recognized by their mannerisms as they appear more like (he opposite sex. It also includes those homosexuals who cross-dress.

(5) **The tea room homosexuals** are those who have temporary sexual relations with many partners, half of them are married and most hide their secrets.

Possible factors in the development of homosexually: A great deal of sexual research suggest that human beings cannot be divided exclusively into heterosexual or homosexual as far as human sexuality is concerned. Human behaviour falls on a continual. Homosexual thoughts are not uncommon in behaviorally heterosexual individuals and heterosexual fantasies are common in behaviorally homosexual persons. According to many experts human beings are 'bi-sexual individuals having potentialities for being heterosexual or homosexual. Some factors that have been found to play an important role in the development of homosexuality are as follows :

(1) **Physiological factors:** According to some investigators genetic and hormonal factors play a very important role in the development of homosexuality. However, many have contradicted this view with their research findings. This area of research remains so filled with contradictory findings that no conclusions can be effectively drawn.

Long ago Kallman (1952) found a concordance rate of 100 percent for homosexuality in a sample of monozygotic twins and a significantly lower rate for dizygotic twins, his findings have not been confirmed by others (Kolb 1963 Mooney & Ehrhardt, 1972). If there is a genetic cause for homosexuality, most theorists now believe that it would be in the form of a predisposition for individuals to become homosexual if they encounter a particular kind of environment.

While the genetic explanation for homosexuality has not received much support, other theorists sharing the biological view have proposed hormonal differences between homosexuals and heterosexuals. They suggest that homosexual men have lower levels of testosterone (the male sex hormone) and homosexual women lower levels of estrogen (the female sex hormone). Some evidence of testosterone deficits in male homosexuals have been found (Kolodny ct. al. 1971, Lovaineet. al. 1970). More recent work has implicated other hormonal substances called luteinizing hormones in the case of female homosexuals (Doerret. al. 1976).

(2) **Psychoanalytic theories**: Psychoanalytic theories view homosexuality in terms of unconscious fears. One major psychoanalytic view is that individual turns to homosexual behaviour because of heterosexual behaviour. The adult avoids heterosexual behaviour because it stimulates unacceptable incestuous feelings which were never resolved in childhood. Some case studies of homosexuals in psycho-analysis lend indirect support to this theory. Bieber et. al. ~1962) compared 106 male homosexuals in treatment with 100 heterosexuals in treatment. The homosexual subjects reported that their mothers were more domineering and demanded more intense emotional relationships with them than was reported for the mothers of the heterosexual males. In addition, male homosexuals reported that their fathers were distant or hostile, and were poor figures for role identification, hence these individuals became homosexuals.

Study by Evans, (1969) of homosexuals who were not in treatment found that some homosexuals (but not all) remembered their mothers as being close binding and-their fathers as being distant and unacceptable. The members of the heterosexual control group in this study were less likely to describe their parents this way.

Freud in his "Three Essays on the theory of Sexuality" suggested that all people were bisexual (attracted to both sexes) at the point in their normal development when they loved both of their parents. Homosexuality is seen as the result of an arrest of normal development at the bisexual (homoerotic) stage, or as a regression back to that stage.

Freud implicated the mishandling of the oedipal stage and the failure of the male child to form a satisfactory relationship with his father as a major cause for the retardation of normal sexual development. Freud believed the presence of a detached, cold and even hostile father, together with a close, binding, seductive mother sets the stage for the development of a homosexual orientation. However, the presence of a truly loving and caring father probably could prevent the development of a homosexual orientation, regardless of what the mother was like.

(3) **Learning Theories:** According to many, homosexuality can be a learned human behaviour. Whenever interactions with a female will lead to unpleasant rejections and on the other hand interactions with male member would lead to positive reinforcement. The individual gradually through such reinforcements learn to become homosexual. Various principles of learning can explain the development of homosexual behaviour.

(4) **Socio-cultural factor**: Many socio-cultural factors have been found to be responsible in the development of homosexual behaviour. Homosexuality is found to be high in certain environments or Socio-cultural settings, for example, researchers have observed homo-sexuality is higher in prison in mates, armed forces personnel and in boys hostel.

TREATMENT TECHNIQUES FOR SEXUAL DYSFUNCTIONS

The treatment of sexual dysfunction has been of concern to mental health experts since a very long time. However, in recent years the study and treatment of sexual dysfunction has received academic as well as research attention. Many new techniques of treatment has been devised as a result of various developments in social, behavioural and physical sciences and these treatment techniques have given good success rate. However, various traditional treatment approaches, including psychoanalysis have been tried with individuals who have had sexual dysfunctions. But the results with these traditional techniques have been very poor. Various behavioral techniques have given good results with respect, to sexual dysfunctions. Some of these techniques are as follows:

(1) **Behavioural approach: Anxiety Reduction Techniques:** Behavioural approach, in which patients arc taught relaxation techniques, or anxiety reduction techniques, are effective in psychosexual dysfunction. Nemetz, Craig and Reich (1978) have successfully treated primary orgasmic dysfunction

(2) **Systematic desensitization**: Wolpe (1958) was among the first to use "systematic desensitization" to treat psychosexual dysfunction, lace (1973) also used systematic desensitization to treat women with orgasmic dysfunction. The basic strategy is to ask the individual to determine at what stage of sexual 'activity anxiety began and then go beyond that point only gradually and in small steps, so that the anxiety is reduced totally. The patient is trained to relax by suggestions. The patient is also asked to practice relaxation technique at home with the help of a cooperative partner. Within 5 to 25 sessions the patient can successfully overcome the sexual dysfunction.

Systematic desensitization, has often been used to decrease the anxiety associated with sexual behaviour, Ince (1973) describes the successful treatment of a woman who was so anxious about sexual intercourse that she had developed orgasmic dysfunction.

The patient was asked to describe the sexual relationship between her and her husband, that is, the lovemaking, in precise detail, and to relate which aspects of it made her anxious. An outline of the sequence of acts, in order of occurrence and also in order of anxiety arousal is as follows :

1. Her husband moves toward her in bed.
2. Her husband kisses her.
3. Her husband embraces her and she returns the embrace.
4. Her husband caresses her breasts and she caresses his penis.
5. Her husband stimulates her vagina while she continues to cares' him.
6. Intercourse, occasionally preceded by oral-genital stimulation.

Systematic desensitization was the treatment method employed. The patient was treated in relaxation by means of suggestion. Within two sessions she was able to completely relax. Then, under conditions of relaxation, the lovemaking sequence was described to her in detail by the therapist. The patient was first directed to indicate to him when she clearly visualized each scene, and also to indicate when she felt anxious by raising her hand. Each time anxiety occurred she was relaxed again prior to continuation of therapy. The patient was also given the task of relaxing herself at home in bed, prior to engaging in sexual relations, and her husband was instructed to postpone his advances until she had done so.

Following the initial desensitization session, the patient had intercourse with her husband and was able to remain relaxed and enjoy the activity. She did not however, experience orgasm. The following night she came the nearest to having an orgasm that she had since she had been married. One Week later she had her first strong desire for sexual intercourse.

Two days later she awakened in the night with a desire for intercourse, awakened her husband and enjoyed the sexual act immensely but did not have an orgasm. One week after that she began to feel as affectionate toward her husband as she had felt prior to her marriage and her sexual desires were "as they had been before.

Within five more days she experienced her first orgasm and from then on reported no more difficulty in reaching an orgasm during her now frequent lovemaking sessions. The entire duration of therapy was one month.

(3) **Masters and Johnson's approach : Enjoyment of Sexual Act** - Most of the treatment approaches to sexual dysfunction are based on work of Masters and Johnson's. Their treatment follows the following stages:

(a) Complete physical examination to find out whether any physical aspect is the cause of the problem.

(b) Once chances of physical causes are ruled out, the client and the partner are taught to enjoy touching and exploring one another's body, without engaging in sexual intercourse. This is called 'Sensate focus'.

(c) After 'sensate focus', the client and the partner are allowed to have intercourse at home.

(d) During all these stages, the doubts, anxiety, misconceptions about sexual activity are clarified by the counsellor from time to time. The therapist continues counselling in a relaxed or less anxious environment, gives knowledge about 'appropriate' sexual behaviour and educative feedback is given. This step-by-step process of reducing anxiety and teaching right behaviour is very effective treatment.

Masters and Johnson's treatment rests on two basic assumptions(1)

The first is that sexual dysfunction is not an individual problem "her" problem or "his" problem but a problem of the marital unit, in which sexual communication has broken down. (2) The second assumption is that in order to reactivate the individual's natural ability to respond to sexual stimuli, the couple must be relieved of all performance pressures. Essentially they must return to a goalless, non-demand "petting" stage in order to rediscover their ability to be "pleasured" by touching and caressing.

(4) **Specific techniques developed by Master and Johnson for specific sexual dysfunction:** In Master and Johnson's program and in other sex therapy programs, the specific techniques that the couple is instructed to use vary with the form of sexual dysfunction involved.

(a) **Premature ejaculation-**For premature ejaculation, many therapists prescribe the so-called pause technique. In this procedure the Woman stimulates the man's penis until he feels ready to ejaculate, at which point he signals her to stop. Once the need to ejaculate subsides, she begins stimulating him again, until he once again signals her to stop. Repeated many times, this technique gradually increases the amount of stimulation required to trigger the ejaculation response, so that eventually the man gains control over the response.

(b) **Erectile dysfunction:** In erectile dysfunction as well as in orgastic dysfunction, to be discussed after this, the basis of treatment is the general formula prescribed by Masters & Johnson : "A high level of stimulation in an atmosphere of low demand". In Erectile dysfunction, the therapist, in order to eliminate anxiety, may actually tell the patient to try not to have an erection while the couples are going through their "petting" exercises. This technique of prescribing the behaviour that the patient is trying to accomplish is called paradoxical instruction. Forbidden to have an erection, the patient may find himself sufficiently free of anxiety that he begins responding to the sexual stimuli and thus has the "prohibited" erection. Once this happens, the therapist permits the couple, in very gradual stages, to proceed further and further towards intercourse, always with the warning that the techniques "work best" if the man can prevent himself from having an erection.

(c) **Orgastic dysfunction** - For orgastic dysfunction, a common procedure is to teach the woman to masturbate, again with no performance demands. First she masturbates alone, possibly with the help of an electric vibrator and/or erotic pictures and reading material (she may also be encouraged to use sexual fantasies to enhance arousal). Next, the man is taught to manipulate her to orgasm. Finally manipulation is paired with intercourse (Lopiccolo and Lobitz, 1972).

(5) **Kaplan's suggestion on treatment of sexual dysfunction**: The successful behavioural treatment approaches all utilize anxiety reduction and behavioural practice. H. S. Kaplan (1975) feels that therapy for sexual dysfunction must go beyond these two factors. Sexual dysfunction occurs in human relationships, most of which have been in existence for many years. Kaplan's approach emphasizes psychotherapy in addition to direct sexual training and anxiety reduction. She feels that if the interpersonal difficulties of the sexual partners are not resolved, the gains of strict behavioural sexual therapy may be undone.

Of all the various treatment techniques available for sexual dysfunctions. Master and Johnson's program appears to be extremely successful in eliminating the disorders of vaginismus (100 percent success). Premature ejaculation (98 percent success) and primary erectile disturbances (70 percent success). When followed up after a year, their clients showed an impressive 80 percent success rate for sexual dysfunctions in both women and men.

METHODS OF TREATING SEXUAL DEVIATIONS

While most people with psychological problems seek help because their symptoms make them uncomfortable and unhappy, that is not necessarily the case in sexual disorders, especially paraphilias. These people may not seek treatment until they are forced to do so by actual or threatened legal action. Needless to say "forced therapy" is difficult in unmotivated and uncooperative clients. Although traditional forms of individual psychotherapy have had inconsistent success in treating such clients.

Among the current therapeutic techniques, behaviour therapy and cognitive behavioural therapy have shown some success. Some of the commonly used treatment techniques used to treat paraphilia or sexual deviation are as follows:

1. Aversion therapy: Individuals with sexual deviations respond better to aversion therapy. Typically, the patient would be shown slides of the stimulus that normally triggered his arousal a little girl, a patent leather shoe, whatever. Then, Once he was aroused, he would be given a mild electric shock, which he could turn off by flipping a switch that changed the slide to one showing a more conventional sexual stimulus, such as a nude woman. This simple technique was reported successful in a number of cases fetishism, masochism, transvestism, and exhibitionism and in some cases of pedophilia and sadism.

2. **Covert sensitization:** Today, the reconditioning aspect of behavioural treatment is often handled through cognitive techniques, such as covert sensitization, in which the patient simply imagines the pairing of aversive stimuli with the unwanted behaviour. For e.g., a pedophile might be instructed to manage himself involved in sex play with a little girl. Once he is aroused, by this fantasy, the story continues. He is asked to visualize himself being caught in the act by his wife and children, then being arrested in front of the neighbours, then seeking his name in a headline and reading a lurid newspaper account of his crime, then loosing his job, and so forth. This technique is often useful in eliminating the unwanted behaviour.

Thus, we see that in covert sensitization, sex objects that initially are positively valued are associated .not with pleasure but with discomfort. For instance, in treating a sadist an image of inflicting pain on another may be paired with images of becoming nauseated soon, through classical conditioning. The image of pain infliction makes the person sick. In this way, the frequency of the deviant behaviour may be reduced. Mahoncy (1974) has concluded that covert sensitization is consistently effective with sexual paraphilias.

3. **Thought stopping technique:** To control sexual fantasizing, a "thought stopping" technique may be used by itself or in combination with covert sensitization. In this procedure the therapist asks the patient to close his eyes and talk about his sexual thoughts. At some point during this process the therapist will shout "stop". After a period of time, the client will be instructed to say "stop" himself each time the unwanted thoughts begin to emerge. Parentean and Lamontague (1981) have applied thought stopping successfully to a number of paraphilias.

4. **Hormonal therapy** has been a recent addition to attempted treatment. In this approach, ant androgens are given to sex offenders to diminish sensitivity to circulating androgens. This reduces erotic arousal and desire. Money and his associates have been major investigators using this approach (Money ct. al. 1975). Usually, the dosage of medication is combined with psychological counselling for a period of 6 months to 2 years. Walker (1977) reports that patients report a sense of relief that their sexual compulsion no longer governs what they do. Money et. al. (1976) found that sex offending paraphiliacs (like exhibitionists and pedophiliacs) who remained for the completion of therapy reported a reduction of erotic imaginary and fewer sex offending incidents than those who dropped out of treatment.

MICROPHALLNEUROSIS

The male's concern about the size of his penis has been called microphallneurosis by Glenn (1972). Such concerns are quite common. Many researches have studied the common ranges of flaccid and erect penis size, and their combined results yield the following data :

The flaccid penis has an average length of about 4 inches, with a common range of 23 inches to 4.5 inches. Erect penis length averages about 6 inches, with a common range of about 4.5 inches to slightly over 8 inches. The circumference averages 4.2 inches. These measurements vary some what from study to study and do not include the unusually small or large penis. An interesting finding (Masters & Johnson, 1966) was that the smaller flaccid penis increased to a greater degree when erect than the larger flaccid penis, and that penis size bears almost no relationship to the male's overall body size. Sexual satisfaction and/or performance is also not affected by the size of penis.

(b) **Strange sexual behaviours:** At the extreme range of low frequency sexual behaviour, there is a broad variety of sexual objects and modes of function which have been described and named as strange sexual behaviours. Some are listed and described below :

1. **Zoophilia** Sexual use of animals through masturbation or intercourse. This disorder is more frequently seen in rural areas, but cases have been described in which household pets have been trained to engage in sexual acts with humans.

2. **Coprophilia:** The need to have faces present either visually or tactiley to enhance sexual satisfaction. An example from Cleckley (1975) follows : "He would go to places where he was not known and there he would visit the public men's rooms of the railroad station in search for pieces of feces. Then he collected them, wrapped them up carefully and carried them around with him, thus experiencing sexual-orgastic relief".

3. **Necrophilia:** Sexual activity with a dead body.

4. **Frottage:** Rubbing against other persons' bodies (typically strangers) to obtain sexual satisfaction; most frequently occurs in public places such as crowded elevators and subways.

5. **Siliromania-**Dirtying or Mutilating female bodies or clothing to obtain sexual satisfaction.

6. **Piquer:** Obtaining sexual satisfaction for stabbing another in the breast

or buttock with a sharp pointed instrument such as a needle or ice pick. The intent is not usually to kill. Fortunately this is an extremely rare behaviour.

7. **Klismaphilia:** Sexual gratification obtained from giving or receiving an enema.

8. **Obscene telephone calls:** These are generally made by males. Roughly speaking about 25 percent of the obscene telephone calls have a sexual content. The sexually oriented calls appear to be made exclusively by males, who are usually lonely, under stress, feels inadequate and obtain a sense of strength and pleasure from the shocked reaction of female who answers the call, especially if the reaction involves outrage.

9. **Satyriasis and Nymphomania:** Compulsive promiscuity, often called "satyriasis" in males and "nymphomania" in women, involves high frequency sexual behaviour of a "driven" quality, which is rarely satisfactory to the individual. While orgasm can occur, and usually does, in males, shortly after the sexual experience the individual is dominated by the need to engage in a sexual act again. In the classic case, the individual is searching for love but feels unlovable and must go from sexual liaison to sexual liaison in an attempt to prove to the self that he or she really is worth loving.

(c) **Sexual behaviour and DSM-III:** The categories of sexual disorder or behaviour in DSM-III (1980) include the following:

A. Psychosexual Dysfunctions:

1. Inhibited Sexual Desire.
2. Inhibited Sexual Excitement.
3. Inhibited Female Orgasm.
4. Inhibited Male Orgasm.
5. Premature Ejaculation.
6. Functional Dyspareunia.
7. Functional Vagnismus.
8. Atypical Psychosexual Dysfunction.

These disorders are equivalent to the psychosexual dysfunctions described by most researchers such as Masters and Johnson, and avoid the somewhat perjoreative term "frigidity" and "impotence".

B. Gender Identity Disorders

1. Transsexuals.

2. Gender Identity Disorder of Childhood.

3. Atypical Gender Identity Disorder.

C. **Paraphilias:** Includes disorders such as transvestism, pedophilia, voyeurism, etc. These disorders were previously called "sexual deviations", and the individuals who manifested them were called "sexual deviates". "Paraphilia" avoids the negative connotations of these terms.

D. **Other psychosexual disorders.**

1. Ego-dystonic Homosexuality.

2. Psychosexual Disorders Not Elsewhere Classified.

"Psychosexual Disorders Not Elsewhere Classified" is a residual, wastebasket term. The use of Ego-dystonic Homosexuality reflects a belief that homosexuality is a disorder only when it causes the homosexual significant psychological difficulty, is not accepted by the ego, not when the individual is accepting and adjusted to his or her sexual orientation.

(d) Masturbation is also called as auto criticism and has been one of the most misunderstood aspect of sexuality.

The word Masturbation comes from the latin word "Masturbare" which itself is derived from two latin words "Manus" hand and "stubrare" (to defile), giving the sense of "to defile with hand". Masturbation means manipulation of the genital organs of oneself or others to derive sexual arousal, stimulation and gratification. When one plays with his sex organs and derives stimulation and satisfaction from it he or she is said to be indulging in masturbation.

The first real facts about who masturbates were discovered by Kinsey and his associates in 1940s. They reported that 58% of the women and 92% of men had masturbated at some points in their lies.

Hunt's research carried out in 1970i- has shown that masturbation among sexes has increased during the last 30 years.

Hunt's analysis indicates that 60% of women aged 181024 masturbate and by late 20s and early 30s, 80 percent of the women had masturbated. Hunt also found that 70 percent of married men and 60% of married women masturbated.

People of all ages, sex, culture, races, caste, creed, religion and marital status indulge in it.

Masturbation is one method used as an outlet of the sexual urge. This is the only method of sexual excitement, arousal and gratification that is very handy and trouble free.

Masturbation helps one get on much better terms with one's own body and to become more aware of one's own sexuality. It helps one understand different sensitive Zones of one's body so that this knowledge can be of great help during sexual intercourse and foreplay.

For those not initiated into sex, masturbation is a part of a process of self discovery and beginning to feel that one is a man or woman. Masturbation as such is not abnormal and has many beneficial aspects.

Masturbation becomes abnormal under the following conditions :

(i) When masturbation is preferred over intercourse or is associated with sado-masochistic or highly pornographic fantasies.

(ii) When an individual has the choice of several sexual outlets but finds that sexual satisfaction can only be obtained through masturbation-

(iii) When masturbation interferes with sexual intercourse. For many people orgasm is reached only through masturbation but sexual intercourse fails to lead to orgasm. In such cases masturbation as a practice, interfering with heterosexual adjustment become abnormal.

(iv) Compulsive masturbation is also an abnormal practice as it interferes with sexual adjustment.

(v) In many individuals masturbation gives rise to feelings of guilt. Many feel weak and disgusted due to masturbation. It is only when such feelings arise that masturbation becomes abnormal.

6

Personality Disorders

The study of personality disorders has not received due attention. It is one of the most neglected topics in the field of Abnormal Psychology. Our limited knowledge of Personality Disorders has been due to the limited research generated on these topics. In recent years, however, this topic has received a great deal of attention, especially with its inclusion in DSM-III.

According to Allport personality disorders can be defined as relatively enduring characteristics of personality that leads to subjective discomfort or/and makes individual adaptation to his environment difficult and leads to maladaptive forms of behaviour.

Today, we find that personality Disorders are grouped into different categories. This was, however, not the case a few decades ago. Different personality disorders were lumped together under a general heading like "antisocial", "Psychopathic", "Sociopathic" or "social" personality disorders etc. Personality Disorders were given more emphasis in DSM-II and were listed as a separate diagnostic entity in it. DSM-III also clarified the picture by distinguishing between personality traits and personality Disorders.

According to DSM-III personality traits are defined as enduring patterns of perceiving, relating to and thinking about the environment and on self that are exhibited in a wide range of important social and personal contexts. It is only when personality traits are inflexible and maladaptive and cause either significant impairment in social or occupational functioning or subjective distress that they constitute personality Disorders.

Most of the personality Disorders are manifested during adolescence or earlier and continue throughout most of the adult life, though they often become less obvious in middle or old age.

People with personality disorder generally have disturbances of mood and interpersonal problems which are generally longstanding and ego syntonic i.e. accepted as a part of the self. Most of the individuals with personality disorder don't seek active professional psychological help, unless and until they have trouble with law or are forced to take such help by relative, friends and other responsible persons. The Scientific study of personality disorder began with the 'DSM-III classification which is as follows:

1. Eccentric Cluster

(1) Paranoid personality disorder.

(2) Schizoid Personality Disorder.

(3) Schizotypal personality disorder.

II. Fearful Cluster.

(1) Avoidant personality disorder.

(2) Dependent personality disorder.

(3) Compulsive personality disorder.

(4) Passive-aggressive personality disorder.

III. Erratic Cluster

(1) Histrionic personality disorder.

(2) Borderline personality disorder.

(3) Narcissistic personality disorder.

(4) Antisocial personality disorder.

Besidesthe11categoriesofpersonalitydisorderslistedinthefbovetable, there is yet another category of personality, disorder, in DSM-III called as Atypical, mixed or other personality disorder. In this chapter we would first discuss the definition of personality and personality disorders, obstacles to the study of personality disorder and classification of personality disorder.

Following this we would discuss all the eleven types of personality disorder discussed in the DSM-III.

We would discuss the antisocial personality disorder in great detail including its causes and treatment as this particular disorder has greatly attracted the interest of not only mental health experts but also of law makers, policy makers and general public.

Personality has recently become the prime topic of academic interest, and has reached its acme during the last few decades. It was not until the mid-1930s that the study of Personality became formalized and systematized especially in American Psychology. Nevertheless Schultz (1976) mentioned; "Personality is not the dominant emphasis in Psychology today.......for more than half of Psychology's history as a science it paid relatively little attention to it......" Today Personality Psychology is one of the growing sub fields of Psychology, which is attracting academicians, researchers, clinicians and layman alike. It is a multidisciplinary field drawing heavily from other related areas and contributing towards our understanding of Human Behaviour.

Hall and Lindzey (1957) in the first edition of their handbook on Personality, pointing to the contribution of Personality Theorist remarked "Personality Theorist have been rebels. Rebels in Medicine and in Experimental Science, rebels against typical methods and respected techniques of research and most of all rebels against accepted theory and normative problems....." Similarly, pointing towards the contribution of Personality Psychology very recently Hellema (1979) pointed out, "Traditionally its has always been Personality Theorists, who have opened up II-'VJI perspectives in Psychology, and have led the way in new thinking."

DEFINITION OF PERSONALITY

The word, "Personality," has been derived from the Latin word, "Persona', which was used for the "mask" utilized by the actors to change their appearance but in Roman times it was taken' as a particular character itself. Since then the word. Personality, is used to refer not only to one's character but also to those aspects of individual's behaviour that set him apart from other individuals.

It is not easy to define Personality. Turkat and Levin (1984) recently examining the literature on definitions of Personality noted that they were unable to identify a unifying definition. Years ago Gordon Allport (1937) recounted as many as fifty definitions of Personality. According to Allport (1961), "Personality is the dynamic organisation within the individual of those Psychophysical systems that determine his characteristic behaviour and thought." This is one of the most comprehensive definitions that takes into account the biological as well as the Psychological variables involved in the development of the individual's Personality. The words, "Dynamic Organisation", in the above definition, imply that the individual is an ever changing and developing organism as a result of new experiences and new goals. They also further imply that an individual goes on changing and developing but at the same time maintaining coherence. The word, "Psychophysical" imply that Personality is neither exclusively a Psychological nor an exclusively Physiological Phenomenon. Both these aspects interact and influence each other and in this process our behaviour including our thoughts, feelings, emotions, attitudes and other aspects of our inner self are shaped into a pattern that becomes, "characteristic' of a Particular individual. By the word, "Characteristic", is meant that each individual is unique in itself, however, similar the experiences of two or more people might be. This definition though not oriented towards any particular theory emphasizes heavily on the individual being or represents the person-concerned approach. In contrast to this definition let us examine another definition presented by well-known learning theorist, Walter Mischel (1976). According to him. Personality can be defined as, "the distinctive pattern of behaviour, including thoughts and emotions that characterize each individual's adaptation to the situations of his or her life". This definition implies that Personality is largely confined to terms of the adaptation of an individual to his surroundings. By the word, "Characteristic," Mischel meant that each individual was unique and that Personality was a relatively stable feature of a given individual. His stance largely represented the situational approach. Because it leaned heavily on the role of environment.

Recently Hall and Lindzey (1985) noted that all definitions of Personality can be grouped into five categories. The first was largely used by layman where Personality tended to have an evaluative connotation. It was a measure of a Person's social skills or the reflection of his or her most outstanding characteristic. The other four categories of definition reflected the most common theoretical orientations regarding the structure and functioning of Human Personality. These four categories of definition are biosocial, biophysical, omnibus and integrative. The biosocial definition emphasized the social factors that played an important role in determining an individual's Personality. Mischel's definition discussed above falls in this category. The biophysical group of definitions emphasized the organic, inherent components of Personality. The omnibus definition listed every concept considered of importance in describing the person, where as an integrative definition held that Personality was what gave order and congruence to many different behaviours in which a person engaged. Allport's definition discussed above falls into this last category.

PERSONALITY DISORDER DEFINED

Many abnormal behaviours are characterized by sudden disruptions or changes in pattern of behaviour, mood and thought, but one set of disorders, however, does not happen suddenly. These patterns of behaviour appear to be deeply ingrained and are manifested primarily as exaggerations. These are referred to as Personality Disorders.

The category of Personality Disorder is relatively new. It was introduced by the American Psychiatric Association's Classification in its first Diagnostic and Statistical Manual ((D.S.M.-1) (1952). Before the publication of this manual, Personality Disorders were largely termed as "Character Disorders". D.SM. -11 (1967) (the second edition) defined Personality Disorder as "deeply ingrained maladaptive pattern of behaviour that are perceptibly different in quality from psychotic and neurotic symptoms. Generally these are life long patterns often recognizable by the time of adolescence of earlier." The D.S.M.-III (1980) has given due importance to Personality Disorders. It has classified Personality Disorders on a separate Axis. i.e. Axis II. It distinguishes between Personality "Traits" and "Disorders" as follows:

"Personality Traits are enduring patterns of perceiving relating to and thinking about the environment and one's self, and are exhibited in a wide range of important social and personal contexts. It is only when Personality Traits are inflexible and maladaptive and cause either significant impairment in social or occupational functioning or subjective distress that they constitute Personally Disorders.

Thus, Personality Disorders are a heterogeneous group of deeply ingrained, usually life-long, maladaptive patterns of behaviour in which there is an absence of true neurotic or psychotic symptoms. Although these persons cause themselves and others much unhappiness their behaviour is usually Egosyntonic and there is little motivation for change (Arkema, 1981).

In conclusion, we can say that Personality Disorders are learned life-long consistent patterns of characteristic behaviour which impair an individual's occupational, interpersonal and social functioning, and which lead to problematic behaviour both for the individual and for those around him.

All Personality Disorders share some common characteristics. Vaillant and Perry (1985) listed following four characteristics to be common in almost all Personality Disorders:

(1) an inflexible and maladaptive response to stress - Persons with Personality Disorders had difficulties in facing stressful situations. These indi-

vidual in stressful situations behaved in ways which were considered as abnormal by their fellow beings.

(2) a disability in working and loving relationships which is generally more serious and always more: persuasive than that found in Neurosis-On Scale of Mental Health, individuals with Personality Disorders fall in the category between Neurosis and Psychosis. Patients with Personality Disorders have interpersonal difficulties. They find it difficult in getting along with others. They are inadequate in the "give and take" relationship. Most of them are demanding in nature, cither in tern's of modest requests or in terms of manipulative threat. With regard to work history, they are poor and have adjustment problems. The D.S.M.-111 (1980) mentioned that individuals with Personality Disorders are generally dissatisfied with his or her in ability to function effectively.

(3) elicitation by interpersonal conflict-Personality Disorder generally arise in an interpersonal context. The behaviour of such individuals annoys other people which results in their being labelled as "sick" or "bad". 'These people lack in empathy. They cannot see themselves with others as others see them. The D.S.M.-111 (1980) mentioned that "frequently individuals with Personality Disorders are dissatisfied with the impact his or her behaviour was having on others,"

(4) Individuals with Personality Disorder have a peculiar capacity to get under the skin of others- According to the D.S.M.-(111) (1980), besides these above characteristics, all Personality Disorders have in common disturbances of mood, frequently involving "depression" or "anxiety".

OBSTACLES TO THE STUDY OF PERSONALITY DISORDER

In the history of the Study of Psychopathology, Personality Disorders have been a neglected and little understood topic. They "......have historically been in 3 tangential position among diagnostic syndromes, never having achieved a significant measure of recognition in the literature of cither Abnormal Psychology or Clinical Psychology" (Millon, 1981).

Personality Disorders has not been a much research topic in academic circles as can be seen from the very few controlled experimental studies or exemplary clinical reports (Turkat & Levin, 1984). Neither are practitioners much interested in them because as noted by Vaillant & Perry (1985), Patients with Personality Disorders continually demonstrate to mental health professionals the limit of their expertise. The neglect of the study of Personality Disorder or our little understanding of the Personality Disorders can be attributed to the following factors:

(1) There is no common agreement upon definition of what constitutes Personality and hence what is a Personality Disorder, is difficult to define.

(2) The lack of an operational definition of Personality has led to difficulties in preparing a valid and reliable Classification System for Personality Disorders, which has led Psychologists and other Mental Health Experts, to misdiagnose Personality Disorders. Turkat and Levin (1984) in their review of the literature of Personality Disorders concluded that the-principles of science were not rigidly utilized in the study of Personality Disorders. The persistent finding of their review was the lack of appropriate diagnostic practice with regard to Personality Disorders, which made them remark "if Clinical Psychology is to make a significant contribution to the understanding of Personality Disorders then the principles of science must be rigidly utilized.

(3) Psychiatrists and other Mental Health Experts till recently did not acknowledge the fact that patients with Personality Disorders were functionally more disabled than the neurotics.

(4) Patients with Personality Disorders Were not considered as lying within the realm of Psychiatry or Psychology, because Personality Disorders constituted a large percentage of the jailed population, welfare recipients and General Practitioner patients (Vaillant and Perry, 1985).

(5) Patients with Personality Disorders like neurotics or psychotics; do not *a* frequently come to the attention of Mental Health Experts, either on their own or through their relatives. Only when they have conflict with the Law or with the Societal norms that they are forced to seek the help of Mental Health Experts.

(6) Patients with Personality Disorders arc found to be irregular in treatment and follow-up and poor in terms of prognosis, which again has led majority of the Mental Health Experts not to take them so seriously as other patients and to treat them in a prejudiced manner. A combination of all these factors has been responsible for the lack of appropriate understanding about Personality Disorders. However, in recent years, the topic of Personality Disorders have received a lot of attention. Diagnostic and Classificatory Systems for Personality Disorders have been developed and improved upon and a great deal of research is underway to study the causes, treatment, family background, personality profile, etc., of patients exhibiting Personality Disorders.

CLASSIPICATION OF PERSONALITY DISORDER

Classifying Personality Disorders is a difficult task, difficult because to define Personality operationally is difficult. Since it is difficult to define Personality operationally, a reliable and valid Classification System of Personality Disorders has also become difficult. Turkat and Levin (1984) noted that the Classification of Personality Disorders suffers from a lack of valid and reliable Classification System, which was noted by Frances (1980) and by Spitzer, Forman and Nee (1979).

Difficulties inherent in classifying Personality Disorders are best illustrated by Vaillant and Perry (1985) '.in the following statement:

"Classifying Personality Disorders poses the basic problem of whether to focus more on the term, "Personality", which is best conceptualized in terms of dimensions, or whether to focus more on the term, "Disorder", which is best viewed as the presence or absence of pathological state or disease".

In this section, we will examine the D.S.M.-111 (1980). Classification of Personality Disorder not only because it is the common current classification in psychiatric practice but also because it is used by a large majority of Mental Health Experts. Besides, some personality disorders like the Borderline Personality Disorder was first given formal recognition by this Classification System.

For our convenience we can divide the DSM-III classification of personality Disorder into the following three broad Clusters:

I. Eccentric Cluster

1. Paranoid Personality Disorder.
2. Schizoid Personality Disorder.
3. Schizotypal Personality Disorder.

II. Fearful

1. Avoidant Personality Disorder.
2. Dependent Personality Disorder.
3. Compulsive Personality Disorder.
4. Passive-Aggressive Personality Disorder.

III. Erratic Cluster

1. Historionic Personality Disorder.
2. Narcissistic Personality Disorder.
3. Antisocial Personality Disorder.
4. Borderline Personality Disorder.

ECCENTRIC CLUSTER OF PERSONALITY DISORDER

According to DSM-III there are three types of personality disorders classified under the eccentric cluster. These three types of personality disorders are as follows:

1. Paranoid personality disorder.
2. Schizoid personality disorder, and
3. Schizotypal personality disorder.

These three types-of personality disorders generally show certain eccentricities of behaviour and parallel quite clearly the paranoid and schizophrenic psychoses. Many researchers consider these disorders to be a varient of schizophrenic disorder.

I. Paranoid Personality Disorder It is characterized by pervasive and unwarranted suspiciousness and mistrust of people, hypersensitivity and restricted affectivity. These symptoms are not due to paranoid disorder or Schizophrenia. Paranoid personality disorder, therefore, should be distinguished from Paranoid Disorder and Paranoid Schizophrenia. The latter are psychotic disorders and severely disabling, involving reality testing disturbances. In contrast paranoid personality disorder is not disabling. Here a person becomes suspicious in almost all situations and with almost all people. If any one presents him with convincing contradictory evidence about his/her suspiciousness the individual with the paranoid Personality Disorder may even become suspicious of one who challenges her or his suspicious ideas. Transient ideas of reference are very common in this disorder i.e. they think that others are taking special notice of them, or saying vulgar things about them.

Individuals with this disorder are usually argumentative and exaggerate difficulties. They are critical of others and have difficulty in accepting criticism themselves. Their affectivity is restricted and they do not get emotionally attached with people. They lack soft, passive, sentimental and tender feelings. This disorder is more commonly diagnosed in men.

DSM-III's Diagnostic criteria for Paranold Personality Disorder

(A) Pervassive, unwarranted suspiciousness and mistrust of people as indicated by atleast three of the following:

(1) Expectation of trickery harm from others.

(2) Hyper vigilance, manifested by continual scanning of the environment for signs of threat, or taking unneeded precautions.

(3) Guardedness or secretiveness.

(4) Avoidance or accepting blame when warranted.

(5) Unquestioning the loyalty of others.

(6) Intense, narrowly forced searching for confirmation of bias, with loss of appreciation of total context.

(7) 0verconcern with hidden motives and special meanings.

(8} Pathological jealousy.

(B) Hypersensitivity as indicated by atleast two of the following:

(1) Tendency lo get easily provoked and quickness to take offence.

(2) Exaggeration of difficulties, e.g. "making mountains of mole hills".

(3) Readiness to counterattack when any threat is perceived.

(4) Inability to relax.

(C) Restricted affectivity as indicated by atleast two of the following:

(1) Appearance of being "cold" and unemotional.

(2) Pride taken in always being objective, rational and unemotional.

(3) Lack of the sense of humour.

(4) Absence of passive, soft, tender and sentimental feelings.

(D) The above characteristics are not due to any other mental disorder such as schizophrenia or a paranoid disorder.

Thus, from the above DSM-III description we see that to obtain the diagnosis of paranoid personality disorder, people must show an interpersonal style characterized by rigidity, unwarranted suspicion, Jealous, envy, hypersensitivity, and anger. Generally these people are argumentative and tend to blame others for their problems. (Million, 1981). However, inspite of the fact that they are usually loners, and have few if any close friends, Lion (1981) notes that they often have a recognizable sense of humor. This humor may be cutting, self-deprecating, and sardonic - a style that Lion feels characterizes some very successful comedians. Paranoid personality style also may be seen in some bigots or overly jealous spouses.

Weintraub (1981) describes the paranoid personality as more interested in mechanical devices than people, although sensitive to the power and rank of others. The paranoid personality's hypersensitivity to others can make interpersonal interaction tense and uneasy.

People with paranoid personality disorder arc rarely treated in psychotherapy because they tend to avoid initiating interactions 'with mental health systems. Generally, they may be brought into psychotherapy by other family members but, characteristically, because they sec others and not themselves as responsible for whatever problems are occurring, they may leave therapy early. These are cold, unpleasant people whose limited affect, suspiciousness, and lack of responsiveness drives others away, thus confirming their view of the world as made up of people who do *not* care.

2. **Schizoid Personality Disorder:** Like paranoid personalities, schizoid personalities are associated with symptoms that parallel psychotic syndromes. Early mention of the schizoid personality disorders can be found in the writings of the European psychiatrists Bleuler, Kretschmer, and Kraepelin who believed there was a specific personality out of which schizophrenia developed. Later the term "Schizoid" came to mean a personality profile that designated a more general population of people characterized by social withdrawal. Schizoid people appear to be aloof and reserved. They do not seem to need emotional ties with others, preferring to be quiet, distant, and reclusive. If they adjust, it appears they adjust on the periphery of society in lonely jobs that most others do not want. In some cases, they can show a great deal of interest in such projects as astronomy, philosophical movements, or health fads, but only as long as they involve minimal interaction with others.

People with schizoid personality disorder spend much of their time fantasizing about being owerful and overcoming others. They seem to have great difficulty expressing anger and usually channel such feelings through daydreaming and fantasy. However, even though they may appear sullen and hostile, they rarely act out their anger.

Thus we see that in this disorder an individual lacks the capacity to form social and interpersonal relationship. They lack warm, tender feelings for others and are indifferent to praise, criticism or feelings of others. Such individuals are loners', seclusive, reserved and lack close friendship with people. They usually appear to be 'cold' and aloof.

Individuals with this disorder are not clear cut in their goals, are indecisive in their actions and usually indulge in day-dreaming. Science they lack the capacity to form interpersonal relationship they rarely marry and whenever they marry, marital problems are common. The sex-ratio of the disorder is unknown but, in general, it is more commonly found in men. Nothing specific is known about the prevalence of this disorder. Heston. found that 3.0% of the general population has this disorder; on the other hand Rosenthal observed that schizoid disorders may encompass 7.5% of the population. DSM-III's Diagnostic Criteria for Schizoid Personality Disorder, is as follows:

(A) Emotional coldness and aloofness and absence of warm, tender feelings for others

(B) In difference to praise or criticism or to the feeling of others

(C) Close friendship with no more than one or tow persons including family members.

(D) No eccentriatics of speech, behaviour or thought characteristic of schizotypal personality disorders

(E) Not due to psychotic disorder such as Schizophrenia or Paranoid disorder.

(F) If under 18, does not meet the criteria for schizoid disorder of childhood or Adolescence.

3. **Schizotypal Personality Disorder** Sometimes referred to as simple or latent schizophrenia in the past, scilizotypal disorders represent a connection between schizoid personality disorder and schizophrenia. Typically, their behaviour is "odd" and they may claim clairvoyance or other special powers of thought. Like the schizoid personalities, schizotypal individuals are socially isolated, but in addition they manifest a marked tendency for loose thinking and communicating. Affective stimuli, be they, positive or negative, can cause schizotypal individuals' speech to become digressive and incoherent. They seem to be on the verge of becoming schizophrenic should they experience even a moderate amount of stress. The authors of DSM-UI appear to assume that there is some sort of biologically based genetic component in this disorder.

In this disorder there are various oddities of thought, perception, speech and behaviour. These are not so severe enough to meet the criteria of Schiozophrenia. Like the Borderline and Narcissistic personality disorders, to be discussed ahead, this is also one of the newer entities to be included for the first

time in DSM-III.

The epidemiology, prevalence and sex-ratio of this disorder is still unknown, although some authors suggest that it may be more prevalent than Schizophrenia. In 1981 Kendler ct. al. suggested, in their family and adoption studies ofS chizophrenics, that Schizotypal personality Disorder is more common in the biological relatives of chronic Schizophrenics than in controls.

The clinical features of a Schizotypal personality Disorder represent the borderline between schizoid personality and Schizophrenia. In Schizotypal personality disorder, perceiving, thinking and communicating arc disturbed. The individual's speech may be strange with poorly expressed concepts, odd word usage or vagueness. Speech may be circumstantial or over-elaborate or metaphorical. Social isolation, constricted effect and suspiciousness is common. More research is needed on this disorder to clarify our understanding of it, which is lacking at present.

DSM-III's Diagnostic Criteria for Schizotypal Personality Disorder

(A) At least four of the following are present:

(1) Magical thinking e.g. superstitiousness, clairvoyance, telepathy,"6th sense", "others can feel my feelings" (in children and adolescents, bizarre fantasies of preoccupation).

(2) ideas of reference.

(3) social isolation, e.g. no close friends or confidants, social contacts limited to everyday tasks. actually present (e.g. "I felt as if my dead mother were in the room with me"), depersonalization or derealization not associated with panic attacks.

(5) odd speech (without loosening of associations or incoherence) e.g. speech that is digressive, vague, overlabored, circumstantial, metaphorical.

(6) inadequate rapport in face-to-face interaction due to constricted or inappropriate effect e.g. aloof, cold etc.

(7) suspiciousness or-paranoid ideation.

(8) undue social anxiety or hypersensitivity to real or imagined criticism.

(B) Docs not meet the criteria for Schizophrenia.

DIFFERENT TYPES OF PERSONALITY DISORDERS

Fearful cluster of personality disorder includes four different types of personality disorder. These are:

(a) Avoidant Personality Disorder.

(b) Dependent Personality Disorder.

(c) Compulsive Personality Disorder, and

(d) Passive-Aggressive Personality Disorder.

The single most salient symptom in all the above personality disorder is anxiety and fear. This particular symptom may be expressed differently depending on the particular personality disorder.

We would discuss the above personality disorders in brief.

(a) Avoidant Personality **Disorder** It is characterized by hyper- sensitivity to potential rejection, humiliation or shame. There is unwillingness to enter into relationships unless given strong assurance of uncritical acceptance. There is social withdrawal in spite of the desire for affection and acceptance. Individual having avoidant personality disorder has low self-esteem. Thus, like Schizoid Personality Disorder, Avoidant Personality Disorder is marked by social withdrawal, however, the Avoidant Personality Disorder withdraws not out of the desire to be alone but out of the fear of rejection.

Avoidant persons are more commonly labelled shy, reticent, reserved and timid in social situations. In addition to withdrawal, avoidant people are characterized by a typical set of cognitive "distortion" such people experience much fear of negative evaluation from others, combined with a tendency to evaluate their own behaviour too negatively. They experience a great deal of self-conscious and self absorption, which limit their ability to process and to respond appropriately to feedback from others. Avoidant people usually complain of low self-esteem, which appears to be a natural result of their chronic tendency to devalue themselves.

Avoidant Personality Disorder is generally associated with depression, anxiety and anger at oneself, for their lack of inability to develop social relationship.

The prevalence of the disorder is unknown. Though it is considered to be common, no information is available on its sex ratio and familial pattern. The course and prognosis of this disorder are also unknown.

DSM-III's Diagnostic criteria for Avoldant Personally Disorder

(A) Hypersensitivity to rejection, e.g. apprehensively alert to signs of social derogation, interprets innocuous events as ridicule.

(B) Unwillingness to enter into relationships unless given unusually strong guarantee of uncritical acceptance.

(C) Social withdrawal, e.g. distances self front close personal attachments, engages in peripheral social and vocational persona] attachments, engages in peripheral social and vocational roles.

(D) Desire for affection and acceptance.

(E) Low-self-esteem, e.g. devalues self-achievement and is overtly dismayed by personal shortcomings.

(F) If under 18, does not meet the criteria for Avoidant Disorder of childhood or adolescence.

(b) **Dependent Personality Disorder:** This is also a relatively new category of diagnostic entity appearing in DSM-III and is roughly equivalent to Passive-aggressive personality. Dependant type which appears in the DSM-I.

In this disorder individual passively allows others to assume responsibility for major areas of his or her life because of lack of self-confidence and an inability to function independently. The individual with this disorder subordinates his or her own need to those of others on whom he or she is dependent, such individuals leave major decisions to others for e.g. marriage, choice of a job etc. Generally, individuals with this disorder do not make demands on the people they depend for the fear that their relationship may break.

Pessimism, doubt, passivity and fears about expressing sexual and aggressive feelings characterize the behaviour of the persons with this disorder. The individual has learned to externalize may problems in such a fashion that in any relationship the patient becomes a passive member. Most of the theories of the cases of dependent personality disorder are largely psychosocial.

This disorder is apparently common and is diagnosed more frequently in women. No information is available with regard to familial information, course id prognosis of this disorder.

DSM-III's Diagnostic Criteria for Dependent Personality Disorder

(A) Passively allows others to assume responsibility for major areas of life because of inability to function independently (e.g. let spouse decide what kind of job he or she should have).

(B) Subordinates own needs to those persons on whom he or she depends in order to avoid any possibility of having to rely on self e.g. tolerates abusive behaviour.

(C) Lacks self-confidence e.g. sees self as helpless, stupid.

Persons with dependent personality disorder often will come into psychotherapy when the people they depend on leave. They present special problems to therapists because, as they arc prone to do outside of therapy, they become excessively dependent. This dependency often can stand in the way of therapeutic progress.

(c) **Compulsive Personality Disorder:** Is a term that has been used in the psychological literature for over 60 years and is characterised by preoccupation with rules, order, organization, efficiency and detail. There is rigidity and inability to express warm emotions or take pleasure in normal pleasurable activities.

According to Chapman compulsive personality evidences excessive orderliness, frugality and cold mechanical quality in his relationship. They cannot tolerate disorder and uneconomical quality in their relationships. They cannot tolerate disorder, dirt and incomplete tasks. Such individuals can decompensate into depressive or marked anxiety.

The prevalence of compulsive personality disorder is unknown because the point at which the compulsive personality traits, which are common become a disorder is not clear. Compulsive personalities are found frequently in vocations that value accuracy, orderliness and moral rectitude, more than warmth and sociability. Many observers have anecdotally noted the tendency for a compulsive personality to be most common in oldest children and more common in men than in women.

DSM-III's Diagnostic Criteria for Compulsive Personality Disorder

At least four of the following arc present:

(i) restricted ability to express warm and tender emotions e.g. the individual is cold conventional, serious, formal and stingy.

(ii) perfectionism that interferes with the ability to grasp "the big picture e.g. preoccupation with trivia] details, rules, order, organization, schedules and lists.

(iii) insistence that others submit to his or her way of doing things and lack of awareness of the feeling elicited by this behaviours, e.g. a husband stubbornly insists his wife complete errands for him regardless of her plane .

(iv) Excessive devotion lo worn and productivity to the exclusion of pleasure are the value of interpersonal relationships.

(v) Indecisiveness decision-making is cither avoided, postponed or protracted, perhaps because of an inordinate fear of making a mistake, e.g. the individual cannot get assignments alone on time because of ruminating about priorities.

Vaillant and Perry (1980; 1985) listed nine traits from most to least .important that describe the compulsive disorder: emotional constriction, orderliness, parsimony, rigidity, strict conscience, perseverance, obstinacy, indecisiveness, and a lack of sexual provocativeness. Above all, compulsive personalities are organized, through, serious, and slaves to their schedules.

Unlike most other personality disorders, people with compulsive patterns are aware of their suffering and will seek treatment on their own (Saizman & Thaler, 1981). Psychotherapy with compulsive people may be characterized by a fight for control of the therapeutic relationship. The client may either be very compliant or may attack the therapist's intelligence and/or fairness. While difficult, therapy can be successful if the therapist can give support and not be drawn into the role of an adversary (Weintraub, 1981).

(d) **Passive-aggressive personality Disorder:** Relative to other personality disorders, passive aggressive personality disorder has received scant empirical attention, although considerable psychoanalytic theory on the disorder exists. In passive-aggressive personality disorder an individual indirectly expresses resistance to demands made by others in either social or occupational functioning. The resistance is expressed indirectly rather than directly through such maneuvers as procrastination, dawdling, stubbornness, intentional inefficiency and "forgetfulness".

Individuals with this disorder are not lazy or experience dissatisfaction with job or studies, instead passive-aggressive manoeuvering is a cover for an underlying hostility toward other people. For e.g. and student who bates the teacher will purposely not do her homework or will oppose whatever the teacher will say.

No information with regard to prevalence, sex ratio and familial pattern is available on this disorder.

DSM-III's Diagnostic criteria for passive-Aggressive Personality Disorder

(A) Resistance to demands for adequate performance, in both occupational and social functioning.

(B) Resistance expressed indirectly through atleast two of the following:

(1) Procrastination (2) dawdling (3) stubbornness (4) intentional inefficiency (5) "forgetfulness".

(C) As a consequence of A and B, pervasive and long standing social and occupational ineffectiveness (including the roles of housewife or student).

(D) Persistence of the behaviour pattern even under circumstances in which more self-assertive and effective behaviour is possible.

(E) Does not meet the criteria for any other personality Disorder and if under age 18 docs not meet the criteria for oppositional disorder.

Thus, from the above discussion, we see that more than the other personality disorders, passive-aggressive personalities tend to mix anger with their anxieties. DSM-III classification of passive-aggressive personality describes people who resist demands of others to perform certain tasks by procrastination, dawdling, stubbornness, intentional inefficiency, or forgetfulness. Although these people are not assertive, they can find fault in those who are in authority or on whom they arc dependent.

Generally, interacting with passive-aggressive personalities can be an unnerving experience. Most people are unaware of the ability of- passive-aggressive individuals to manipulate them into a hostile interaction. It is unsettling to find oneself becoming angry at someone and not be aware of why. Passive-aggressive personalities have a knack for drawing people close to them And then responding with anger-eliciting behaviours.

Psychotherapy with passive-aggressive personalities can be very complex. As Vaillant and Peiry (1980; 1985) point out, to fulfill their demands, supports their disordered way of interacting to refuse their demands is tantamount to rejection. After rejection, passive-aggressive people have been known to choose suicide as a way of escaping their feelings of emptiness and abandonment.

PERSONALITY DISORDERS LISTED IN THE ERRATIC CLUSTER

Erratic cluster of personality disorders represents those personality disorders in which there is dramatic, emotional and erratic behaviours. Individuals having any one of the disorder belonging to this cluster seek to be the center of attention. There are four types of personality disorders that belong to erratic cluster of personality disorders. These are as follows:

(a) Histrionic Personality Disorder.

(b) Narcissistic Personality Disorder.

(c) Borderline Personality Disorder, and

(d) Antisocial Personality Disorder.

We would discuss the first three personality disorders in this section. Antisocial Personality Disorder would be discussed in the next section.

(a) **Histrionic Personality Disorder** is a disorder of personality that belongs to the erratic cluster of personality disorder. It is usually characterized by overtly dramatic reactive and intensely expressed behaviour which often disrupts their interpersonal relationship. Such behaviour is aimed at attracting attention and sympathy from others.

Considerable range of behaviour is associated with the diagnosis of this disorder. Individuals always draws attention to themselves, they throw irrational angry outbursts or tantrums. They are emotionally labile and generally behave in an exaggerated manner. Such individuals also display disturbed ability to maintain deep, long lasting attachments.

Inspite of being creative and imaginative these individual have little interest in intellectual achievement and analytic thinking.

This disorder is more commonly observed in females than in males and is more common among family members than in general population.

When diagnosed among males, it is sometimes associated with a homosexual arousal pattern. Although histrionic patients sometimes seem naively unaware of their sexual display, their-dress is seductive, provocative or even exhibitionistic in manner.

Individuals with this disorder tend to be impressionable and easily influenced by others or by facts: However, their interpersonal relationships are usually stormy and ungratifying because these individuals use emotional displays, both to obtain attention and desired goals and to evade unwanted external responsibilities and unpleasant inner effects.

DSM-III's Diagnostic Criteria for Histrionic Personality Disorder:

(A) Behaviour that is overtly dramatic received and intensely expressed as indicated by atleast three of the following:

(i) Self-dramatization e.g. exaggerated expression of emotions.

(ii) Incessant drawing of attention to oneself.

(iii) Craving for activity and excitement.

(iv) Overreaction to minor events.

(v) irrational angry outbursts.

(B) Characteristic disturbances in interpersonal relationships as indicated by atleast two of the following :

(i) Perceived by others as shallow and lacking emotions eyen if superficially warm and charming.

(ii) Ego-centric, self-indulgent and inconsiderate of others.

(iii) Vain and demanding.

(iv) Dependent, helpless, constantly seeking reassurance.

(v) Prone to manipulative, suicidal threats, gestures or attempts.

Millon (1981) refers to histrionic people as showing a "gregarious pattern". They share with dependent disorders the need to be with and depend on others, but where dependent people quietly attempt to ingratiate themselves to a few others, the histrionic people put on a "show" often laced with sexual innuendo and ploys to please and manipulate others. The constant emotional displays, fickleness in feelings and relationships, sexual provocativeness, although at first interesting and exciting, soon wear thin and lead to disturbances in relationships. Histrionic people tend to be vain, egocentric, shallow, and inconsiderate of others, needs. Their inconsiderate behaviour occurs in spite of the fact that histrionic individuals have what Millon calls "an exquisite sensitivity to the moods and thoughts of those they wish to please".

Treatment is difficult with histrionic individuals because they generally are unaware of their own feelings and have trouble expressing emotions honestly. Although infrequent, when they do seek therapy it is usually because they have experienced some sort of social disapproval or interpersonal deprivation. Their motivation for long-term therapy is usually low and environmental management medication, and behavioural management appear to be minimally effective (Millon, 1-981).

(b) Narcissistic Personality Disorder have been a subject of discussion in the psychoanalytic literature for at least 50 years. Indeed, the concept of narcissism is nearly as old as psychoanalysis itself, having been introduced by Freud in several early papers. However, narcissistic personality disorder has recently been accorded the status of a distinct nosological entity.

This is one of the new categories added to the DSM-III and is more commonly used in the psychological writings. Narcissist Personality Disorder is characterized by grandiose sense of self-importance or uniqueness, preoccupation with fantasies of unlimited success, exhibitionistic need for constant attention and admiration and characteristic disturbances in interpersonal exploitativeness, relationship that alternates between the extremes of over-idealization and devaluation and lack of empathy.

Depressed mood in response to minor events is extremely common in this disorder. Self-esteem is unstable in these patients who are preoccupied with how well they are doing and how well others regard them. Individuals with this disorder are overtly grandiosed and are preoccupied with their own attributes, accomplishments and fantasies. Individuals with this disorder may also meet the criteria for histrionic, antisocial or borderline personality disorder.

In general literature on narcissistic personality disorder consists primarily of contradictory theoretical discussions of psychoanalytic concepts.

The incidence, prevalence, sex ratio and familial pattern of the narcissist personality disorder have not been investigated. Anecdotally, among those who seek treatment, the disorder is more common in men.

DSM-III's Diagnostic Criteria for Narcissistic Personality Disorder.'

(A) Grandiose sense of self-importance or uniqueness e.g. exaggeration of achievements and talents focus on the special nature of one's problems.

(B) **Preoccupation with fantasies** of unlimited success, power, brilliance, beauty or ideal love.

(C) **Exhibitionism**-the person requires constant attention and admiration.

(D) Cool, indifference or marked feelings or range, inferiority, shame, humiliation or emptiness in response to criticism, indifference of others or defeat.

(E) Atleast two of the following characteristics of disturbances in interpersonal relationships:.

(1) Entitlement exception of special factors without assuming reciprocal responsibilities e.g. surprise and anger that people will not do what is wanted.

(2) Interpersonal exploitativeness, taking advantage of others to indulge in own desires or for self-aggrandizement, disregard for the personal integrity and rights of others.

(3) Reliability that characteristically alternates between the extremes of over idealization and devaluation.

(4) Lack of empathy, inability to recognize how others feel e.g. unable to appreciate the distress of someone who is seriously ill.

Narcissistic personalities share with the histrionic personality, a tendency to be demonstrative, dramatic, and at times seductive. However, where the histrionic person is playful and warm, the narcissistic person is naughty and cold (Akhtar & Thompson, 1982). To be diagnosed as a narcissistic personality, people must show a grandiose sense of self-importance, a preoccupation with fantasies of power and ideal love, demands for constant attention in the form of admiration, and a response of feelings of rage or emptiness to criticism. Further, in their interpersonal interactions with others these people show a remarkable inability to empathize. Although exploiting others is a common pattern, narcissistic people often are surprised and upset when others do not meet their wishes (Vaillant & Perry, 1980; 1985).

There is considerable disagreement among the major theorists about whether the pattern actually comprises a separate diagnostic entity. Kohut (1977) sees narcissistic personality as separate from other personality disorders, while Kemberg (1975) argues that it is a variant of borderline personality disorder. Others have attempted to resolve this apparent disagreement by offering other perspectives that describe narcissistic and borderline personality disorders as parts of the same dimension (Adier, 1981), but differing primarily in the way they present themselves to others (Rothstein, 1979). At this point, the eventual status of this "new entry" into the diagnostic system is unclear.

(C) **Borderline Personality Disorder:** Borderline personality disorders, in recent years, have received a great deal of research attention and is a term which has undergone many changes. It was earlier known as Borderline personality organization, pseudoneurotic Schizophrenia, Borderline patient, Borderline syndrome, Borderline Neurosis, "asif" personality etc. This term was introduced for the first time in DSM-III and is characterized by instability in mood, behaviour and self-image. There is instability in behaviour, unpredictable and physically self-damaging behaviour is present. There is also affective instability and identity disturbances. Individuals have problems of tolerating being alone or get depressed when alone.

No systematic studies on the epidemology of this disorder has been carried out but it is more commonly diagnosed in women. Individuals who display this disorder also show many features of other personality disorders, such as histrionic, Schizotypal, Narcissistic and Antisocial Personality Disorder.

Most of the individuals with this disorder are intelligent but usually function below their level. Gunderson and Singer (1975) reviewed the entire literature on Borderline personality disorder and found that most authors seem to characterize most Borderline patients as having following six features :

(1) Presence of intense affect usually of a strong hostile or depressed nature.

(2) A history of impulsive behaviour which may take episodic acts like self-mutilation, drug abuse etc. or may display more chronic behaviour patterns like promiscuity, self-destructive behaviour etc.

(3) They display superficial adaptiveness beneath which there is disturbed identity camouflaged by rapid and shifting identifications with others.

(4) Brief psychotic experiences which generally have a paranoid quality and is often provoked by abuse of illicit drugs.

(5) On psychological testing Borderline patients demonstrate abnormal responses on structured tests like WAIS.

(6) Disturbed interpersonal relationships which arc either transient superficial or excessively intense.

DSM-III's Criteria of Borderline Personality Disorder:

(A) At least 5 of the following are required :

(i) Impulsivity or unpredictability in atleast two areas that are potentially self-damaging e.g. Spending lavishly, sex, gambling, substance abuse, shoplifting, over-eating, or such other physically self-damaging acts

(ii) A pattern of unstable or intense interpersonal relationship e.g. marked shifts of attitude, idealization, devaluation, manipulation (consistently using others for one's own ends) etc.

(iii) Inappropriate intense anger or lack of control of anger e.g. frequent displays of temper, constant anger.

(iv) Identity disturbances manifested by uncertainty about several issues relating to identity, such as self-image, gender identity, long-term goals or carrier choice, friendship, patterns, values and loyalties e.g. "who am I", "I feel like my sister when I am good".

(v) Effective instability, marked shifts from normal mood to depression, irritability or anxiety, usually lasting a few hours and only rarely more than a few days, with a return to normal mood.

(vi) Intolerance of being alone, frantic efforts to avoid being alone, depressed when alone.

(vii) Physically self-damaging acts e.g. Suicidal gestures, self-mutilation, recurrent accident or physical fights.

(viii) Chronic feelings of emptiness and boredom.

(B) If under 18, does not meet the criteria for identity disorder.

PERSONALITY DISORDER

It has been known since a long time but different labels were used to refer to this disorder. In this disorder the rights of others are violated. Individuals with this disorder find themselves in confrontation with the laws and norms of society. This-disorder starts before the age of 15, poor work history, interpersonal difficulties, impulsive behaviour, conflicts with social values and norms and aggressive, assaultive behaviour are the characteristic features of this disorder.

This is relatively one of the most studied and researched disorder. This disorder is more common in males than in females. It is estimated that about 3% of American men and less than 1% of American women suffer from this disorder. The sex difference with regard to antisocial personality disorder may be due to the fact that minimal brain dysfunction, attention deficit disorder and overt childhood behaviour problems, which contribute to the etiology of antisocial personality are more often found in boys than in girls. Another reason that might contribute to sex differences in antisocial behaviour is due to the socio cultural differences and child-rearing practices. In most of the Cultures girls are taught right from childhood to suppress their anger **and** to be more confirming to societal norms.

Besides sex differences, sociocultural differences with regard to this disorder too exist. It is more common, in lower class populations due to poverty, upbringing and other socio-cultural factors. With regard to familial pattern this disorder is more common in the fathers of both males and females.

We will now examine the DSM-III criteria for antisocial personality disorder and some of its shortcomings.

DSM-III's Criteria of Anti-Social Personality Disorder:

(A) Current age least 18.

(B) Onset before the age 15 as indicated by a history of three or more of the following before that age :

(1) truancy (positive if it amounted to atleast five days per year for atleast two years, not including the last year of school).

(2) Expulsion or suspension from school for misbehaviour.

(3) Delinquency (arrested or referred to Juvenile court because of behaviour).

(4) Running away from home overnight atleast twice while living in parental or parental surrogate home.

(5) Persistent lying.

(6) Repeated sexual intercourse in a causal relationship.

(7) Repeated dninkenness or substance abuse.

(8) Thefts.

(9) Vandalism.

(10) School grades markedly below expectations in relation to estimated o know IQ (may have resulted in repeating a year).

(11) Chronic violations of rules at home and/or at school (other than truancy).

(12) Initiation of fights.

(C) At least four of the following manifestations of the disorder since age 18:

(1) Inability to sustain consistent work behaviour as indicated by any of the following:

(a) Too frequent job changes (e.g. three or more jobs in five years not accounted for by nature of job or economic or seasonal fluctuation).

(b) Significant unemployment (e.g. six months or more in Five years when expected to work).

(c) Serious absenteeism from work e.g. average three days or more of lateness or absence per month).

(d) Walking off several jobs without other jobs in sight (Note similar behaviour in an academic setting during the last few years of school may substitute for this criterion in individuals who by reason of their age or circumstances have not had an opportunity to demonstrate occupational adjustment).

(2) Lack of ability to function as a responsible parent as evidenced by one or more of the following :

(a) Child's malnutrition.

(b) Child's illness resulting from lack of minimal hygiene standards.

(c) Failure to obtain medical care for a seriously ill child.

(d) Child's dependence on neighbours or non-resident relatives for food or shelter.

(e) Failure to arrange for a caretaker for a child under six when parents are away from home.

(f) Repeated squandering, on personal items, of money required for household necessities.

(3) Failure to accept social norms with respect to lawful behaviour as indicated by any of the following :

Repeated thefts, illegal occupation (Pimping, prostitution, fencing, selling drugs), multiple arrests, a felony conviction.

(4) Inability to maintain enduring attachment to a sexual pattern as indicated by two or more divorces and/or separations (whether legally married or not), desertion of spouse, promiscuity (ten or more sexual partners within one year).

(5) Irritability and aggressiveness as indicated by repeated physical fights or assaults (not required by one's job or to defend someone or oneself) including spouse or child beatings.

(6) Failure to honour financial obligations, as indicated by repeated defaulting of debts, failure to provide child support, failure to support other dependents on a regular basis.

(7) Failure to plan ahead, or impulsivity as indicated by travelling from place to place without prearranged job or clear goal for the period of travel or clear idea about when the travel should terminate, or lack of fixed address for a month or more.

(8) Disregard for the truth as indicated by repeated lying use of aliases, "conning" others for personal profit.

(9) Recklessness as indicated by driving while intoxicated or recurrent speeding.

(D) A pattern of continuous antisocial behaviour in which the right of others are violated, with no intervening period of at least 5 years without antisocial behaviour between age 15 and the present time except when the individual was bed-ridden or confined in a hospital or penal institution).

(E) Antisocial behaviour is not due to either severe mental retardation, Schizophrenia or manic episodes.

In the above DSM-III's diagnostic criteria of this disorder, we find several important factors, which many mental health experts use to characterize this order, missing. Some of which are as follows :

1. Lack of anticipatory anxiety.
2. Inability to learn from experience.
3. Lack of guilt and remorse over transgressions, and
4. Lack of Loyalty to others.

DSM-III's Diagnostic criteria also neglect the differences between primary and secondary types of antisocial personality disorders. Primary antisocial personality disorder is described most clearly by Harvey Cleckely in his book "mask of sanity" which is symptomatic of anxiety associated is a reaction and inner conflict. The behavioral pattern displayed by secondary type f antisocial personality disorder is less and severe as in the primary type.

The following are the 16 indicators of Antisocial personality disorder as identified by Cleckley.

1. Superficial charm of good "intelligence".
2. Absence of delusions and other signs of irrational thinking.
3. Absence of "nervousness" or psychoneurotic manifestations.
4. Unreliability.
5. Untruthfulness\and insincerity.
6. Lack of remorse or shame.

7. Inadequate motivated antisocial behaviour.

8. Poor judgement and failure to learn from experiences.

9. Pathological egocentricity and incapacity for love.

10. General poverty in major effective reactions.

11. Specific loss of insight.

12. Unresponsiveness in general interpersonal relations.

13. Fantastic and uninviting behaviour with drink and some times without.

14. Suicide rarely carried out.

15. Sex life impersonal, trivial and poorly integrated.

16. Failure to follow any life plan.

Some of the most salient characteristics of anti-social personality, have been briefly elaborated, besides those given in the table.

(1) Individuals with antisocial personality disorder have a tendency and a history of indulging in illegal behaviour or behaviour that is socially disapproved. Repeated thefts, illegal occupation like pimping, prostitution drug pedding etc. are common. There is a history of multiple arrests. Promiscuity, history of exposures, homosexual acts etc. are frequent in them.

(2) Such individuals fail to carry out the responsibility with regard to sexual relationship. Parenthood and financial obligations. Such individuals will not look after the health and well-being of their children properly, they will borrow money from others by using any means e.g. by selling ornaments, telling lies or through cheating. They will also not support other family members who are dependent on them.

(3) Hostility, aggressive and assaultive behaviour is more frequently present in individuals having this disorder. Physical fights are more common among such individuals. A minor controversy or a small little problem can make them indulge into serious fights or homicial acts.

(4) Impulsive and a moral behaviour is another characteristic feature of this disorder, they lack value and respect for others. They have a tendency to betray others. Their behaviour is aimless, thrill-seeking. They are hedonists and guided by the pleasure principle. Their feelings and emotions are superficial and fleeting.

(5) They exhibit lack of empathy, guilt and loyalty with others. Such individuals cannot understand the emotions and feelings of others. When they

commit something wrong they do not feel guilty. Perhaps their superego is not that well developed to control the instinctual wishes. They also cannot keep sustained relationship for a prolonged period of time.

ETIOLOGY OF ANTISOCIAL PERSONALITY DISORDER

Antisocial personality disorder generally arises as a result of the combination of many factors operating together. Biological factors especially heredity or genetic factors, cortical correlates and autonomic under arousal have been found to be associated with antisocial behaviour. However, one cannot deny the role of psychological and socio cultural factors.

BIOLOGICAL THEORIES OF ANTISOCIAL PERSONALITY

(a) **Heredity:** The hypothesis that heredity or genetic factors play an important role in the causation of antisocial personality 'disorder' is not new and has been supported by a great deal of research evidence. Since last one decade there is a revival of interest in this area and a great deal of research has been carried out. Investigations of possible genetic transmission .of antisocial characteristics have most often involved study of twin off-springs of psychopathic and/or criminal parents and the adopted children of psychopaths or criminals. Reviewing the results of the concordant studies, Eysenck and Eysenck (1978) concluded that 55% of monozygotic twins are concordant for criminal conduct as opposed to 13% of dizygotic twins, whereas Cloninger et. al. (1978) pointed out concordance rates as high as 70 for monozygotic twins and 28 for dizygotic twins. Recent evidence from United States adopted studies also supports the possibility of an inherited predisposition in antisocial behaviour.

One of the strongest support for the genetic theory of antisocial personality disorder comes from the discovery of chromosomal abnormality called "XYY", which results in the birth of a male child. Such individuals are also called as "super males". Such individuals have low intelligence coupled with aggressive behaviour and criminal tendencies. Individuals with XYY chromosomes are found frequently in penal institutions or prisons and mental hospitals. However, it is still not known that aggressive behaviour is due to genetic deformity or due to the abnormal physical stricture which these individuals develop as a result of genetic abnormality, which leads to problems in social adjustment and subsequent aggressive behaviour. More research is needed to clarify our understanding of it.

(b) **Cortical Correlates:** Many investigators have studied the EEG (Electroencephalographs) records of individuals showing antisocial personality disorder and have discovered some EEG abnormality in many of the cases.

Ellington, long ago, found that 31 to 58% of such individuals display some EEG abnormality. Most of the EEG abnormalities arc of slow wave activity and positive spike phenomena from temporal lobe is seen. Such findings point out to two things:

(1) mutational retardation, and (2) uninhibited impulsive aggressive behaviour both of which arc common characteristics seen in antisocial personality disorder.

(c) **Autonomic** Nervous System **under arousal:** The autonomic nervous system of the individuals having antisocial personality disorder is not aroused to the same degree as that of the normals. Such individuals are not aroused autonomically upto an optimal level. It seems that their Autonomic Nervous System is inhibited due to certain biological defects. It is this that gives rise to the characteristic features found in individuals having antisocial personality disorder. It is this under arousal which give rise to adventurous risk-taking behaviour of such individuals because ordinary behaviour does not arouse them upto an optimal level.

PSYCHOSOCIALTHEORIES OF ANTISOCIAL PERSONALITY

(A) Psychoanalytic Theory-Psychoanalysis gave one of the first psychological interpretation regarding the etiology of this disorder. It pointed out that such individuals fail to develop an adequate superego control which allows its forces to dominate individual's behaviour. Lack of adequate development of the superego in such individuals is traced to the family conflicts, wrong parental model and inappropriate parent-child relationship. Psychoanalysis was the first to point out that parental deprivation, through family conflicts, broken homes, separation or divorce and the child fails to internalize the parent's socio-culturally accepted values which leads to the poor development of its superego as a result of which it forces dominate and the ego cannot regulate the behaviour in a socially desired manner. However, direct support does not exist for psychoanalytic theorizing about antisocial personality disorder.

(1) The first is the role of modelling. Bandura and associates have done , a lot of work in this area and in general the conclusion of various studies carried out is that modelling can teach aggressive behavaiour and trigger specific aggressive acts. By modelling, we mean imitating i.e. learning by observing others. Parents and other significant persons in the family serve as models for the growing children.

(2) The second important factor, according to the behavioural theorists, is the role of reinforcement.-They (Antisocial) have not been conditioned

appropriately with regard to reinforcement. Reinforcement history of antisocial individuals reveals that they have not been negatively reinforced for antisocial behaviour, besides, the reinforcement that the parents provide is generally non-contingent reinforcement. Children of such parents perceive no connection between their behaviour and the treatment they receive and hence gradually over a period of time such children become desensitized to social stimuli like norms, rules, laws etc. which regulate our behaviour. Antisocial behaviour can also be learned through direct positive reinforcement. Any antisocial act attracts parents or teachers' attention whereas honest and sincere act goes unnoticed. In order to seek such an attention individuals may engage in antisocial behaviour.

Theories of Socio-cultural view-point: These point out to the fact that changes in our socio-cultural environment and relationship gives rise to a aggressive and antisocial acts. The present age has seen the rise of alienation, loneliness, frustration and such other evils which have given rise to antisocial behaviour. Changing values have added to our confusion about what is wrong and what is right. Most of our traditional norms have undergone changes drastically. What was considered abnormal or deviant yesterday has become a normal practice today. These socio-cultural changes have not been in the right direction, and give rise to a state of formlessness which is called as 'anomie'. This socio-cultural view-point points out that changes in our social system and institutions are required if we have to overcome this problem and control antisocial behaviour.

7

Schizophrenic Disorders

Schizophrenia -is a major mental disorder. It is classified among psychotic Disorders and affect about 1% of the population at a given period of time. It is estimated that about 2/3rd of the patients in mental hospital suffer from this disorder.

Schizophrenia refers to a group of psychotic disorders in which there are certain characteristic disorders like disturbances in reality testing, hallucination, delusion, withdrawal from society etc.

The recent history of schizophrenia dates back to 1850's during which time benedict Augustin More, described a case of a young boy and labeled him as suffering from dement precoce.

Kahibaum described two different types of schizophrenia called as hebephrenia and catatonia. In 1896 Kraepelin further classified schizophrenia disorder.

In 1911 Eugene Bleuler coined the term Schizophrenia, the developments in diagnostic-classification systems like ICD and DSM added to our understanding of this disorder.

In this section we would first describe schizophrenia and discuss some of the most important symptoms found among schizophrenics. There are some characteristic disorders or symptoms in schizophrenics like disorder of thought and communication, disorder of perception, motor behaviour, affect

etc. which we would discuss in detail with examples.

Following this we would discuss the various types of schizophrenic disorders.

We would then discuss the etiology or causes of schizophrenia. What causes schizophrenia has become a very controversial question. Some researchers emphasize the role of hereditary, genetic & biochemical factors whereas, others emphasize the role of teaming, family interaction & socio-cultural factors.

The treatment of schizophrenia is a long drawn process. The prognosis, i.e. the recovery from illness depends upon the duration and the type of schizophrenia one has. There are wide variety of treatment techniques available, some have become more controversial than others. For example Electro Convulsive Therapy (E.C.T.) has become more controversial and some researchers advocate that it should be banned. We would discuss the various treatment techniques available to treat schizophrenia.

We would then end this chapter with a few short notes.

chizophienia is a major mental disorder having a characteristic set of symptoms. Schizophrenia most closely approximate what most of us think as "craziness" Schizophrenia ranges from mild to intense.

Its most severe form involves a major personality disorganization and estrangement from what most of us consider "reality". Personality disorganization or decomposition means that the person who exhibits schizophrenic behaviour shows a deterioration from a previous level of functioning. He or she can no longer perform life tasks as well, as before the onset of the disorder. Work suffers, social relationships become stormy, all the individual's social roles become difficult and disorganized.

The disorganization and deterioration of behaviour is particularly problematic for such person's relatives i.e. spouse, children and parent and has an impact on friends and acquaintances, employers and supervisors, teachers, strangers and frequently the police. Most of us may never have close contact with an individual who has schizophrenic disorder, unless we go into one of the helping professions. Schizophrenic behaviour occurs in about I in 100 persons.

DISORDERS AMONG SCHIZOPHRENIC

The specific behaviour seen in the schizophrenic disorders are quite varied. Some of the characteristic disorders found among schizophrenic are as follows:

(1) Disorder of thought and communication.

(A) Form of thought (B) Content of thought

(A) Form of thought is of 4 types:

(i) Cognitive slippage was a term that was used by Paul Meehl to describe the process of looseness of association. Eugen Bleuler (1980) has used the term derailment. In this process ideas shift from one subject to another which may be only slightly related or which appear totally unrelated. Frames of reference may change and in extreme cases totally unrelated ideas may be lumped together.

(ii) In addition to loose manner in which thoughts and concepts are associated, Schizophrenic thinking may also be characterized by **extreme concreteness & literalness.**

(iii) **Autism** is another thought disorder found in Schizophrenia. It means that they live primarily within themselves. Their thinking is dominated by their wishes, fears, fantasies and inner life to a greater extent than in the normal person.

(iv) The Final problem in the Schizophrenic thought process is **the apparent lack of normal logic in reasoning.**

(B) **Content of thought:** Content of thought is usually of two types :

(i) Schizophrenic has **poor insight.** They think that their problems are outside. Most schizophrenia have little or no awareness that their difficulties are of their own making. They deny that their problems are internal. They see them as imposed by outside agencies or other people.

(ii) Second type of problem in the *content of thought* is the maintenance of *false belief or delusions.* Delusions or false belief must be one which the person's culture does not accept and it must be maintained inspite of evidence to the contrary. Delusional beliefs are fixed so that the individual maintains them '*even* then others prove they arc not correct. True delusions often begin as vague unformed ideas that something is "not quite right" and may be preceded by ideas of reference. An idea of reference is a belief or feeling that events in the environment have a special reference to the individual.

For example, a man at a party sees several person across the room having a conversations. Without any evidence, he concludes that they are talking about him. To take another example. If an individual is standing in his balcony and if he sees that far away on the road three people are talking to each other he would conclude that they are talking about him, criticizing him or planning to murder him. The delusion reported by Schizophrenic is described as "chaotic and unsystematised". Compared to the Logical complex and systematic delusion seen in paranoid individuals.

Delusions of the following types have been identified as important aspects of problems in the content of thought. There are many types of delusional beliefs, some of them include :

1. Delusion of persecution

2. Dclusion of reference

3. Grandiose delusions

4. Delusions of influence and control, which can be manifested in any of the following forms.

(a) Thought broadcasting (b) thought insertion (c) thought withdrawal and (d) external control.

(i) **Persecutory delusions**-These false beliefs involves the notion that some person or agency is plotting against the subject, manipulating events, spreading lies, trying to kill the individual, and so on.

(ii) **Delusions of reference-** The belief that others arc talking, about oneself, that one is being included in TV shows or plays or referred to in news articles, and soon.

(iii) **Grandiose delusions-** The belief that one is a very special person, for example, God, or a new Messiah or that one has done or knows something particularly significant such as how to cure cancer. Such a delusion may be combined with persecutory ideation, as in the patient who knew the "secret to world peace", but was being kept locked up by "warmonger capitalists, pinkos, and Fidel Castro".

(iv) **elusions of influence and control:** These delusions are considered very common and characteristic of schizophrenia. They are among the symptoms emphasized by the German psychiatrist Kurt Schneider (1959), who called them first-rank symptoms, and contrasted them with second rank symptoms, which are less unique to schizophrema and are often seen in Other diagnostic groups.

(a) **Thought broadcasting:** The belief or experience that one's thoughts are broadcast into the external world where others can hear them as they occur. One subject experienced this visually as a shimmering in the air as her thought! left her head.

(b) **Thought insertion:** The belief that thoughts are being inserted into one's mind by an external agency. The thoughts are often "bad". One subject asked his therapist to call the subject's uncle to ask that the uncle stop putting thoughts about homosexual behaviour in the subject's head.

(c) **Thought withdrawal:** The experience that thought are being taken away or stolen. A patient reported that her thoughts were disappearing like "Popping soap bubbles", and that this was being done by "invisible acupuncture".

(d) **External control:** The belief or experience that feelings, impulses, actions, or thoughts are not under one's control, but are imposed by an external source. In one or more of these areas, the patient experiences no self-violations and feels unable to prevent the occurrence or to take responsibility for it. In are extreme example, a woman reported that the devil filled her with hate and made her kill her children, while she was helpless to stop herself.

Some common patterns of delusional thought are listed in the following

Some common patterns of delusional Thought

Delusion of Influence	A belief that others are influencing one by means of Wires, TV, and so on, making one do things against one's will.
Delusion of grandeur	The belief that one is in actuality some great person or historical Figure, such as Napoleon, Queen Victoria, or the President of the united states.
Delusion of persecution	The belief that one is being persecuted, haunted or interfered with by certain individuals or organized groups.
Delusion of reference	The belief that others are talking about one, that one is being included in TV shows or referred to in news articles, and so on.
Delusion of bodily change	A belief that one's body is changing in some unusual way for example, that the blood is turning to snakes or the flesh to concrete.
Delusion of nihilism	A belief that nothing really exists, that all things are simply shadows; also common is the idea that one has really been dead for many years and is observing the world from afar.

Besides the above characteristics of thought and communication schizophrenic thinking also has the following aspects :

(a) Their speech is characterized by **Incoherence** the realizations of schizophrenic are totally incoherent. The sentence structure used may be appropriate, with the proper use of nouns, verbs and the like, but the meanings of the words themselves have a bizarre flavour and arc difficult to comprehend.

(b) Neologism is another characteristic of schizophrenic thought many a times the schizophrenic will make up-a new word that has no meaning to the listener.

(c) Clang Association is one type of thought disturbance seen among schizophrenics. This is a sentence or a statement that consists of a series of rhyming words chained together not on the basis of any logic, but simply because they rhyme.

(d) Word Salad is a disturbance and thought seen among schizophrenics. When there is a complete break down of coherence, so that there are no associative links between words or thoughts, not even clang associations, then the schizophrenics speech looses all communicative value. This total disorganization of speech is referred to as a word salad.

Cognitive dysfunction or dysfunction of thought is an important aspect of schizophrenia. Some examples of cognitive dysfunction in schizophrenia are summarized in Table given below.

Table – Some Examples of Cognitive Dysfunction in Schizophrenia.

Mystical-magical thinking: Confusion between fantasy and reality. "I think that I am invincible, therefore I am going to jump off this building and not be hurt".

Concretization: Abstraction is not possible so Figurative thoughts and actions become literal. If asked to tell the meaning of a proverb like "A stitch in time saves nine", a schizophrenic might say "I should sew nine buttons on my coat".

Overinclusion: Inability to exclude irrelevant stimuli and cues. Reading this table, a schizophrenic might be unable to "tune out" the color of the room, the feel of the chair under him, or the sound of his own breathing.

Inability to hold a set: Schizophrenic people cannot use a "Ready!" signal to improve performance on tasks like reaction time. So "Ready, Set ! Go !" may result in the same speed of response as just plain, "Go !"

Sudden blocking of stream of thought : Often the schizophrenic person's thought will suddenly stop in mid sentence. After a few seconds or minutes of seeming confusion, he or she may begin an entirely new topic.

(2) **Disorder of perception and sensation:** One of the most dramatic disorders seen in schizophrenic behaviour is changes in perception. These changes include distortion of real stimuli (illusion), and perception in the absence of external stimuli (hallucinations), such distortions may occur in all sensory areas.

Other perceptual experiences may include distortions such as changes in odour or the taste of food (e.g. food does not taste or smell right). Sonic experience distortion of touch (feeling numbness or tingling sensations).

More intense distortions of perception, called illusions, may occur. In an illusion, the individual misinterprets real stimuli. Hallucinations consist of perceptions in the absence of any external stimuli. They have often been compared to dreaming while awake.

Hallucinations may occur in any of the sensory realm although auditory hallucinations seem to be the most frequent, and visual hallucinations, the second most common. Auditory hallucinations usually consist of hearing voices which speak to or comment about the persons.

Visual hallucinations may be frightening or pleasant. An individual may see a vision of a religious figure or demon. When hallucinating, people may become frightened or angry and respond behaviorally.

In a comparative study of newly admitted schizophrenic and no schizophrenic patients, Freedman & Chapman (1973) found that Schizophrenics reported a significantly greater number of changes in their perceptual functioning including, visual illusions, disturbing acute auditory perception, inability to focus attention, difficulty in identifying people, and difficulty in understanding the speech of others. Schizophrenics have also reported of factory changes, complaining that their own body odour is more pronounced and more unpleased.

Second these reports arc confirmed by standard laboratory perceptual tests which indicate that Schizophrenics do poorly on perceptual tasks such as size estimation, time estimation and proprioceptive discrimination (i.e. discrimination of the orientation of their bodies in space, where their hands & feels are etc.)

(3) **Disorder of Affect and Emotions**: Both Kreaplin and Bleuler have found the disorder of affect in the schizophrenic individual. Schizophrenic individual displays different disorders of effect or emotions. Some of which are as follows :

(a) **Anhedonia** : It is the inability to experience pleasure. Harrow et. al. (1977) have found that Anhedonia is most characteristic of people having long term schizophrenic behaviour rather than acute first episode disorder. Meehl (1962) considers anhedonia to be one of the primary deficits of schizophrenia.

(b) Individuals with a schizophrenic disorder appear to have quantitative differences in affect. They too have **shallow or blunted affect.** This term refers to a reduced emotional responsiveness. Such individuals may be described as stony or cold. When this affective disorder become severe, these persons are often said to have flat affect, they appear to be apathetic or indifferent, and show virtually no emotional response. Individuals with shallow or blunted affect seem very similar to a showroom model or a robot.

(c). Another disorder of affect is **inappropriate affect.** These individuals may laugh, grin, or giggle when discussing events that normally arouse emotions of sorrow or sadness, such as the death of a loved one, or they may break into tears when talking about neutral events, rage and anger may also be inappropriately expressed.

(d) A fourth disturbance of affect seen in many schizophrenics is .an exaggerated ambivalence. Ambivalence is a term used to describe a state in which two conflicting emotions are experienced towards an object, event or persons at about the same time.

The degree of affective disorder, particularly anhedonia and blunted or flat affect has been considered by some to be a significant indicator of the severity of the schizophrenic disorder.

(4) **Disturbances in motor behaviour** are obvious physical manifestations that can be observed visually. Most disorders of motor behaviour are not dramatic.

Some common disorder of motor behaviour include unusual mannerism. This includes stereotyped behaviour, agitational immobility, echolalia and echopraxia. In echopraxia, an individual echoes the behaviour of another person. If some one scratches, so does the Schizophrenic. When manifested verbally, this mimicking is called as echolalia (The person may parrot other speech). A more common behaviour manifested in long term schizophrenic disorder is stereotyped behaviour in which the individual engages in a unusual repetitive behaviour.

(5) **Disorders of Socialization**: Many schizophrenic individuals manifest disorders of socialization. The most common being social withdrawal and ideation. Social withdrawal and ideation may result because of the above mentioned disorders. Many Schizophrenic individuals also display socially inappropriate behaviour. The most common being the absence of socially inappropriate behaviour. Many schizophrenic also avoid health care and personal hygiene.

Besides the above characteristics.-

Bleuler identified two groups ' of symptoms which he called as Fundamental symptoms and secondary symptoms.

These symptoms are as follows :

(1) **Fundamental Symptoms** : (Also called as four A's)

(i) affect (flat, blunted or inappropriate),

(ii) associations (loose, derailed or fragmented),

(iii) ambivalence (usually to an extreme degree),

(iv) autism (unusual, self-centred thinking).

(2) Secondary Symptoms include

(i) Hallucinations

(ii) Grandiosity

(iii) Paranoid thinking and

(iv) Hostility and belligerence.

Besides the above symptoms researchers have also found cross-cultural differences in the symptomatology of schizophrenia. Twelve major symptoms of the Schizophrenics are as follows :

(1) Restricted affect

(2) Poor insight

(3) Thought broadcasting

(4) Absence of early waking

(5) Poor rapport

(6) Absence of depressed appearance.

(7) Absence of elation

(8) Widespread delusions

(9) Incoherent speech

(10) unreliable information

(11) Bizarre illusions

(12) Nihilistic delusions

Researches have also found that, When exact criteria are used the disorder can be diagnosed with fair accuracy. Also, schizophrenia is shown to occur with approximately equal frequency in various parts of the world and show many of the same symptoms.

TYPES OF SCHIZOPHRENIC DISORDERS

It was Kraepelin, who categorized schizophrenia into different types. He divided schizophrenia into different subtypes on the basis of the behaviour characteristics. He identified 3 sub-types on schizophrenia, (a) Hebeiphrenia (b) Catatonic and (c) Paranoia. Eugene Bleuler added the simple type to this list. These above mentioned categories of schizophrenic sub-types have persisted since that time. Recently, DSM-III has categorized schizophrenia . into the following 5 types.

1. Disorganized type
2. Catatonic type
3. Undifferentiated type
4. Paranoid type
5. Residual type

(1) **Disorganized type:** Disorganized type was earlier called as hebephrenic. This disorder developed slowly, gradually, over a long period of time and is marked by incoherence and flat, blunted, inappropriate or silly affect. Such individuals appear to have regressed to infantile levels of behaving. They are among the most impaired individuals who develop a schizophrenic disorder. Onset is usually early (i.e. in adolescence) and the disorder progresses slowly with behaviours becoming more and more disorganized as time passes. Delusion and hallucination, when present, are fragmented and simple. This disorder is severe having poor prognosis.

(2) **Catatonic type:** Catatonic type is the second major category of schizophrenic disorder given by DSM-III. Catatonic Schizophrenia A characterized primarily by psycho-motor disturbance. There may be a stupor, physical rigidity, excitement, posturing or oppositional behaviour (in which the person does the opposite of what is desired). The individual may rapidly swing between withdrawn face and excitability. Mutism (the absence of speech) is common in this group. The onset of these symptons may be quite sudden. One may sec waxy flexibility.

Thus we sec that catatonic schizophrenia is of 2 type.

(a) Stuporous Catatonia

(b) Agitated Catatonia

Stuporous catatonia is marked by is marked by mutism, automatic obedience and waxy flexibility. Mutism refers to absence of speech. Automatic - obedience refers to the persons tendency to follow all instructions, even the most absurd (e.g. pat your head and stand on one foot). In waxy flexibility there is compliance of a more passive sort in that the person can be placed in a wide variety of awkward postures and may even remain in that position until moved out of it

Agitated catatonia is chaiacterised by motor excitement in which the patient manifests wild, uncontrollable behaviour which is unceasing and often very destructive.

(3) **Paranoid type**: The Paranoid sub-type is one of the most commonly diagnosed schizophrenic disorder. The individual often have had a fairly well organised personality before onset of the disorder and usually do not become as disorganised as the catatonic or disorganized type. They are, however, often suspicious, angry and hostile. People with this disorder may occasionally act on their delusions or respond to their hallucinations in violent manner. Most individual with this disorder have a poor prognosis.

Paranoid type of Schizophrenia differs from the other types in several important ways. Typically, these people show minimal impairment in functioning and few affective symptoms and manifest the disorder later in life as compared to with the other sub-types.

(4) **Undifferentiated type**: The essential feature of this type of Schizophrenic disorder is that it cannot be classified in any category previously listed or that meet the criteria for more than one of the above mentioned schizophrenic disorder.

(5) **Residual type**: This term is used to categorize an individual who has had Schizophrenic episode in the past, but who now has no prominent psychotic symptoms. However, such cases manifest some continuing deficits such as blunted affect, withdrawal or illogical thinking.

With respect to types of schizophrenia, it is worth noting here that there are three more types of schizophrenia noted in DSM-III these are as follows

A. Brief Reactive psychosis.

B. Schizophreniform disorder.

C. Schizoaffective psychosis.

We would discuss these in brief.

A. **Brief Reactive psychosis**, is characterised by sudden onset and duration lasting from a few hours to a maximum of 2 weeks. The symptoms include bizarre ideas, mutism, inappropriate affect, silliness and transient hallucination

& delusions. Most often the disorder is precipitated by some severe psychosocial stressor such as death of a loved one, severe accident and injury, or combat experience the rapid onset, however, also is typically followed by a rapid remission and recovery to the premorbid level of functioning in common parlance, the brief reactive psychosis are probably best known as "nervous breakdowns".

B. **Schizophreniform disorder**: If the symptoms of schizophrenia last longer than 2 weeks but less than six months, the diagnosis of schizophreniform disorder would most likely be applied. This short lived psychosis differs from the schizophrenia not only in duration but in the fact that essential recovery to premorbid adjustment again is more likely. Further, there does not appear to be as clear genetic link for the schizophreniform psychosis as with the schizophrenia.

C. Schizoaffective psychosis sometimes the diagnosis of schizophrenia is complicated by the presence of manic and/or depressive symptoms is construction with the basic signs of "true" schizophrenia. In DSM-III it is assumed that as long as the presence of affective (emotional) components are secondary, schizophrenia still may be diagnosed. However, there are instances in which affective symptoms are so strong that a diagnostician cannot decide whether the pattern is one of Schizophrenia with strong affective psychosis (such as depression or mania) with significant schizophrenic involvement. It is for these cases that the DSM-III category of schizoaffective disorder is reserved.

THEORIESOFSCHIZOPHRENIA

There are a wide variety of factors that may lead to development of Schizophrenia.

These factors are as follows:

(1) Psychoanalytic Theory; (2) Interpersonal communication or family Theories (3) Schizophrenia as a learned behaviour, (4) Socio-cultural theories of Schizophrenia; (5) Biochemical Theories; (6) Heriditary factors; (7) Schizophrenia as an arousal and motivation dysfunction; (8) Phenomenological Existential theory; (9) Diathesis stress model of schizophrenia.

2. **Psychoanalytic theory:** The psychoanalytic view of Schizophrenia is very much speculative because Freud was not particularly concerned with schizophrenia as his focus was on individuals who manifested less severe disorders. According to Freud in Schizophrenia the individual's ego does not develop enough to mediate successfully between id, superego and environment. Subsequently when sexual or aggressive id impulses threaten to overwhelm the individual, the fragile ego crumbles and the massive regression occurs, which

leads to symptoms of schizophrenia.

Psychoanalytic theory assumes that there are two major causes for the schizophrenic's regression and resultant break with reality, (i) The first is an increase in the strength of id impulses, especially infantile sexual impulses seeking erotic gratification, *(it)* The second is a concomitant increase in anxiety and guilt brought on by these socially unacceptable and forbidden impulses. To alleviate the anxiety and guilt, the ego attempts to defend against the expression of the forbidden impulses. When everything else fails, and the ego perceives that it can no longer effectively inhibit the expression of these undesirable impulses, the defense mechanism of regression is employed to return the individual to an earlier developmental stage. By regressing back to the oral stage before the ego has been differentiated from the id, the individual can in effect reject reality. By rejecting reality, the individual can avoid the anxiety and guilt associated with the temptation to express infantile sexual and aggressive impulses. It was assumed that individuals who were fixated at the early oral stage of development were predisposed to demonstrate this regression and the resultant break with reality.

Carl Jung, a Freudian associate, did not develop any specific theory of schizophrenia but the opposed Kraplelin's views on schizophrenia and proposed that an organic disorder did not result in Schizophrenia. Jung said that the mechanism was actually the reverse. He proposed that the emotional disorder of schizophrenia produces an abnormal that the emotional disorder of schizophrenia produces an abnormal metabolism which causes physical damage to the brain.

Sullivan, a neofreudian explained the development of schizophrenia on the basic of interpersonal relationship. Sullivan believed that distorted interpersonal relationship lead to anxiety and regression. Sullivan uses the word parataxic distortion to refer to disturbed relationship between parent and child.

When parents treat children inconsistently or over punitively or overindulgently, the child may experience "a disaster of self-esteem". To defend against this disaster, the person uses parataxic distortion; that is, the individual distorts subsequent interpersonal interactions. This distortion consists of an identification of one person (such as girl friend) with another real person (such as mother), or fantasy person. When parataxic distortion is not corrected, the individual loses consensual validation, the recognition by others of the appropriateness of the .person's thinking and behaviour. Lack of consensual validation makes interpersonal relationships even more difficult, leading to more parataxic distortion. The individual spirals down into the distorted human relationship which we call schizophrenia.

2. Interpersonal communication and family theories of Schizophrenia: Emphasize the relationship between individual as an important determinant of Schizophrenia. Sullivan's theory discussed above is one type of interpersonal theory. According to these theorist Schizophrenia is due to a pathological communication pattern which Bateson and his colleagues have **called it Double Blind.**

In this communications, the child or adult child is emotionally dependent on the parent and the relationship is so intense that it is extremely important that the parental message be understood, since if they are not, psychological or physical punishment will follow. The parent, however, expresses two conflicting messages at the same time. Because of the importance of the relationship, the child or adult child cannot confront the parent's conflicting message, comment upon the conflict, ignore it or escape from it. The individual is caught in a situation from which escape is impossible and in which punishment is likely, the contradictory messages thus lead to development of symptoms that we call schizophrenia.

Related to interpersonal theory, many researchers have found that family relationship plays an important role in the development of schizophrenia.

Arieti (1974) sees the schizophrenic family milieu as one in which the child is deprived of all security and is submerged in an atmosphere of anxiety and hostility.

Lidz *(1973)* claims that great number of Schizophrenic children come from families that fall into one of two categories : **the** schismatic family, in which parental discord has divided the family into opposing factions and the 'skewed family, which remains reasonably calm but only beaus one spouse is totally dominated by the other. In both situations the child is denied the emotional support necessary for a sense of security and self worth. Furthermore, role modification may become extremely problematic, particularly in the schismatic family, where identification with our parent might antagonize the other and thus cause even greater hostility.

The noted psychoanalyst Freeda Fromm Reichmaim (1952), introduced the term Schizophrenogenic to denote a particular type of mother which schizophrenics were sometimes observed to have. These mothers were described as extremely overprotective and intrusive. They were continually intruding into the life of their child, even when the child was an adult. The mother had to know exactly what her child was doing, thinking, and feeling at each moment. Such maternal behaviour has been thought to prevent the child from developing a separate identity; and the offspring's lack of identity and lack of separateness are believed to lead to schizophrenia.

Theodore Lidz, Flech and Comelison (1965) have found that mothers of individuals who have developed schizophrenia are often unstable, intrusive women. They found that the fathers were also disturbed either paranoid and aggressive, or passive, ineffectual, and distant.

Wynne &Binger (1963), and Singer & Wynne (1965) identified two from of schizophrenic communication (a) amorphous style and(b) fragmented style. In amorphous style communications are very vague, loose and indefinite for example "you can go or not, it's Ok, I'am not sure what you want to do". In fragmented style there is a marked' disruption and lack of closure. A typical statement of this type might be, "I told you to stop or I' will...... oh, go ahead and do it, but........ wait.... I'll tell you what I think later.

After the initial work of Wynne & Singer, data from other studies have supported the position that deviant family communication is associated with. schizophrenia. In reviewing these studies. Lien (1980) has concluded that "of all" aspects of family life, disordered communication is the most likely to be associated with the development of schizophrenia".

There have been virtually hundreds of studies examining family dynamics and schizophrenia. However, the great majority of these have significant methodological flaws in experimental design that make the results impossible to interpret meaningfully. Fontana (1966) reviewed a great number of these families studies and found only five that met the methodological criteria he deemed necessary for interpreting results with any degree of certainty. On the basis of these five studies, be felt that only two broad conclusion could be made concerning the family patterns of schizophrenics :

(i) There is much more conflict present between the parents of normals.

(ii) Communication between the parents of schizophrenics is less clear than that between parents of normal individuals. That is, according to Fontana, conflict and lack of communication between parents of schizophrenics seem to be more closely associated with the occurrence of this disorder than any other family interaction pattern.

(3) **Schizophrenia as a learned behaviour disorder**: Some inter personal theorists imply that Schizophrenic behaviour is a learned behaviour disorder which is learned from parents.

The social learning theorists Albert Bandura, Leonard Ullman and Leonard Krasner arc among those who have suggested possible mechanism.

Albert Bandura (1968) has proposed that hallucinations, delusions, ideas of reference and other disorders seen in Schizophrenic develop through a process of learning, modelling and reinforcement. According to Bandura's formulation, the disturbed parental models arc present in the families of those who become schizophrenic. Bandura also suggests that cognitive processes are quite important in learning to be Schizophrenic.

The theorists who have most strongly advocated a learning model of schizophrenic behaviour are Ullman and Krasner (1975).they take the position that Schizophrenic behaviour is primarily due to the "extinction of attention to social stimuli to which normal people respond". According to these researchers. If one is not reinforced for attending to normal, usual social stimuli and instead attends to unusual external stimuli or, internal stimuli, such as one's own autistic thoughts then one will manifest "loose associations" and strange speech patterns. The lack of attention to the social stimuli presented by other people will result in behaviour of aloofness and social isolation.

The disorders of affect present in schizophrenia are seen by Ullman and Krasner (1975) as being due to a life long absence of reinforcement for emotional expression. That is, they believe that some Schizophrenics have not been reinforced for laughing, smiling or crying. Inappropriate affect in others occur because the individuals were not taught to discriminate between stimuli. According to Ullman and Krasner hallucinations are learned by watching these types of behaviour being modelled in popular movies, reading about them and seeing others manifest them.

Strange beliefs became delusional according to Ullman and Krasner. when the person discovers that.

(a) talking about such ideas obtains attention,

(b) the attention of other is found to be reinforcing, and

(c) other more normal behaviours are not effective in gaining reinforcing social attention.

Ullman-and Krasner (1975) have been extraordinarily successful a conceptualizing a theoretical-framework for explaining Schizophrenia from socio psychological framework. However, their concepts are not well documented with experimental evidence.

(4) **Socio-cultural theories of Schizophrenia:** Ayllon et. al. have focused attention on the social role behaviour of schizophrenics. They have raised the question of the degree to which the bizarre behaviour we see in Schizophrenics is due to societal expectations of what a " crazy" person is "supposed" to be like. The idea that schizophrenia is a social role that people enact, rather than an illness is shared by some other theorists, (e.g. Pomicci 1974, Schaff 1975).

Thomas Schaff (1975) believes that Schizophrenia is simply a label applied to deviant behaviour. The individuals behave "as if sick". Sarbin (1969) Suggests that schizophrenia consists of an individual behaving in a manner which meets the expectations of society.

Socio-cultural theories also .emphasize, on the incidence rate of Schizophrenia which has been reported to vary from culture to culture for example one study found the incidence of Schizophrenia per thousand adults to be 3.5 for Chinese adults and 13.1 for traditional French-Canadian community. This substantial variation suggests that differences in these culture may have influenced the amount of Schizophrenia present.

The importance of socio-cultural factors in the development of Schizophrenia has received support from studies of the incidence of Schizophrenia in various socio-economic classes. In one classic study Fairs and Dunham (1939) found higher rates for mental disorder in lower-class inner-city areas. The rates of Schizophrenia decreased in higher-status areas at the fringe of the city. These findings have been frequently replicated.

Several studies have generated data that the higher proportion of people with schizophrenia in the lower socio-economic classes may be due to the drifting of middle and upper class Schizophrenics to lower Socio-economic neighbourhoods after their Schizophrenia develops.

(5) **Biochemical theories of Schizophrenia:** There are many biological factors that give rise to schizophrenic behaviour.

(a) Health and his colleagues (1958) implicated **abnormal Plasma proteins (gama globulins)** in the blood as a causative agent. They isolated such a substance called taraxein in the blood of schizophrenics. In a startling experiment, they injected this substance (Obtained from the blood of Schizophrenic patient) into normal subjects (volunteers), who then displayed schizophrenic behaviour. Although, it created a major stir, this study has never been successfully replicated.

(b) Another example of a substance once implicated in the development of schizophrenics is nicotinic acid (part of Vitamin B complex).

Hoffer et.al. (1957) concluded that schizophrenia may be due to Vitamin deficiency. Hoffer (1966) administered large dosages of Vitamins to schizophrenics and found that a large percentage improved in their behaviour.

(c) More recent research on the biochemistry of schizophrenics has focused on the biochemical activity involved in the transmission of nerve impulse.

(d) **Dopamine theory:** According to many researchers Dopamine, one type of a neurotransmittor plays an important role in the causation of schizophrenia. Excess of dopamine theory comes from the study of amphetamine psychosis. According to some researchers excessive production of dopamine is less likely to be the issue than is an excess Sensitivity to dopamine at the receptor site.

(c) **Psychomimetic drugs:** One chemical known to stimulate schizophrenic-like behaviour is the hallucinogenic drug mescaline. It resembles adrenalin, a chemical occurring naturally in the body. Osmond and Smythies (1952) and Hotter (1964) suggested that an adrenalin-like substance, adrenochrome, and one of its metabolites, adrenolutin, are responsible for psychotic behaviour. Research has shown that in schizophrenics a greater amount of adrenolutin was metabolized (manufactured) from adrenochrome, while in normal individuals adrenochrome was metabolized into another substance called dihydroxy-N-methyl indole. It is assumed that adrenolutin, which acts like mescaline, is responsible for symptoms of schizophrenia some studies, however, have failed to find such differences between schizophrenics and normals (Holland, Cohen, Goldenberg, Sha & Leifer 1958), making this biochemical hypothesis inconclusive.

Another well-Known psychomimetic drug that has been investigated is LSD (lysergic acid diethylamide). The chemical cell structure of LSD closely resembles that of serotonin, a neurotransmitter substance found in the brain. Wooley (1962) has reported than an excessive amount of serotonin causes agitation like that produced by LSD, while an insufficient supply of serotonin caused suppression of activity like that in catatonic states. It is assumed that serotonin and other similar chemical, known as tryptamine (both of which are classified as indolamines), are chemically altered in an abnormal manner to form hallucinogenic compounds. Again, however, this biochemical model has not yet been adequately tested.

These similarities between symptoms of schizophrenia and those produced by drugs such as mescaline and LSD initially prompted many investigators to suggest that the biochemical underpinnings might be the same. However, schizophrenia and the so-called "model psychoses" produced by such drug differ significantly from one another, not only in particular symptoms but in overall symptom patterning as well.

The biochemical theories of schizophrenia are quite complicated and difficult to understand unless one is well versed in. biochemistry.

(6) **Hereditary theories of schizophrenia:** Since the pioneering work of Bleuler and Kraepelin many researchers pointed out that schizophrenia has a

hereditary base. Researchers in order to find out the role of hereditary in the causation of schizophrenic disorder has focussed their attention on the following different types of studies.

(a) Family studies, (b) Twin studies and (c) Adoption studies

(a) **Family studies**: In 1961, Rudin published the first of the family studies of Schizophrenia. In a family study, the relatives of a person with Schizophrenia are studied to determine if they have a greater incidence of the disorder than the general population. If they do, the data are taken to indicate that the disorder has a genetic component.

Rosenthal (1970) and Slater and Cowie (1971) have demonstrated that the general population risk is 1% whereas closer relatives show a higher risk which is graded on the basis of relationship.

Many family studies have found that even though most relatives of schizophrenics do not manifest schizophrenia, they do manifest Schizophrenia spectrum disorders which include Schizoid and inadequate personality disorder and "borderline" Schizophrenia.

(b) **Twin studies:** Two types of twins are studied one is monozygotic (or identical) and second is dizygotic (or fraternal). Identical twins have an identical inheritance and fraternal twins are genetically, no more similar than ordinary siblings. If Schizophrenia has a similar genretic components than Identical twins, but nor fraternal twins should be concordant, if he or she had the same dignosis. Concordance rate is significantly higher 'for identical twins than for fraternal twins indicating the role of genetic factors in Ac development of Schizophrenia.

(c) **Adoption Studies**: Most of the adoption studies especially those carried out by Heston (1966) and that by Kety et.al. (1976) has shown that genetic factors play an important role in the causation of schizophrenic disorder.

Heston found that out of the 47 children born to Schizophrenic mothers which were given away for adoption soon after birth, 10% became schizophrenic. None of a control group of children of normal mothers developed schizophrenia. Also the children of Schizophrenic mothers were more inclined to be mentally retarded, sociopathic or neurotic.

All the above mentioned studies indicate that hereditary factors play an important role in development of Schizophrenic disorder.

(7) **Schizophrenia as an Arousal and Motivation Dysfunction:** In recent years many researchers have focussed attention on arousal and motivational dysfunction among schizophrenics. Today there is sufficient data implicating specific difficulties in arousal and motivation among schizophrenics. Motiva-

tion theorists generally perceive schizophrenia as and inability to receive, process, or respond to internal and external stimulation (Nuechterlein & Dawson, 1984a).

One arousal theorist, Mednick (1958), believes that prodromal schizophrenia is characterized by excess arousal in the form of a massive anxiety. Because of stimulus generalization, a great number of ordinarily ignored stimuli become associated with this massive anxiety. Therefore more rd more environmental and internal stimuli have the power to make the person anxious and fearful. A vicious circle may then develop in which more and more stimuli arc associated with anxiety. Soon the person is so aroused that he or she responds with anxiety to nearly every event or experience. According to Mednick, when this point is reached, the person may seen as suffering from acute schizophrenia.

To cope with the intense anxiety of acute schizophrenia, the person tries to find way to reduce the aversive feelings. One way to do this is to stop responding to the real work and to attend to small numbers of tangential, irrelevant events and stimuli. The physiological result of this attentional shift is a dramatic reduction in arousal to a lower-than-normal level; the person's behaviour is now consistent with that of an under aroused and nonresponsive chronic schizophrenic. Research evidence for poor arousal levels among schizophrenia maybe exemplified by the work of Zahn (1975);

(8) Phenomenological-Existential Theory : R.D. Laing (1967) has been the most influential advocate of a phenomenological-existential model of schizophrenia. In this approach, schizophrenia is construed as resulting from society's imposing unreasonable restrictions on an individual, blocking attempts for personal growth and autonomy and demanding conformity. The schizophrenic individual is seen here as one who attempts to escape from a stressful, unbearable world by changing his or her inner representation and interpretation of reality. Laing also insists that schizophrenia is not "insanity", but merely a rcflection of an individual who cannot suppress his or her instincts and emotions to conform to an abnormal society. He views schizophrenia is as a retreat from the painful, mad reality of the external world, and as an existential search for meaning and personal autonomy. The "mad reality", according to Laing, is usually a stressful and distorted family system. Rather than trying to eliminate the patient's schizophrenic behaviour, Laing suggests that the experience should be viewed as potentially meaningful and beneficial for personal growth. Therapy should therefore be directed at helping the client make the "trip" from the external world to inner reality as a means of developing greater personal enlightenment, much as an individual helps another through a psychedelic drug trip. Also, Laing uses family therapy, with schizophrenics.

Laing's approach to schizophrenia assumes that it is not necessarily a serious psychological disorder, but merely a disruption of social relations that results in the search for the real meaning of one's life. In certain way's this view is similar to aspects of Ullman and Krasner's learning theory approach (discussed above). Schizophrenia is viewed as a form of behaviour learned in order to deal with unacceptable environmental demands. However, inherent in Laing's early writings is the idea that the schizophrenic experience is a potentially good, positive, growth process. There is little evidence, though, to indicate that individuals who have undergone schizophrenic episodes are any better off or more enlightened than before.

(9) **Diathesis-stress Model**-Looking at the results found in family studies, twin studies, and adoptee studies as a whole, one is led to conclude that genetic factors play an important role in the etiology of schizophrenia. However, the fact that there is never an exact relationship (e.g., less than a 100% concordance rate in twin studies) suggests that the involvement of additional factors in this disorder. Currently, a widely held position proposes a diathesis-stress formulation of schizophrenia. That is, some individuals genetically inherit a diathesis (predisposition) toward the development of schizophrenia, but schizophrenia will only actually develop in those predisposed individuals who are exposed to particular stressful experiences for which they have not developed effective coping behaviours. Meehl (1962) has proposed such a model. He suggests that the genetic predisposition that potential schizophrenics inherit is a neutral defect which he calls shcizotaxia. In schizotaxic individuals, Meehl assumes, the common everyday stresses and strains of living produce a slightly peculiar personality structure or makeup that he labels schizotypy. If this schizotype happens to be raised in a positive, nonstressful environmental, he or she will remain relatively normal, although possibly demonstrating certain slightly eccentric behaviours. But if by bad fortune, this individual is realised in a highly stressful environment, then he or she will develop schizophrenia

A more comprehensive diasthesis-stress model has recently been proposed by Zubin and Spring (1977). They introduce the concept of vulnerability as a "common denominator" that takes into account genetic, physiological, developmental, learning, and stress factors in the etiology of schizophrenia. This vulnerability model suggests that everyone is endowed with some degree of vulnerability for developing schizophrenia which, under suitable circumstances, can trigger an episode of the disorder. Numerous factors, ranging from inborn genetic characteristics to acquired learned propensities, contribute to a person's degree of vulnerability. The highly vulnerable person is one who encounters a great many factors, which are sufficient to produce a schizophrenic episode. Others, because of their genetic makeup and lack of other risk factors, have a low degree of vulnerability and in all likelihood will not develop the disorder. The attractive feature of this model is that it proposes means of measuring vulnerability. Such diathesis-stress models show great promise for better understanding of this disorder.

TREATMENT APPROACHES FOR SCHIZOPHRENIC DISORDERS

When the behaviour disorder is Severe (as often it is) the individual is usually treated in a residential setting, a public or private mental hospital. However, many Schizophrenic individuals are treated in a community set up or in an out patient department.

The various treatment methods of Schizophrenic individual can be grouped into two broad categories.

1. Biological treatment consisting of (a) Chemotherapy and (b)E.C.T and

2. Psychosocial therapeutic approaches consisting of (a) individual psychotherapy; (b) Behavioural approaches (c) community therapy approaches.

1. Biological treatment: The current biological therapies used for treating Schizophrenia were not developed from research based on specific biological theories the reversed occurred. Many theories were initially developed because these biological treatments worked. Later research was based on the theories and new treatment have been developed as a result of this theory based research.

(a) **Chemotherapy:** In 1950s a revolutionary change in the treatment of Schizophrenic individuals occurred as a result of the development of antipsychotic drugs. The most commonly used antipshchotic drug is phenothiazines called Chlorpromazine which is sold under the brand name Thorazine. These drugs have been so important that the National Institute of Mental Health (1975) considers them one of the two most significant discoveries in the 25yrs from 1950 to 1975.

The phenothiazines were among the earliest antipsychotic drugs used and continue to be the most commonly prescribed, drugs.

The Phenothiazines can reduce psychomotor excitement, agitation, delusion and hallucinations, tensions, hostility, negativism, poor sleep patterns and social withdrawal.

However, they do not seem to lead to much improvement in insight, judgement, memory or orientation.

Spohn and associates (1977) found that, with phenothiazine the treated group improved significantly whereas control group became worse. Further they found that eight week follow up period of medication led to following specific changes.

(1) The treated group was better able to attend to visual tasks requiring continuous concentration. (2) the treated group's ability to correctly perceive visual stimuli under varying lengths of presentation improved. (3) the treated group's physiological response to stressors decreased. Many studies have found similar results, which suggest that the antipsychotic drugs help the patient to filter out distracting stimuli. Most theorists (and much research) suggest that these drugs act by decreasing the activity of the dopaminergic system of neuro-transmitters.

Much of the credit (or criticism) for the tremendous decrease in mental hospital populations since the mid-1950s must go to the antipsychotic drugs.

Antipsychotic drugs have many side effects. Use of the drugs can result in many problems. There may be drowsiness, dry mouth, blurred vision, impotence, allergic reactions, weight gains, and uncontrollable trembling of the extremities. The disorder tardive dyskinesia sometime occurs in people who take the drugs over long periods. This disorder is apparently irreversible and consists of repetitive in voluntary facial movements such as smacking and licking of the lips, sucking movements, chewing movements, rolling and protrusion of the tongue, blinking, grotesque grimaces, spasms of facial muscle, and body movements such as jerking of the fingers, ankles, and toes, and contractions of neck and back muscles. Other side effects of long term use of the antipsychotic drugs are yet to be discovered.

Before we end our discussion on chemotherapy We should briefly discuss ~the work of Lehmann (1966).

In his review of the effectiveness of chemotherapy, Lehmann (1966) concludes that drugs are usually the treatment of choice for schizophrenia because they are far superior to any other treatment procedure in rapid effectiveness, sustained action over a period of time, and ease of administration with both acute & chronic schizophrenic patients.

Even though Lehmann points out the effectiveness of chemotherapy in alleviating major symptoms, he at the same time indicated that it does not provide a cure for this disorder. The use of chemotherapy alone without any attempt to deal with possible situation/interpersonal factors involved may not lead to any permanent long-term improvement of most behaviour disorders. Chemotherapy usually needs to be used in combination with psychological treatment techniques to ensure that one adequately deals with factors that might prompt a possible reoccurrence of the schizophrenic breakdown.

(b) **E.C.T. stands shock therapy or Electro Convulsive Therapy**: It was developed in 1938 and since then it is used with a wide variety of Schizophrenic patients.

E.C.T. task force (1975) *found* that about 25% of psychiatrist consider E.C.T. as an appropriate treatment for schizophrenia and about 60% do not consider it to be so. E.C.T. has declined in popularity today but still it is used in private hospitals and by psychiatrists in private practice.

In the E.C.T. treatment, the subject lies prone, electrodes arc placed on one or both temples, and a "dose" of 70-130 volts is given from I to 5 seconds. The subject immediately becomes unconscious. With the use of muscle relaxant drug, the sezure is only minimally noticeable as tremors in the hands and feet. After the treatment, the subject experiences a period of confusion and may. Have a memory loss of events preceding the treatment. Treatments are usually given several times per week until the problem behaviours disappears during a period of two to three weeks.

E.C.T. has become a very controversial form of treatment approach. Some considering it to be a boon to schizophrenic patients others considering it to be unethical and barbaric form of treatment.

In recent well controlled double blind study of E.C.T. Tailor and Fleminger (1980) found that patients treated with E.C.T. were more greatly improved after 6 treatments and at the end of the therapy (8-12 treatments) than the control patients, who had not received E.C.T.

(2) **Psychosocial Treatment**: Many clinicians are convinced that Psychosocial treatments have much to contribute to the treatment of Schizophrenia. However the application of these treatments to Schizophrenia is an extremely difficult task.

We would now discuss the following psychosocial treatment

(a) **Individual Psychotherapy**: Traditional psychoanalytic approach is not only difficult but also impossible with Schizophrenic as it is difficult to establish rapport with them.

Two noted therapists who have applied psychoanalytic concepts to the treatment Of Schizophrenia with some success are (1) Frieda Fromm Reichmann (1952) and (2) Hary Stack Sullivan (1953).

Psychodynamic psychotherapy with individuals who have a schizophrenic disorder is a challenge. One noted the rapist who specialized in this technique was Elvin Semrad. Semrad's approach has been reviewed by G. Adier (1979) aftd can be condensed into three basic points :

1. The therapist's empathic understanding allows the individual with schizophrenia to. make human contact and this contact interferes with the schizophrenic process. 2. Therapy must assist the patient in dealing with a previously unbearable reality, and is recognizing his or her own responsibility for the dilemma. 3. The therapist must both support and frustrate the patient. This creates a setting in which the therapist can help the patient focus on recognizing feelings. Once recognized, the patient's feelings can begin to be integrated into the rest of the personality. As the various aspects of the personality become reintegrated, the therapist can begin lo withdraw from the relationship. The primary issue for the therapist is to create an atmosphere of devoted acceptance and trust in an effort to "reach" the patient. The patient in this atmosphere restrains himself or herself to establish communication with others and to relinquish bizarre individualist ways of living. With an increased ability to communicate, the patient, through the therapist, gains insight into the genetic and dynamic nature of his or her disorder, and gains self-esteem (Aricti, 1966, 1980). Other individually oriented psychotherapeutic approaches differ somewhat (e.g., the approach of Carl Rogers), but .all share the goals of creating a trusing relationship between therapist and patient. When applied to schizophrenics, this goal requires active intervention by the therapist.

A great deal of research work has been carried out to test the effectiveness of psychoanalytic therapy with schizophrenic patients. Mosher and Keith (1979) have reviewed the major outcome studies on psychosocial approaches to Schizophrenia and have found conflicting results. After reviewing the same studies as Mosher and Keith, Donald Klein (1980) concludes that "there is little evidence to support the ideas that psychosocial treatments to Schizophrenia are of any clinical significance in reversing or ameliorating the course of the disorder". At the same time he suggest that such treatments may be significant in helping people with a Schizophrenic disorder to maintain themselves outside hospitals or to avoid psychiatric hospitalization.

(b) **Behavioural approaches:** Learning theory approaches have been found to be very useful in changing many undesirable behaviours seen in Schizophrenics.

One of the pioneering work on behavioural approaches with Schizophrenics has been represented by the work ofAyllon et. al. Ayllon's work resulted in the developmental of Token Economy approach for the broad scale treatment of Schizophrenic patients in hospital settings. In token economy approach desirable behaviours are reinforced by providing tokens which can later be exchanged for certain material goods or privileges, whereas undesirable behaviour is treated by the withdrawal of positive reinforcement or by punishment such as fines.

It has been observed that token economy approach has been found to be very effective. Atthowe and Krasner (1968) found that token economy approach led to less apathy, widened patterns of interest, more communication, less bizarre behaviour and increased levels of self-care skills.

Specific problem behaviours have also been modified through the application of behavioural principle. The basic principles of reinforcement are applied just as in token economy, but with focus on one specific behaviour in one specific individual.

The successful application of behavioural principles for treating Schizophrenic requires great deal of planning, specification of techniques and consistency in applications.

Learning principles do not appear to be of use in modifying the primary deficit of Schizophrenia, however they do .help the Schizophrenics in changing many types of behaviour which create great difficulties for them.

(c) **Community Approaches:** In recent years many community approaches have been developed lo help the Schizophrenic individual adjust and readjust better in society. Family therapy with the aim of increasing better interpersonal relationship has been found to be highly effective with Schizophrenics. Community awareness programmes through mass media can also go a long way in helping Schizophrenics adjust better in society.

(d) **Millieu Therapy:** In place of individual psychotherapy, group/social therapy techniques have been used with some success in treating Schizophrenia. With in the institutional setting, milieu therapy is used, in which the entire clinical facility is used as a therapeutic community, with as few restraints as possible placed on the freedom of patients. Patients are urged to regulate their own activities, take part in a wide variety of activities, and develop socially appropriate interpersonal relationship. An attempt is made to develop a constructive environment in which an individual can learn more about herself or himself and more effective ways of responding to individuals, situation, and stress.

One of the significant advantages of milieu therapy is that patients are treated by the staff as responsible human beings who are capable of, and ex pected to, produce behaviour change. It is a more humanistic approach than traditional custodial approaches (which are, unfortunately, still used in many hospitals today).

A slightly different type of milieu therapy is a form of residential community initially developed by R.D. Laing in London in 1965. This community, called Kingsiey hall, is one in which little distinction is made between patients and staff. The residence is set up as a group of people helping .one another. In keeping with Laing's (1967) theory of Schizophrenia, the Schizophrenic reaction that a person is going through is not viewed as a breakdown, but merely as an experience that the person is going through which is both valid and meaningful for him or her. The goal of the staff is to emotionally support and work with the patient as he or she goes through this experience. In the United States, Soteria House in SanJose, California is an example of a residential community patterned after Kingsiey Hall.

An adequate evaluation of milieu-therapy type programs has not yet been made, so that their clinical effectiveness has not been objectively demonstrated (Mosher 1974). However, they show promise in helping Schizophrenics to progress through their Schizophrenic experiences in a non threatening environment.

DIMENSIONS OF SCHIZOPHRENIA

Early research in Schizophrenia simply compared groups of undifferentiated Schizophrenics with group of normal individuals. But these studies found that Schizophrenic groups were far too heterogeneous for the purposes of certain kinds of research. Hence investigators began searching for dimensions along with a more homogenous subgroups of Schizophrenia can be formed. Researchers for their better understanding, has classified Schizophrenia into the following four dimensions:

(a) Process reactive dimension

(b) The chromic-acute dimension

(c) The non-paranoid Paranoid dimension and

(d) Withdrawal activity dimension

We would now discuss these dimensions in brief:

(a) **Process-Reactive Dimension:** The process reactive dimension of Schizophrenia can be traced back to the work of Kraepelin and Bleuler. According to Kraepelinthe true Schizophrenia always has a deteriorating course. Thus he believed in process dimension, whereas according to Bleuler Schizophrenic individuals recover completely or almost completely. Thus Bleuler believed in reactive dimension. Since then clinicians and researchers have focussed their attention on process-reactive dimension of Schizophrenia, especially with respect to treatment and prognosis.

The process reactive dimension seems to be on a continuum on which people fall rather than two discrete types of onset.

Process Schizophrenia is the type that develop over long periods with deterioration becoming more and more obvious as time passes. It generally has poor prognosis whereas reactive Schizophrenia has a sudden onset of malad justice behaviour. The prognosis for this disorder is generally good.

The process reactive dimension has also been discussed in terms of premorbid competence, the individual's level of adjustment 'before the onset of symptoms. The person at the reactive end of the continuum, has a good premorbid adjustment. This person was relatively competent at dealing with life before the onset of the disorder, and did acceptably well in school, in social relations, in work and marriage. The individual with a poor premorbid personality has a long history of behavioural problems poor social relationship, family trouble, and a poor work history. Such a life style indicated a lack of coping skills. Almost by definition, the process Schizophrenia has a poor premorbid personality. Since the gradual onset of the disorder is likely to begin early in adolescence.

Over the years, the research has been quite convincing that the process reactive, poor premorbid-good premorbid dimensions are related to prognosis or likelihood of recovery.

Many clinicians and researchers have become convinced that the process type is one disorder and reactive Schizophrenia with good premorbid personality is another.

The evidence for these dimensions is so convincing that DSM-IP (1980) now categories the person who has a first episode of Schizophrenia behaviour as having Schizophrenic form disorder, only after the behaviour has lasted atleast six months is the person diagnosed as having schizophrenic disorder.

(b) **Chronic-acute dimension:** The DSM-II includes a category termed acute schizophrenia to refer to those patients who show a very rapid onset of symptoms and bizarre behaviour that seem to be precipitated by some specific emotionally stressful experience. In contrast, chronic schizophrenia is used to characterize those patients who display a more gradual onset of abnormal symptoms that do not appear to be triggered by any particular event. This differential rate of onset is analogous to one of the criteria employed in the process (poor premorbid)-reactive (good-premorbid) dimension.

In current research, the chronic-acute distinction is used somewhat differently, referring to the patient's length of hospitalization. As a general rule, chronic patients are defined as those who have been hospitalized for more than year's, whereas acute patients are those who have had a shorter period of hospitalization. The two-year cut off point is used because the probability of being discharged generally is extremely low if one has been hospitalized for more than two years (Brown 1960). These types usually show quite different symptoms : Those Schizophrenics with shorter periods of hospitalization usually display clear-cut bizarre behaviours. They also have at better chance of being released from the hospital, in contrast to patients hospitalized for longer periods.

(c) **Non paranoid - Paranoid dimension -** The paranoid-non paranoid distinction is based on the presence (paranoid) or absence (non paranoid) of delusions of persecution/grandeur. Paranoid schizophrenics, like reactive and acute schizophrenics, usually have a better prognosis for improvement, brifer hospitalization, and fewer rehospitalizations.

(d) **Withdrawal-Activity dimension**: Venables (1957) was the First investigator to introduce the activity withdrawal distinction of schizophrenia. He also developed an activity rating scale to help researchers studying this dimension. Until recently, however, this dimension has been almost completely neglected in the research on schizophrenia. Depue (1976), though, has demonstrated that it is of potential value, since it appears to be related to a number of behavioural, clinical, brain damage, and neuro physiological factors. The activity-withdrawal distinction appears to represent two different form of schizophrenia. Patients on the "activity" end of the dimension are associated with excessive and impulsive motor and verbal behaviour, greater degree of interpersonal contacts, less flat emotional effect, and lower incidence of delusions and hallucinations than "withdrawal" schizophrenics. They also have shorter institutionalization stays and faster recovery rates. Although there is currently no research comparing this dimension with others, the "activity" schizophrenics have many similarities to the reactive, acute, and paranoid schizophrenics.

PRIMARY VERSUS SECONDARY DEFICITS IN SCHIZOPHRENIA

The major issue in the schizophrenic behaviour is which of the characteristics form primary or basic deficits and which of the behaviours are secondary to basic deficits. In order to find out which disorders are primary and which are secondary psychologists and researchers have fixed their attention on the following two topics:

(a) the study of attention based on reaction time and distraction experiments; and

(b) the role of certain cognitive factors. According to researchers cognitive disorders found in schizophrenic individual arc the result of the secondary disorder, primary disorder .being the disorder of attention and concentration.

David Shakow has studied the phenomenon of alertness and readiness to respond to various stimuli. The results of their studies have pointed out that schizophrenics usually have slower reaction times than normal, and chronic schizophrenics are slower than acute schizophrenics. He also found that chronic or process schizophrenics have decreased attention on tasks. According to Neale this is due to the fact that schizophrenics are unable to avoid attending to distracting stimuli.

Asarnow et. al. also studied reaction time in biological children of mothers who bad schizophrenia. Their study showed that deficits in attention is not due to the presence to symptoms such as hallucinations and affect disorder. The deficit is present even when these symptoms are not present. Cronwell et. al. (1979) consider this deficit to be primary factor in schizophrenic vulnerability, rather than a result of schizophrenic, whereas, on the other hand Meiselman has found that slowed reaction time can be induced in normal subjects if they acted in accordance with the common stereotype of a mentally ill person. Meiselman has interpreted his own finding and that obtained from other researchers suggesting that reaction time deficits are a function of making uncommon associations and uncommon associations are not the primary deficits in schizophrenia.

Many researchers are of the view that thought disturbance in schizophrenia is secondary to the primary disorder of internal mediation. In schizophrenic individual the filtering mechanism which filters irrelevant stimuli are absent, Schwartz place and Gilnore (1980) have suggested, based on their research, that perceptual deficit seen in schizophrenics is due to an inability to organize incoming data at an early stage of perceptual process, resulting in disordered thinking. For e.g. Chapman & Chapman have demonstrated that schizophrenic individuals are less able to ignore non-contextual meanings of words. For e.g. if you ask someone to hand you a screwdriver while you were fastening a board in place, they would hear your request in this context, but associate the term 'Screwdriver' with 'screw' and respond as if you had made a sexual comment or request. Chapman & Chapman see these types of errors by schizophrenics as being a difference in the frequency with which normal 1 associations are made rather than a qualitative difference in thinking, Meiselman suggests that reaction time difficulties are a function of making uncommon associations and uncommon associations are not the primary deficit in Schizphrenia. The difficulty with which schizophrenics modify their associations and the ease with which normals do so suggest that individuals who develcp schizophrenia have a more basic deficit which limits their associative flexibility and results in more autistic associations.

DSM-111 AND SCHIZOPHRENIC

DSM-III, refers to the third edition of the diagnostic and statistical manual of mental disorder. DSM-III was published in 1980 by the American Psychiatric Association. The Primary features of schizophrenia, as defined by DSM-III, are much more specific and includes a number of Kurt Schneider's First rank symptoms.

The DSM-III diagnostic criteria for schizophrenia is as follows :

A. At least one of the following during a phase of the illness.

(1) Bizzare delusions (content is potently absurred and has no possible bais in fact), such as delusions of being controlled, thought broadcasting, thought insertion or thought withdrawal.

(2) Somatic, grandiose, religious, nihilistic or other delusions without persecutory or jealous content.

(3) Delusion with persecutory or jealous content if accompanied by, hallucination of any type.

(4) Auditory hallucinations in which either a voice keeps up a running commentary on the individual's behaviour or thoughts, or two or more voices converse with each other.

(5) Auditory hallucination on several occasions with content of more than one or two words, having no apparent relation to depression or elation.

(6) Incoherence, marked loosening of associations, markedly illogical thinking, or marked poverty of content of speech if associated with at least one of the following:

(a) blunted, flat, or inappropriate affect

(b) delusions or hallucinations

(c) catatonic or other grossly disorganized behaviour.

B. Deterioration from previous level of functioning in such areas as work social relations and selfcare.

C. **Duration:** Continuous signs of the illness for at least six months at some time during the person's life, with some signs of the illness at present. The six-month period must include an active phase during which there were symptoms from A, wither without a prodromal or residual phase, as defined below.

Prodromal phase-A clear deterioration in functioning before the active phase of the illness not due to a disturbance in mood or to a Substance use disorder and involving at least two of the symptoms noted below. ("Prodromal" refers to the period prior to the development of major symptoms).

Residual Phase: Persistence, following the active phase of the illness, of at least two of the symptoms noted below, not due to a disturbance in mood or to a substance use disorder, ("Residual" refers to symptoms that remain after major symptomatology has diminished).

PRODROMAL OR RESIDUAL SYMPTOMS

(1) Social isolation or withdrawal

(2) Marked impairment in role functioning as wage earner, students, or homemaker

(3) Marked peculiar behaviour (e.g. Collecting garbage, talking to self in public, or hoarding food)

(4) Marked impairment in personal hygiene and grooming

(5) Blunted, flat, or inappropriate affect

(6) Digressive, vague, over elaborate, circumstantial, or metaphorical speech.

(7) Odd or bizzare ideation, or .magical thinking, (e.g. superciliousness, clairvoyance, telepathy, "sexth sense", "others can feel my feelings", overvalued ideas, ideas of reference)

(8) Unusual perceptual experiences, (e.g., recurrent illusions, sensing the presence of a force or person not actually present)

8

Paranoid Disorders

Paranoid disorders are an important group of psychotic disorder that has received a great deal of attention from mass media. The paranoid disorders are most frequently portrayed in novels, movies and television dramas. This type of psychosis is also the one most likely to involve violence to others.

The study of Paranoid disorder is net new. Freud developed his theory of Paranoia in 1911. What causes Paranoia is debatable issue. The research support is also lacking with respect to various theories concerning the etiology of paranoia which is discussed later in this chapter.

Through the years, there has been a great deal of debate about whether the various forms of paranoid disorders are sufficiently different to be labelled as categories of psychosis, or are merely variants of the same basic schizophrenic disorder. Infact, these paranoid disorders by themselves are rarely observed in the clinic. One reason is that they are often accompanied by other forms of psychopathology. Another is that the "pure" paranoiac, except for isolated delusions such as those of the individual who feels exploited, the overty jealous spouse, or the fanatically religious person, is usually in contact with reality and can function effectively in society.

Research is needed to determine whether paranoid disorders are distinctively separate from one another and are fundamentally distinct from schizophrenia. DSM-III has classified paranoid disorder into three types, these are (a) paranoia, (b) paranoid state, and (c) shared paranoid disorder (also called as Polie A deux).

The most important symptom of paranoid disorders is the presence of suspiciousness, persecutory delusion, emotional detachment, aloofness, and has touch with reality. In this chapter we will first define paranoid disorders and its Chief symptoms and types.

We would then distinguish between paranoid personality, paranoid disorders and paranoid schizophrenia. We would also discuss whether these three are separate disorders or lie on a continuum.

Following this, we would discuss the causes or etiology of paranoid disorder in detail. There are various theories put forward to explain the development of paranoid disorders. Most of these theories tack empirical support.

Towards the end of the chapter we would discuss the various treatment techniques developed for paranoid disorders.

DEFINITION OF PARANOID DISORDERS

Paranoid disorders refer to a group of psychotic disorders which range on a continuum from mild to severe. Individuals with paranoid disorders have delusions which are rigid and fixed.

The most common delusion experienced by individuals with paranoid disorders is delusion of persecution and reference. Delusion of grandeur may also be present in many cases.

The various delusional beliefs are maintained in spite of the convincing evidence to the contrary.

The reported incidence of paranoid disorder is low. Individuals with this disorder may come to the attention of a social agency when they begin to act on their beliefs, otherwise paranoid individuals can often function reasonably well in society, since their personality is not significantly affected in areas outside the delusional content. Hence they are often able to avoid involuntary hospitalization.

Delusion of various types, cither one or in combination is the cheif and only characteristic of individuals having paranoid disorders. These individuals have strong beliefs that seem impervious to reality. Except for the delusional belief their personality in all areas is intact. They have appropriate and realistic affect, their judgement is good and they are usually appropriately oriented. Hallucinations are generally rare. Individuals with paranoid disorders are capable of maintaining basic economic and minimal social skills.

TYPES OF PARANOID DISORDERS

There arc three types of paranoid disorders which arc as follows :

(1) Paranoia, (2) Paranoid state, and (3) Shared paranoid disorder (also called as Folie A deux).

(1) **Paranoia**: The primary feature of paranoia is the development of delusion or false beliefs. This belief develops progressively and slowly in a subtle and insidious manner. The belief system is unmodifiable. The belief system at the same time is accompanied by clear and orderly thinking especially in areas not related lo the delusion.

Individuals who have paranoia frequently considers themselves to have special powers or abilities and their affect is appropriate to the belief system.

Those who have paranoia are often socially isolated, appear eccentric and seem reclusive, they behave in ways which may harm others, for example their suspicion of others may make them take legal action against others. They may not have problems in their day lo day functioning but these individuals are difficult to live with and they may create turmoil and disruption among family members and others with whom they may come in contact long before they are identified as paranoia.

These individuals are sensitive to reactions of others, are rigid and seem to be unable to or unwilling to develop open, warm and affectionate relationships with others. Some exhibit what has been described as "magical thinking". According to wider magical thinking is "thinking in terms of absolutes in terms or omnipotence (all powerfulness) and omniscience (all knowing-ness) in terms of magic certainties, pleasant and unpleasant.

Individuals who develop paranoia have certain personality characteristics, tend to be arogant and dominating, infused with their own self-importance and unable to accept blame for things that go wrong.

Individuals who develop disorder that we call paranoia gradually become more and more disturbed over time.

(2) **Paranoid** State is a paranoid disorder which develops suddenly. This disorder rarely becomes chronic and is followed by a significant life change which often precedes the development of this disorder. This disorder is most commonly seen in individuals who most deal with a life change such as emigration to a new land, induction in to military, menopause, separation from family for the first time, major disasters and failing health. The symptoms experienced in this disorder are more or less same as that experienced in paranoia.

(3) **Shared paranoid** disorder is also called as "Folie A deux" which in French means insanity of the two people. In this disorder two people share, at least partly, a delusional system. Ordinarily one person develops an established paranoia. A second individual. As a result of a close, dependent, emotional relationship, comes to share portions of the other's delusional system. The individual with the original well established paranoia is usually the dominant member of the relationship, and is generally the more disturbed of the two.

The second person tends to be submissive and less caught up in the delusional system. If separated from the dominant member this person's delusional belief will often rapidly disappear or diminish.

Shared paranoid disorder is found among blood relatives.

According to Potasu and Brunell (1974) the shared paranoid behaviour is an outward projection of intolerably an get and hostility toward each other. The shared beliefs provide a bond that conceals the underlying deep hostility that each person feels towards the other.

Freud delineated 4 manifestation of paranoia on the basis of analysis of Schreber's case, which- has become a classic case inanalytical history. These 4 types of paranoia are delineated on the logic of its symptomatology. These are-

(a) Paranoia involving delusion of persecution.

(b) Paranoia involving erotomania-a condition of hetro-sexual fixation.

(c) Paranoia involving Jealousy and

(d) Paranoia involving denial of core conflict.

We would not go into the detail or Freud's types of paranoia as they fall outside the scope of our present discussion.

IS RARANOID BEHAVIOUR ON A CONTINUM

There is a general disagreement among psychiatrists, psychologists, researchers and others with respect to whether paranoid disorders lie on a continue or not. According to some researchers paranoid disorders are psychotic disorders and hence a variant of Schizophrenic disorders, whereas, according to other researchers like Kendler and associates paranoid disorders or psychoses are distinct from Schizophrenia. The position that psychotic paranoid disorders are distinct from paranoid personality disorder and paranoid Schizophrenia. The position that psychotic paranoid disorders are distinct from paranoid personality disorder and paranoid Schizophrenia .is supported by some interesting recent research. Some researchers like Debray (1975) Watt, Hall and Oiley (1980) have reasoned that if paranoid personality disorder and paranoid disorders are milder varients of paranoid Schizophrenia, then we would expect the frequency of these disorders in biological relatives of people with Schizophrenia to be greater than the frequency in the general population. Since the results of the research studies by above mentioned researchers have not found the paranoid psychoses or paranoid personality disorder to have an increased frequency in the relatives of people diagnosed as having Schizophrenia. These researchers have concluded that paranoid disorders are not a variant of Schizophrenia. In addition Kendler & Hays (1981) have observed that individuals with paranoid psychoses do not have an increased risk of Schizophrenia. Similarly, the Danish adoptions studies have found the same results.

The conclusion that one arrives after going through the above mentioned research studies is as follows:

"While definite conclusions are limited by a small sample size, the various studies cited above suggest that the paranoid psychosis arc distinct from Schizophrenia and is more common that has been believed or reported in the past."

Paranoid disorders should be distinguished from paranoid personality disorder and paranoid Schizophrenia. All three have many similarities in spite of being different disorders. In all three cases there is suspiciousness, hypersensitivity, eccentricities of behaviour and seclusiveness. However, there are important differences which are as follows :

In Paranoid personality Disorder the symptoms consist of unrealistic suspiciousness, hypersensitivity and restricted affect. These are enduring personality traits often recognizable during adolescence and lasting through adult life. Delusional belief are not characteristic of the individuals having paranoid personality disorder.

While some individual with paranoid personality disorder may develop a true paranoid disorder in later life, many do not and some people who do develop a paranoid disorder do not have the signs of the paranoid personality prior to the development of the paranoid.

In paranoid Schizophrenia there are delusions as in the paranoid disorders but these delusions are much more bizzare and fragmented. "The person's thinking and behaviour are much less logical and coherent. Paranoid Schizophrenia occurs in adolescence or early adulthood while the paranoid disorders often begin in middle life.

In paranoid disorders delusions are most characteristic. They have a rigid and fixed false beliefs. They also have delusions of persecution, grandeur or reference or jealousy.

When individuals with paranoid disorders have delusion of persecution they feel as being conspired against, followed, drugged, poisoned or cheated. They may also have delusion of grandeur. These delusions are maintained inspite of the convincing evidence to the contrary. Those with a paranoid disorder can often function reasonably well in society. Since their personality is not significantly affected in areas outside the delusional content.

THEORIES OM THE DEVELOPMENT OF PARANOID DISORDERS

Clinical psychologist, researchers and others have formulated elaborate theories on the causation of paranoid disorders. Most of the theories are based on different theoretical perspectives and do not have much empirical support in their favour.

The following are the most important theoretical formulations of this order.

(1) Freud's Psychoanalytic theory.

(2) Cameron's theory of pseudocommunity.

(3) Lemert's Exclusionary hypothesis.

(4) Paranoid as a learned behaviour disorder.

(5) Shame humiliation theory of Colby.

(6) Additional etiological factor as an explanation.

(1) **Freud's Psychoanalytic Theory:** Freud's theory of paranoid disorder has received a lot of criticism but at the same time is held by a variety of mental health experts. Freud explains the development of paranoid disorder on the basis of defense mechanisms of denial, projection and reaction formation. According to Freud every human being has an unacceptable homosexual impulse which is denied by the conscious mind, this impulse is then hatred an hostility which too is not acceptable to the conscious mind. This opposite emotion of hatred and hostility is then projected on to the motivation of others.

Freud based this view on theory of paranoid disorder on the basis of the analysis of an autobiography of Daniel Schereber who was a judge by profession, who developed paranoid Schizophrenia at the age of 42 and had on off attacks till he died at the age of 69.

Freud's theory 'of paranoid disorder, though widely accepted is also widely criticized because he reasoned from limited data, his generalization were too encompassing and there was lack of empirical foundation to support his theory. Ullman and Krasner (1975), the chief critics of Freuds's views state "while some people might become paranoid from a threat of "latent" homosexuality, it seems unreasonable to suggest that all paranoid behaviours must be by definition a function of this etiology".

(2) **Cameron's Theory of Pseudocommunity**: According to Cameron paranoid disorders develop due to deficiency of basic trust in interpersonal relationship. The cause of this deficiency can be traced to early years in one's life. Cameron found that individual who become-paranoid were unable, in early childhood to, develop a trusting relationship with significant others.

These mistrustful relationships gradually leads to preliminary threat. This preliminary threat can be actual or imagined and leads to selective perceptions which enhance their false belief. This selective perception becomes self-reinforcing *and* gradually leads to preliminary crystallization, whereby the paranoid individual finds meaning in what he perceived to be happening which may actually be an imagined event, phenomenon or relationship. If preliminary crystallization remains for a long period of time it leads to development of pseudocommnunity. The paranoid pseudocommunity is the group of real and imagined people or agencies who the paranoid person perceives as united in a determination to destroy the person's reputation of life. It is a pseudocommunity, because, these people, real or imagined are not actually united against the paranoid. When individuals develop paranoid pseudocommunity they start displaying classic symptosm of paranoid disorders. Paranoid person's responses or actions at this time create problems for others who may direct or compel him to seek psychiatric help.

(3) **Lemert's Exclusionary Hypothesis**: Lemert (1969) has suggested that many paranoid behaviours are to some extent realistic response to real situations. People arc "against me" is not a feeling or belief but is a factual experience which only a paranoid individual experiences due to his certain unique personality traits like cold, aloof, suspicious, hostile, accusatory and blaming etc.

Thus, lemert has drawn attention to the fad that the pàranoid's so called delusion of persecutions may not at all be delusions. His pathological behaviour may not be caused entirely from within. I may not be that he only imagines that people arc against him. The paranoid personality is likely lo be cold, aloof, suspicious, hostile etc. and so thoroughly unlikable. Naturally people avoid aim talk behind his back, confront him to mend his ways or even give him the lable "paranoid". This labelling further spreads his notoriety, and escalates the problem which in turn intensifies his paranoid feeling and behaviours. Thus, according to Lemert the immediate environment around one's self is important in determining whether one will develop paranoid disorder or not.

(4) **Paranoid as a Learned Behaviour Disorder:** Ullman and Krasner have

been the chief proponents of learning theory approach towards the development of paranoid disorders they suggest that paranoid behaviour may have been learned through the process of modelling. This view has also been supported by Bandura and Mischell's Social Learning Theory. According to both of them one learns from one's parents that world is a dangerous place behaves, accordingly so as to avoid hurt. With reinforcement of these behaviours one's sensitivity to environmental stimuli is sharpened. Thus, one misinterprets, when people seem to stare or seem to follow. One's information from the environment is in this way biased through peculiar information processing. Thus, false belief originate through modelling and then become so self-reinforcing that they become ingrained and resistant to change leading towards the development of paranoid disorders.

According to some researchers, individuals who have a 'particular personality traits like cold, aloof, hostile, suspicious etc. can be labelled as "paranoid" by other individuals like friends, relatives or peers and colleagues. The individual usually attracts negative reactions from others in subsequent interactions when once he is labelled as "paranoid" by them, due to the labeling bias and the perceptions of others. This labelling behaviour of others then intermittently reinforce the paranoids delusions of being persecuted. Possible the person generally only imagines that people are having negatively but there is not doubt that sometimes they really are behaving so. This intermittent reinforcement of paranoid's self perception is more powerful than continuous reinforcement would be and the person's delusional belief solidifies leading towards the development of paranoid disorders.

(5) **Shame-Humiliation Theory of Colby**: According to Colby paranoid behaviour is a result of shame and humiliation experience. He proposes that when people are threatened with a possible humiliating experience, they feel shame. The experience of shame also occurs in anticipation of the possible humiliating event and serves as a signal to defend against the humiliation by blaming others. This gradually leads to the development of projection and other behaviours found among paranoid individuals.

Thus, according to Colby people experience shame not only following a humiliating experience but even in anticipation of it, when they are threatened by it. This initial feeling of shame acts as a signal defence against the humiliation by blaming others. In this way he explains defenses against homosexuality and projection of hostile impulses as special cases of the shame humiliation issues. Colby has suggested that parent's use of intense shaming techniques during child rearing is an important factor and therefore, treatment of adult paranoid behaviour should focus on developing a sense of personal adequacy and desensitization to threats of humiliation.

Empirical research in support of this theory is at the present time very sketchy.

(6) **Additional Etiological Factors:** Many researchers have suggested that genetic or bio-chemical factors may play a-n important role in the causation of paranoid disorders. However, little research has been carried out in this area. Some researchers like Synder (1972) have tried to associated biochemical disturbances with paranoid behaviour for e.g. the individual who abuses amphetamines, may develop paranoid like delusions, stereotypic behaviour, visual or auditory hallucinations. Manschrock and Petri (1978) have pointed out that organic issues may be involved in the development of paranoid disorders for e.g. sensory losses, such as deafness, seem at times to be precipitating factor for paranoid ideation. Paranoia is common in elderly, having sensory disorders or disturbances.

TREATMENT OF PARANOID DISORDERS

According to Cameron paranoid disorders are considered among the least amenable to treatment. The major reason for this is that since paranoid individual lack insight, has poor motivation and cannot form trustful relationship with a psychotherapist, treatment for them becomes difficult to carry out. Paranoid individuals become involved in treatment usually at the insistence of some other person or agency a spouse, child, parent, a court or some other social, agency. Therapist may also encounter paranoid individuals in treatment for another issue (e.g. in Couple's therapy or Family Therapy).

Paranoid individuals even in therapy have a reluctant and suspicious restraint to therapy.

Tranquilizers may be prescribed to reduce anxiety but the paranoid person may refuse them due to the suspicion that they are poisons.

Psychotherapy which requires trust building with such patients is difficult, therefore, it is essential that the therapist must be non-threatening, permissive and extremely truthful and honest.

According to Cameron the following factors are important in psychotherapy of paranoids : (1) reduction of anxiety, (2) a detached but interested therapist, (3) an absence of argumentation about the folly of the belief, (4) presentation of a differing viewpoint about reality, and (5) the development of a trusting relationship.

Ullman and Krasner (1975) report Successful attempts to modify paranoid behaviour using approaches based on learning theory, including systematic desensitization and verbal conditioning. Davison (1966) used a verbal labeling process successfully, in which the subject learned relaxation techniques and renamed his experience from "pressure points" to "sensations". In the process of this individual's treatment, major changes seem lo have occurred spontaneously:

Reattribution techniques have also been fruitfully employed in changing delusional behaviour (Johnson, Rosoor Mastrin, 1977). By attribution theory, people attribute "causes" for their own and other's behaviour that are experienced or observed. Sometimes through ignorance, events are attributed to unrealistic or irrational causes. In this techniques the person is helped to reattribute events lo his real and rational causes, and delusions have thus been seen to disappear. However, whether long-standing and insidious delusions can thus be removed is yet to be seen.

9

Affective Disorders

Affective disorders constitute one of the most important and frequently encountered disorders in clinical practice. They range from mild subjective depression to severe psychotic depression or suicidal behaviour. The term "affect" is roughly equivalent to mood or emotion. Inappropriate mood, either extreme elation (as in manic disorder) or depression, is common ineffective disorder. Affective disorders are not new to us, they have been described in the early writings of Egyptians, Greeks, Chinese etc. and are aim commonly described in the literary works of Indian and Foreign authors. Affective disorders have been classified in many ways.

Throughout history, depressive disorders have been noted in literature and described by authors such as Dostoevsky and Shakespeare, as well as by a number of famous historical figures.

Affective disorders have been recognized and written about since the beginning of the history of medicine, Mania and Melancholia was described by Hippo crates in the 4th century B.C. and as early as first century AD. TheGreekPhysicianAretaeusobservedthatManiaanddepressioncanoccurinone individual. Pinel wrote a compelling account of depression. Freud, Kraepelin and Bleuler also wrote on depression and distinguished it from Schizophrenia. The central symptoms of depression are 'sadness, pessimism, and self-dislike, along with a loss of energy, motivation, and concentration." In addition, the depressed individual may often experience crying spells, loss of appetite, weight, sleep, and sexual desire, and a desire to avoid people.

Because of the prevalence of this disorder, and its association with suicide, there has been a recent increase in research directed at delineating its courses and possible treatment. This research, however, has been greatly handicapped because of the lack of a precise and clear definition of depression.

We would first discuss the term 'depression' and describe the symptomatology of depressive disorder including the manic disorder.

Following this, we would discuss the DSM-III classification of depressive disorder. Along with DSM-III we would also discuss the various dimensions or categories of depression which today are no longer classified in DSM-III but which are of historical importance. Among these we would discuss the concept of Involutional Melancholia, the concept of Neurotic-psychotic, endogenous - exogenous depression etc.

Suicide is one important outcome of depression and very often is fatal. We would discuss the nature of suicide and some myths about suicide. We would also discuss the types of suicide and the theoretical viewpoints about the **causes of** suicide.

We would then discuss the various theories of affective disorder. Among the various theories of affective disorder, biological, cognitive and learning theories are important and have come empirical support We would also discuss the Psychoanalytic theory of affective disorder.

Affective disorders can be treated with a wide variety of therapeutic approaches ranging from medical, electro convulsive therapy (ECT) to chemotherapy to psychodynamic and behavioural approaches of psychotherapy. Generally, today the biological, behavioural and psychological approaches are combined together to alleviate depression.

We would discuss these various therapeutic approaches to deal with affective disorders.

We would end this chapter with a few short notes.

DEFINITION OF DEPRESSION

Depressive disorders or depression is one of the most common disorder seen in psychiatric practice. These disorders are more prevalent as compared to Schizophrenia.

Depression involved the disorders of mood, emotion or affect. In this disorder an individual displays mood or emotional disturbances which may range from mild to severe.

In affective (also called as mood disorder or depression) disorder a person experiences a wide variety of symptoms ranging from crying spells, guilt feeling and loss of appetite to suicidal acts and aggressive outbursts.

Depression or affective disorder can be manifested in a wide variety of dimensions and may take many forms. The various dimensions we would discuss in the next section. Here we would describe the symptoms of depression expressed in the depressive phase as well as in the manic phase.

Depressive disorders were once called as Manic depressive disorder, term coined by Kraepelin to characterize all cases in .which there was an abnormally high degree of affect, either Mania alone, depression alone or the combination of two. This term underwent a change and in DSM-III it is called a Major Depression (or major affective disorder) which also may be termed unipolar affective disorder or bipolar affective disorder which can involve episodes of major depression intermixed with episodes of manic (or highly energized) behaviour.

CHARACTERISTIC FEATURES OF DEPRESSIVE DISORDER

We would now the characteristic features of this disorder. The signs and symptoms, vary, depending upon the severity and duration of the disorder.

1. **Disturbances of Mood and Thought** : Some of the most common symptoms of mood and thought disturbances are as follows.

(a) Sandess of mood, (b) Negative self-concept, (c) guilt feelings, (d) Suicidal ideas/threat, (e) feelings of helplessness, worthlessness and hopelessness, (f) difficulties in concentration and thinking etc.

The most prominent features of the manic episode, according to them are as follows:

1. **Elevated mood:** This is the essential "diagnostic" feature of a manic episode. Typically, manic feel wonderful, see the world as a wonderful place, and have limitless enthusiasm for whatever they are doing or plan to do. This euphoria is usually mixed with irritability and in some cases may be overshadowed by it.

2. **Hyperactivity:** The expansive mood is usually accompanied by in-

creased activity physical, social, occupational and often sexual.

3. **Sleeplessness:** The manic episode is almost always marked by a decreased need for sleep. Manics may sleep only two or three hours a night and yet have twice as much energy as those around them.

4. **Talkativeness :** Manics tend to talk loudly, rapidly, and constantly. Their speech is often full of puns, irrelevant details, and jokes that they alone find funny.

5. **Flight of ideas and distractibility :** Thoughts race through the minds of manic patients. (This is one reason for the rapid-fire speech). Furthermore, they are easily distracted. While talking of one thing, they will notice something else in the environment (e.g., a magazine cover, the clothing of a passerby) and abruptly begin talking about that instead.

6. **Inflated self-esteem :** Manics, as noted earlier, tend to see themselves as extremely attractive, important, and powerful people, capable of great achievements in fields in which they may in fact have no talent whatever. Thus, they may begin composing symphonies, designing nuclear weapons, or calling the parliament with advice on how to run the country.

7. **Reckless behaviour:** The euphoria and grandiose self-image of manics often lead them into flamboyant and ill advised actions that they would never have considered in their premanic state: buying stress, reckless driving, careless business investments, sexual indiscretions, and so forth. They usually become quite indifferent to the needs of others and think nothing of yelling in restaurants, spending the family savings on diamond rings, or calling their friends in the middle of the night.

8. **Irritability:** From the heights of their euphoria, manics often see other people as slow, doltish spoilsports and can become quite irritable, even hostile, especially when someone tries to interfere with their behaviour. In some cases irritability may be the manic's dominant mood, with euphoria either intermittent or simply absent (DSM-III, 1980).

Bootzin and Acocella, with respect to depressive disorder have pointed out that the course of a major depressive episode follows a smoother curve than that of a manic episode. Though in some cases a severe psychological trauma may plunge the individual into' depression overnight, the onset is usually gradual, occurring over a period of several weeks or several months. The episode itself topically lasts longer then a manic episode and then ends, as it began, slowly and gradually.

As in a manic episode, the person entering a depressive episode undergoes a radical change in all aspects of his or her functioning not just mood, but also motivation, thinking, and physical and motor functioning. The following are the characteristic features of the major depressive episode according to Bootzin and Acocella:

1. **Depressed mood:** This is the diagnostic feature of the major depressive episodic. Almost all severely depressed adults report some degree of sadness or unhappiness (Beck. 1967), ranging from a mild melancholy to total hopelessness. This dejection may be described by the individual as utter despair, loneliness, or simply boredome. Mildly or moderately depressed people may have frequent crying spells; more severely depressed patients often state that they feel like crying but cannot (Mendels, 1970).

2. **Feelings of worthlessness and guilt :** Depressives are dismayed not only by life but also by themselves. Typically, they regard themselves as deficient in whatever attributes they value most: intelligence, physical attractiveness, health, social skills. Their frequent complaints about loss whether of love, material possessions, money or prestige may also reflect their sense of personal inadequacy (Breed, 1967).

Such feelings of worthlessness are often accompanied by a profound sense of guilt. Depressive exaggerate their present and past failings and seem to search the environment for evidence for problems that they have created. If a child has trouble with school work or the car has a flat tire, it is their fault. Depressives see themselves not only as worthless and guilty but also as lost causes. Deeply depressed people generally regard their condition as irreversible (Sarwer-Foner, 1966); they cannot help themselves, nor can anyone possibly help them. This way of thinking has been characterized as the helplessness-hopelessness syndrome (England,1968).

3. **Reduced motivation :** Depression is almost invariably accompanied by reduced motivation, a loss of interest and pleasure in formerly valued activities. Working, caring for children, even conversing with friends or going to the movies such things no longer seem worth doing.

4. **Disturbances of appetite;** sleep, and sex drive: Depression disrupts not only learned behaviours but also instinctive behaviours above all, sleeping, eating, and sexual responsiveness. Most depressives have poor appetite and lose weight; some, however, especially those who have previously been dieters, react by eating more and putting on weight (Poliyy and Herman, 1976). Insomnia is also common in depression. Awakening too early and then being unable to get back to sleep is the most characteristic pattern, but depressed people may also have trouble falling asleep initially, or they may awaken repeatedly throughout the night. And in some cases, the sleep disturbance, like the appetite disturbance, takes the form of excess rather than deficiency, with the patient sleeping. Fifteen hours a day or more. As for the disturbance or sexual responsiveness that accompanies depression, it is almost invariably in the form

of deficiency. Depressives lose interest in sex just as they lose interest in so many other formerly valued activities.

5. **Psychomotor retardation or agitation :** Depression can usually be "read" immediately in the person's motor behaviour and physical bearing. In the most common pattern, called retarded depression, the patient seems overcome by a massive fatigue and shows little spontaneous activity. Posture is stooped, movement is slow and deliberate, gestures are kept to minimum, and speech is low and halting, with long pauses before answering. In severe cases, depressives may fall into a mute stupor. Much more rarely, the symptoms may take the opposite form, called agitated depression, marked by incessant activity and restlessness-hand writing, pacing, fidgeting, complaining, and moaning.

6. **Reduced energy** : As the characteristic psychomotor retardation suggests, depression is usually marked by a severe reduction in energy level. Without having done anything, the depressed patient may feel exhausted all the time.

7. **Difficulties in thinking:** In depression, mental processes, like physical processes, are usually slowed down. Depressives tend to be- indecisive, and they often report difficulties in thinking, concentrating, and remembering.

8. **Recurrent thoughts of death or suicide**: Not surprisingly, in view of their emotional state, many depressives have recurrent thoughts of death or suicide (Beck, 1967; Harder, 1967; Pichot and Lemperienre, 1964). Often they will say that they (and everyone else) would be better off if they were dead, and as we shall see, some depressed people do in fact kill themselves.

TYPES OF AFFECTIVE DISORDER

The classification of affective disorder has had a long history. The recent history of affective disorder can be clearly traced from the DSM-II. It classified affective disorder into Evolutional Melancholia and major depressive illness. It also distinguishes between psychotic. depressive reaction and depressive neurosis. As contrast to DSM-II, DSM-III (Diagnostic and Statistical Manual of Mental Disorders, 3rd edition) classifies affective disorders into following groups:

(1) **Major Affective Disorders :** In this, there is a full blown affective syndrome. Major affective disorder is a sort of Bipolar disorder in which elation and/or Depression arc characteristic symptoms which are further distinguished by whether or not there has ever been a manic episode.

(2) **Other Specific Affective Disorders** are those disorders where there is only a partial affective syndrome of atleast 2 years duration. Other specific disorders include Cyclothymic Disorder and Dysthymic Disorder.

(3) **Atypical Affective Disorders** is a category for those affective disorders that cannot be classified in .either of the two specific subclasses mentioned above.

Internally or externally caused depression are no longer a major classification, and distinction between neurotic and psychotic depression has been eliminated. In place of Neurotic-Psychotic distinction, DSM-III specifies severity of depression from mild to severe. Also, in DSM-III, Involutional Melancholia is no longer separate diagnosis of depression caused by mid-life changes known as climatic changes.

We would now discuss the following dimensions or types of depression:

(a) Normal grief and psychopathological depression.

(b) Depression-continuity V/s Discontinuity.

(c) Exogenous V/s endogenous depression,

(d) Primary and secondary depression.

(e) Dysthymic disorder.

(f) Unipolar and Bipolar depression.

(g) Involutional Melancholia.

We would discuss the above disorders in brief:

(a) **Normal Grief and Psychopathological depression:** Some degree of depression is an essential and necessary aspect of our life. Complete absence of depression is also one sign of abnormality. Temporary grief reactions to a major loss are considered normal and even healthy. Depression becomes abnormal only when it is experienced to an unproportional degree. In other words a psychopathological condition is considered when the grief reaction leads to excessive self-dislike, inordinate self-blame or a prolonged preoccupation with one's problems. A psychopathological condition is also considered when a grief reaction continues long after its initial onset. The criteria used to distinguish between normal and pathological depression are:

(1) The depth of depression,
(2) The duration of depressive disorder,
(3) The extent to which the depressive reaction is associated with feelings of guilt, worthlessness, delusion and/or hallucinations and (4) The extent to which depression interferes with the normal day-to-day life activities of the individual and his interpersonal relationships.

(b) **Depression - Continuity** V/s **Discontinuity** : There are many controversies with regard to the topic .of depression which has divided psychologists, researchers and psychiatrists to a great extent. One such controversy is with regard to the Continuity V/s Discontinuity theory of e depression. Continuity theorists consider depression as a unitary disorder that occurs in various degrees of severity. The neurotic V/s psychotic controversy theory of depression belongs to continuity theory.

Discontinuity theorists distinguish among different types of depression. The endogenous V/s exogenous controversy of depression belongs to discontinuity theory. We will discuss more about endogenous V/s exogenous depression in the latter section.

Beck (1967) tested the continuity and discontinuity hypothesis by analyzing psychiatrists rating of 50 persons diagnosed as-suffering from neurotic depression and of 50 others suffering from psychotic depression. Two ratings were obtained :(i) First, the psychiatrists rated whether each of the 17 clinical signs was present or absent in each case and (ii) secondly, they rated whether each of the 17 clinical signs was present or absent to severe degree.

Discontinuity theory predicts that the clinical signs present in neurotic depression should differ from those present in psychotic depression. Continuity theory predicts that same clinical signs should be present in both neurotic and psychotic depression but psychotic depression should be associated with the presence of those signs into a more severe degree.

Beck found that all 17 signs of depression were present in both neurotic and psychotic depression and that psychotic depression is a more severe disorder. These findings support continuity theory.

Proponents of discontinuity theory claim support for their position both from factor analytic studies of symptomatology and from therapy outcome studies. They also claim support from clinical reports that different therapies have different degrees of effectiveness for neurotic and psychotic depression. Electro-convulsive therapy for e.g. is reported to be more effective for psychotic depression than for neurotic depression and some drugs are reported to be more effective for neurotic depression than for psychotic depression. The evidence for the differential effects of treatment is unconclusive at present.

The continuity-discontinuity debate seems likely to continue until knowledge about etiologies is more conclusive. It seems that the continuity position would be confirmed if neurotic and psychotic depressions have common etiologies. Similarly, the discontinuity position would be confirmed if they have different etiologies.

(c) **Exogenous V/s Endogenous Depression :** Exogenous depression is presumed to be caused by external factors originating outside the body. External factors generally include financial or personal losses. It can be death of a dear one, loss of employment, business, divorce etc. Sometimes exogenous depression is also called as reactive depression, because it occurs as a reaction to some environmental cause.

Endogenous depression arises from within the individual and has no external factor contributing to it. In other words, the term endogenous depression refers to relatively severe depressive behaviour that is neither preceded by a predisposing nor precipitating environmental stress nor influenced by subsequent changes in the environment. According to Winokur (.1979) endogenous depressions are primarily due to dysfunctions of physiology and biochemistry.

Some believe (Klerman and Paykel 1970) that endogenous exogenous distinction, like the psychotic-neurotic primarily reflects severity rather than any real difference in kind.

(d) **Primary and Secondary Depression**: This is another distinction with respect to depression. Robins and Guze (1972) and Winokur (1972) have proposed that depression should be classified as primary V/s secondary.

Primary depression is diagnosed when depressive episodes occur in persons with no previous history of psychopathology except for previous episodes of mania or depression. The primary category provides a group that is symptomatically pure for depression.

Secondary depression is diagnosed when depressive episodes occur in persons with a previous history of psychopathology other than depression or mania. Such a distinction helps the diagnosticians and other mental health experts to plan appropriate therapeutic interventions.

(c) **Dysthymk Disorder** is a term that is synonymous with the term "neurotic depression". The term dysthymic disorder originated from DSM-III. Mehr (1983) considers this term to be very obscure, The essential feature in this disorder is a chronic disturbance of mood involving either depressed mood or loss of interest of pleasure in all, or almost all, usual activities and pastimes. Dysthymic Disorder is of moderate symptomatology. Psychotic symptoms are not present, and there is little likelihood of other severe symptoms such as motor retardation and psychomotor retardation.

The Diagnostic Criteria for Dysthymic Disorder as given in DSM-III are as follows:

A. During the past two years (or one year for children and adolescents)the individual has been bothered most or all of the time by symptoms characteristic of the depressive syndrome but that are not of sufficient severity and duration to meet the criteria for a major depressive episode.

B. The manifestation of the depressive syndrome may be relatively persistent or separated by periods of normal mood lasting few days to a few weeks, but no more than a few months at a time.

C. During the depressive periods there is either prominent depressed mood or marked loss of interest or pleasure in all, or almost all usual activities and pastimes.

D. During the depressive period at least three of the following symptoms are present:-

(i) Insomnia or hypersomnia.

(ii) Low energy level or chronic tiredness.

(iii) Feelings of inadepuacy, loss of self-esteem or self-depreciation.

(iv) Decreased effectiveness or productivity at school, worker home.

(v) Depressed attention, concentration or ability to think clearly.

(vi) Social withdrawal.

(vii) Loss of interest in or enjoyment of pleasurable activities.

(viii) Irritability or excessive anger (in children) expressed towards parents (or care-takers)

(ix) Inability to respond with apparent pleasure to praise or rewards.

(x) Less active or talkative than usual or feels slowed down or restless.

(xi) Pessimistic attitude towards the future, brooding about past events or feeling sorry for self. .

(xii) Tearfulness or crying.

(xiii) Recurrent thoughts of death or suicide.

E. Absence of psychotic features such as hallucinations, delusions, incoherence or fear of loosening of associations.

(F) **Unipolar and Bipolar Depression** :

(a) *Unipolar Depression* : In unipolar depression, the individual experiences only depression with no other type of mood change or with no manic phase. When an individual suffers from unipolar depression, he displays all those symptoms of depression that are mentioned in Q 11.1 of this chapter under the title characteristics of affective disorders, depressive disorder. Please refer to it. Unipolar depression can be exogenous or endogenous. Exogenous depression is also called as reactive depression and occurs as a reaction to environmental or external factors. Endogenous depression arises from factors within the body and is primarily due to dysfunctions of physiology and biochemistry. Unipolar depression has a good prognosis.

(b) *Bipolar Depression :* Falls in the category of Major Affective Disorder. Whereas Major depression is confined to depressive episodes. Bipolar disorder, as the name suggests, involves both manic and depressive episodes.

In the usual case bipolar disorder will first appear in the form of a manic episode. The subsequent episodes may occur in any one of a number of different patterns.

Bipolar affective disorder was earlier called as Manic Depressive Psychoses, a term introduced in 1899 by Kraeplin, who described the disorder as a series of attacks of elation and depression with periods of relative normality in between and generally a favourable prognosis. Bipolar disorder can be mixed, having only manic or depressed clinical behaviour. The symptoms of depressive phase are more or less similar to what we have seen in unipolar depression. The following are the most common symptoms found in manic phase of Bipolar Disorder.

(1) There is a feeling of optimism and elation, speeding up of thought processes. He is energetic, loud and boisterous.

(2) He shows impaired ability to concentrate, is easily distracted and changes rapidly from one trend of thought and activity to another.

(3) Judgement is impaired, sexual and other behavioural restraints are lowered and the individual tends to be extremely impatient With any attempts to restrain his activities.

(4) Delusions of grandeur is also common symptom in many manic individuals.

Coleman considers manic behaviour to be of three types depending upon its severity. These three type of manic behaviour are hypomania, acute mania and . delirious mania.

(g) **Involutional Melancholia** : Involutional Melancholia is a depression of middle and later life which may be manifested in worry, guilt, anxiety, agitation, or paranoid and other delusional ideas. These reactions are often accompanied by gastrointestinal or other somatic complaints which may progress to delusions.

About 4 per cent of all first admissions to mental hospitals are diagnosed as involutional reactions. The disturbance is found more frequently in women than in men; it accounts for 7 per cent of female first admissions, and 2 per cent of male first admissions. The median age at admission is fifty-one for women, and fifty-five for men. A range from forty to sixty five years covers 90 per cent of all first admissions with this psychotic reaction.

While the onset of the disease is usually gradual, it may be precipitated suddenly by some distressing experience. The patient is depressed, expressing ~ persistent fears concerning both his past and future. Hypochondriacally and nihilistic delusions may be present, and there is substantial danger of attempted suicide. Patients may have delusions of guilt over unpardonable sins and may blame themselves for the evils of the world. They are restless, anxious, sleepless, and have unprovoked spoils of weeping. Their intellectual ability is not noticeably affected:

Agreement on the causation of involutional reactions is lacking, though several theories have been offered. A list of theories follows:

1. Involutional melancholia and the menopausal syndrome occur at the same time, but the biological factors play an aggravating role rather than a causative one. This is evident from the fact that no physiological changes have been observed in patients with involutional reactions that are not found in normal people during the climacteric.

2. Of primary psychological importance arc the patient's reactions to his loss of social status and personal security, which may be dependent on physical vigor and arc therefore, threatened by the physical decline during the involutional period.

3. The involutional reaction is more likely to occur in persons having a certain constellation of personality traits (shyness, rigidity, frugality, over consciousness, and inhibition). Such persons usually have a compulsive sense of duty, a narrow range of interests, few friends, and overly strict moral principles.

4. Involutional melancholics usually show a history of failure or unsatisfactory achievement, with the feeling that life is "almost over" and there is no "second chance." Major differences between invointional melancholia and the other types of affective psychosis lie in the age of onset of depression and the lack of significant history of depressive episodes (Akiskal & Webby 1983). Occurring three times more frequently in females between the ages of 50 and 60 and males between the ages of 60 and 70. 'In women, the onset of the disorder usually follows menopause by a maximum of seven or eight years.

Generally, as involutional melancholia develops, people begin to experience periods of insomnia and feelings of inner tension. They may become easily fatigued, both mentally and physically, and show a reduced need for food or sexual activity. Fears for personal health and complaints of a continuous headache arc frequent. Gradually, the person with involutional melancholia may develop a sense of despondency accompanied by constant weeping and loss of interest in favourite activities. As involutional melancholia deepens, insomnia worsens, weight loss increases, and numerous bodily ills may be imagines. The person typically presents a picture of extreme sadness mixed with agitation, often in the form of hand-writing, pacing, repeated pleas for help, and self-deprecating statements. In severe cases, the person may experience, delusions of guilt and bodily changes.

NATURE OF SUICIDE

Suicide is one outcome of affective disorder and is on the increase. Suicide is not only a result of depression it can also occur due to many other factors or causes.

There is a difference between 'suicide' and 'attempted suicide'. In the former, individuals succeed in this act and take their lives, whereas, in the attempted suicide they are not killed. As compared to men, women attempt more suicide, whereas, men actually succeed and kill themselves more than women, violent methods are more likely to be used by men than women. Accurate statistics on suicide are difficult to obtain because many suicides are shown as accidental deaths. In recent years suicide has increased in the younger age group, especially those between 15-24 years.

FACTORS RESPONSIBLE FOR SUICIDE

Psychologists and other observe is have suggested a number of factors that may be responsible for suicide. These factors are:

(a) rising divorce rate,

(b) The effect of parental divorce on adolescent,

(c) fear about the future (i.e. marriage, unemployment, housing problem etc.,) and

(d) stress stemming from school or parental pressure. Garfintel et.al. (1982) on the basis of their study of suicide attempts recently concluded- that suicidal young people often have real problems, and these problems very often have their roots in their parent's problems. In their study they found that suicide attempiers had more experience with substance abuse, more history of psychiatric disorder and more prior psychopathology. In addition, the families of the attempters had more psychiatric disorder, more history of suicide, more parental unemployment and more parental absence whether through death or divorce.

SOME MYTHS OR MISCONCEPTIONS ABOUT SUICIDE

Through the years a number of popular misconceptions have evolved concerning suicide. Investigators such as Pokorny and Shrieidman have listed a number of these. Some of them areas follows :

(1) *If people talk about committing suicide, they will not do it.* The fact is that in roughly three-quarter of all successful suicides the person communication his or her intent beforehand, within a few months of the fatal attempt.

(2) Another misconception completely opposite of the above is *if people think of committing suicide they are likely lo do it.* Majority of the people who think of committing suicide do not necessarily take their lives.

(3) *Whenever depressed people begin to feel better, the risk that they will kill themselves decreases.* Recently Faiberow (1974) pointed out that suicides sic often initiated when the persons begin to recover from a severe depression. A great many people, especially deeply depressed c patients attempt suicide after their mood appears to be getting better.

(4) *People have to be psychotic to kill themselves* is one of the most irrational myths that may people have. Even though most individuals who commit suicide are extremely unhappy, the majority of these individuals are in touch with reality are irrational and are not psychotic.

(5) *People who have attempted suicide and failed were not serious about ending their lives.* Studies have shown that in about 75 per cent of completed suicides, attempts or threats had been earlier.

(6) *Suicides occur much more frequently at certain times of the year such as Christmas, during stormy weather or during the full moon:* There is as yet no conclusive evidence to substantiate such claims.

(7) *Suicide is inherited:* This is another misconception. Many believe that suicide runs in families for e.g. If a mother has committed suicide it is assumed that her children are also likely to commit suicide.

(8) *Suicides are usually committed without warning :* Shriedman argues that many warning sings exist, including depression, statement that the world would be better off without the potential suicide victim.

(9) *Religion is a protection against suicide :* This is another most common myth. Many believe that religious people are less likely to commit suicide as compared to those who are not much religious or who arc atheists.

(10) *To commit suicide is a sign of insanity.* Even though most individuals who commit suicide are extremely unhappy: the majority of these individuals are in touch with reality, are rational, and arc not psychotic.

(11) An *individual with a terminal physical illness is unlikely lo commit suicide :* The awareness that one is going to die soon does not preclude the possibility of suicide. In one study of patients with malignant tumors, Farberow, Shneidman, and Leonard (1963) found that suicides are committed by patients who may have only a few hours or days to live.

THEORIES OF SUICIDE

Suicidal behaviour has been explained from a wide variety of theoretical perspectives. Some of the theories areas follows :

(a) **Psychoanalytic theory :** Psychoanalysts employ an extension of the psychoanalytic theory of depression to account for suicide. It is assumed that when an individual loses someone for whom he or she had ambivalent love-bate, feelings; and with whom he or she has partially identified, the hate feelings and resultant aggression may be directed inward. If these hate feelings are strong enough, the resulting "anger-in" may prompt an individual lo commit suicide.

The individual is not so much killing himself or herself as killing the other person. The ambivalence of many suicidal individuals about taking their own lives is assumed to be the result of the ambivalent love-bate feelings toward the lost person and, as a result of introjection, toward themselves. Such hostility- aggressive impulses were believed to be produced by the thanatos, or death instinct, which, if directed inward, would prompt an individual to take his or her own life.

This psychoanalytic view of suicide has not, however, been demonstrated to be valid, and has not led to the development of an effective treatment procedure "for dealing with suicide.

(b) **Menninger's view of suicide**: The influential and highly regarded psychiatrist Karl Meninger wrote a book in the 1930s entitled "Man Against Himself", which, among other things, describes bow the act of suicide is on a continuum with lesser self-destructive behaviours such as self-mutilation, persistent abuse of alcohol and dangerous drugs, and disregard of personal health requirements. With this viewpoint, the concept of suicide is not confined to self-murder. Ending one's life is simply the ultimate and quickest form of self-destructive behaviour. There are degrees or levels of self-destructive behaviour, with a variety of life-threatening acts that are less lethal, and slower-acting, than suicide.

Menninger (1963) later elaborated on the psychological motives for suicide. Regarding the kinds of suicide, he wrote:

"There are accidental suicides, there are suicides which are substitutes for murder, there are suicides which are a cry for help, and suicides which are miscarriages of an attempt to get oneself rescued. But some suicides are also expressions of total despair and ruthlessly directed at one's own self annihilation. The essence of this ultimate form of suicide is the disintegration of the ego and the overwhelmine of the organism with self directed destructiveness."

Menninger indicates that suicides are frequently acts of revenge. He suggests that the suicidal individual may wish to make the survivor feel guilty and remorseful over the suicide (e.g., "Now you will be sorry that you weren't kinder to me"). Suicide may also be a response to anticipated rejection, a flight from humiliation and feelings of inadequacies. Finally, Menninger indicates that there are certain suicides motivated by the belief that death will result in a "magic revival" or a rebirth.

These views are based on clinical impressions. It will be necessary to determine whether they are empirically supported and can lead to the development of a comprehensive model to use for the prediction, prevention, and or treatment of suicidal behaviour.

(c) **Sociological perspective of suicide** : The French sociologist Emile Durkheim (1897) made one of the first extensive assessments of suicide. He suggested that suicide should not be viewed as the act of an isolated individual, but as an act of an individual within a social context. He analyzed the records of suicide from various countries and during different historical periods. On the basis of his analysis, he categorized three different types of self-destructive behaviour. (i) Anomic suicide occurs when there is a sudden change in the normal functioning of an individual's society. For example, following the wall Street stock marketcrash in 1929, many persons affected by this financial disaster committed suicide because they believed they would no longer be able to continue the lives they had grown accustomed to. *(ii)* Egoistic suicide is committed by an individual who is not integrated into the society. For example, the "longer" who has no ties with others in society lacks social support during periods of stress that might precede a suicidal attempt. Feeling alone and isolated, this individual sees no other alternative but to take his or her own life. *(iii)* Altruistic suicide is committed in response to an accepted and value system of the individual's culture. The practice *of hara-kiri* in Japan and the suicide missions of Japanese Kamikaze pilots during World War I belong to this category. More recently, the self immolations of Buddhist monks during the Vietnam War also fit this category.

Durkheim's sociological framework, while providing a useful descriptive and categorization system, is limited because it does not adequately explain the different reactions of individuals who are exposed to the same demands and stressors within a given society. Not all the people who were financially ruined by the wall Street crash committed anomic suicide. Likewise, not all Buddhist monks committed altruistic suicide during the Vietnam War. Durkheim did recognize the importance of taking into account individual differences, and proposed that the temperament or emotional state of a person would interact with social factors to produce suicide. However, he did not make a systematic attempt to delineate those individual temperament factors proposed to be important. As a result, the sociological orientation cannot be used to predict which of many individuals will commit suicide in response to the same social situation.

(d) **The Behavioural Perspective** is best represented in the work of Ullman and Krasner (1975). According to them self destruction is the result of a particular shift in the persons pattern of reinforcements. The essential feature of this new "suicidal" pattern is the person's estimate of his or her current life situation as having no adequate source of reinforcement. Thus, suicide results from the real, anticipated, or fantasized loss of highly valued reinforcers-job, health, friends, family, and so on.

At the same time that such persons except no further reinforcements from their lives, they may find the thought of death possively reinforcing, in that it will make-the people they leave behind feel sorry for them and will punish with remorse those they feel have hurt them. In other words, such persons may see death as bringing them a number of things they want: attention, pity, and revenge. Thus, from a behavioural standpoint, suicide appears less of an enigma than it does to the Freudians. Like any other behaviour, it involves a movement away from non-reinforcing situations and toward reinforcing situations. In accordance with this interpretation, the behaviourists would treat the suicidal patient, like the depressed patient, by attempting to increase his or her rate of reinforcement.

(f) **The Humanistic Existential Perspective**: The humanists and existentialists place great emphasis on the individual's confrontation with death. Infact, May (1958) suggests that death is the fact that gives life absolute value. He quotes a person in therapy: "I know only two things - one, that I will be dead, someday, two, that I am not dead now. The only question is what shall I do between those two points". In other words, our knowledge of the inevitability of death allows us to take life in earnest and use it to pursue our greatest potential. Suicide, in this view, is an act of waste and defeat, for it eliminates the possibility of realizing one's potential. Indeed, Boss (1976) claims that all "suicides are proceeded by "an existential partial suicide" in which individuals isolate themselves from others, abrogate their responsibilities, and cease pursuing genuine values in life. Thus, the actual suicide is simply the last in a series of inauthentic choices.

Humanistic-existential therapy-for suicidal patients would focus on bringing them to at till realization of their current existence, in the hope that they would find enough meaning in their lives to begin living more authentically. The therapist would also try to draw patients' attention to their potentialities and thus give them some reason to go on living.

VARIOUS THEORIES OF AFFECTIVE DISORDER

A great deal of research, today, is underway to find out and clarify the etiology of Affective Disorders. Number of theories have been put forward. Some important among them are as follows :

(1) Psychoanalytic theory (2) Lewinsohn's learning theory (3) Seligman's theory of depression of learned helplessness (4) Beck's cognitive theory or depression (5) Genetic theory or depression (6) Biochemical factors in 3 affective disorder (7) Integrative view of Affective Disorder.

(1) **Psychoanalytic Theory:** Abraham, in 1911, attempted to interpret depression through psychoanalytic theorizing. In 1917 Freud wrote a classic paper titled "Mourning and Melancholia". This paper was an elaboration of Abraham's view.

Freud and his student Karl Abraham proposed that the major difference between normal mourning and depression is emotional self-centredness, Freud ' assumed that the cause of serious depression develops during the oral period, if an infant's needs are frustrated. Freud proposed that cither deprivation or overindulgence could arrest personal development at oral dependent state. As a consequence of oral fixation, Freud believed, the person would be dependent on others for self-evaluation. In addition Freud assumed that the dependent personality, coupled with later loss of a loved one. would generate serious depression.

Freud proposed that following the actual or symbolic loss of a loved one, oral dependent individuals identify with the lost person and incorporate the grief, love and anger into themselves. He argued that identification, with lost loved one leads to self-blame, self-hate and depression. Thus Freud conclude that anger and grief at the loss are turned inward and the person punished himself or herself by guilt and depression.

Later psychoanalytic writers have greatly modified Freud's early conceptions. Many have stressed the concept of self esteem. These later psychoanalytic theorists have conceptualized depressive individuals as one, who have not fully differentiated themselves from introjected objects (parents) and who cannot maintain their self-esteem unless it is continually bolstered from outside sources (symbolic of the support of the parent in childhood). When these external sources of self-esteem are lost, the individual no longer has a sources of value and becomes depressed.

There has been little or no research assessing the validity of psychoanalytic theory regarding depression. Of the small amount of research that has been conducted, Mendels (1970) has found little evidence to support any of these approaches. In spite of the lack of supporting research the psychoanalytic conception of the affective disorder particularly for the dysthymic and cyclothymic disorders- remains influential in the thinking of many clinicians.

(2) **Lewinsohn's Learning Theory:** Frester was on the first learning theorists to point out the depression is a "function of inadequate or insufficient reinforcers". He further points out that depressed people have a low frequency of behaviour which is most likely to be elicited by positive reinforcement.

In recent years Lewinsohn (1974) has been actively involved in empirically testing and extending the reduced reinforcement conceptualization of depression. Lewinsohn also points to the importance of a lack of appropriate social skill in the development of depression. He defines social skills as the "emission of behaviours which are positively reinforced by others" and notes that if an individual lacks social skills it will significantly limit the availability of positive reinforces in his or her immediate environment leading to depression.

(3) **Seligman's Depression and Learned Helplessness Theory:** The learned helplessness theory of depression is in many ways analogous to cognitive theory except that it incorporates some learning principles. Seligman and colleagues have proposed that the central feature of reactive depression is a fatalistic belief that the central feature of reactive depression is a fatalistic belief that there is nothing one can do to control the important events in one's life i.e.

person's belief that control over environment is impossible.

There is a major difference between Seligman's learned helplessness model and Lewinsohn's learning model, which emphasizes a reduced positive reinforcement concept of depression. Lewinsobn's model is evidentially noncognitive in nature and assumes that mood is directly related to how overt behaviour is reinforced. In contrast, Seligman's mode] is more cognitive because it emphasizes the person's perception of the controllability of events in the environment.

(4) **Beeks Cognitive Theory of Depression :** In recent years many theorists including Albert Ellis, Valins and Nisbett, Aron T. Beck etc. have viewed depression as a result of negative cognitions or thoughts.

Beck points out that depression is a result of cognitive disorder. According to him affective, psychomotor and motivational disturbances of depression are secondary consequences of a primary cognitive disturbance.

Beck (1967) described the predisposing conditions in depression as a primary trial of cognitive patterns which are as follows :

(1) Tendency to interpret interaction with the environment as representing defeat, deprivation or disparagement. The person exaggerates minor setbacks as total failures.

(2) A second cognitive factor is that of low self-esteem, a tendency to view oneself as inadequate, unworthy of love, or otherwise defective in physical, mental or moral attributes.

(3) A third cognitive pattern is that of helplessness and hopelessness. Depressed people tend to view their suffering as unavoidable and see the future as a life of unending hardships and failures.

Such a triad of cognitive patterns makes an individual vulnerable to stresses such as. criticism, failure, setbacks etc. and leads to depression.

Beck has further pointed out that as a result of certain enduring illogical thought processes, individuals develop "depressogenic schemeta" which makes depression a vicious circle. Early in the childhood we develop certain false, irrational and perfectionist attitudes and ways of behaviour which control our present thought processes and make our perceptions and thinking disturbed leading to self blame, self-devaluation and low self-esteem which Causes depression.

Beck described several logical errors committed by depressed people in interpreting reality. They are:

(a) *Arbitrary Inference* : Depressed people draw conclusions in the absence of sufficient evidence or of any evidence at all. A student, for e.g. who gets a second class in the annual exams even after studying very hard and extensive coaching concludes that he will never get first class and that he is worthless person or to take another example, a girl whose husband dies within a week of her marriage, concludes that she is unlucky.

(b) *Selective Abstractions on* the basis of a minor incident or detail a person draws certain sweeping conclusion ignoring the whole context or experience. For-e.g. if a person is not able to give one answer properly in the exam he concludes that his exam was not good and he has done very poorly or perhaps he may not succeed in clearing the exam. In other words person focuses overtly on his minor fault and ignores other important relevant details.

(c) *Overgeneralization* is very much related to selective abstraction. Depressed persons have a tendency to draw an overall sweeping conclusion on the basis of a single, perhaps trival, event. For e.g. if a girl asked for a date which the boy turns down, the girl concludes that she is not attractive.

(d) *Magnification and Minimization :* Depressed people have a tendency to minimize strengths and magnify their weaknesses.

(e) *Inexact labelling* 'Depressed individuals tend to lable events or experiences, in exaggerated term life I am the 'worst', 'weakest', 'stupid', 'biggest failure' etc.

Most of the supporting evidence for Beck's approach is correlational. Many studies have consistently demonstrated that depressives conceptualize their experiences and themselves in these illogical ways.

(5) Genetic theory of depression: There has been a number of studies that suggest the presence of genetic factors in affective disorders, especially in Manie Depressive psychoses (new called as Bipolar Disorder II).

In the early 1950s Kallmann (1953) asserted that there was a genetic basis for affective disorder but soon afterwards, interest in genetic research seemed to wane. However, recently, a number of investigations point out to the possible influence of genetic mechanisms in the causation of affective disorder.

Research on the genetic factors in depression has very often used the twin and family methods and has typically focused on bipolar and unipolar depression.

Long ago, Winokur (1967) found that affective disorders occurred with greater frequency, in the first degree relative (parents, children and siblings) of a group of patients with affective disorders than they did in a control group. Rosenthal (1970) reviewed a series of studies in which it was found that first degree relatives were approximately ten times more likely, than the members of the general population, to be diagnosed as manic-depressive. Also in are view of genetic research on manic depressive psychoses in twins, Price (1927) reported that 66 out of 97 monozygotic (identical) twin pairs were concordant (i.e. who suffered from the disorder) for this disorder, while only 27 out of 119 dizygotic (fraternal) with pairs were concrordant for the disorder. Alien et. al. in 1974 remarked that "many investigators have found a much higher prevalence of affective disorders among close relatives of individuals who suffer affective disorder than in general population". Although these Findings are not conclusive evidence, they do strongly suggest that some genetic factor may play a role in the development of affective disorder, especially in the manic depressive disorders.

(6) Biochemical Factors in Affective Disorders : Growing research evidence points out to the fact that biochemical changes may be one of the major causes of affective disorders because administration of certain substances in certain proportions increase or decreases manic or depressive symptomatology.

At present there are three major theories that point out that affective disorder is a result of changes in our biochemistry.

(1) The first is that depression may be due to imbalances in the level of hoimones and particularly of sex hormones. For e.g. Mendels (1969) argues that the fact that involutional melancholia occur at a time of change in the sex-hormone levels would be seem to indicate a link between affective disorder and these hormones. Reports that oral contraceptives, which contain sex hormones, known to have a sedative effect on the central nervous system, have caused depression in some women, have been cited in support of this hypothesis.

(2) A second theory is that depression may originate in imbalances in sodium and potassium levels. It appears that the proper transmission of electrical impulses from neuron to neuron within the nervous system depends on a highly delicate balance in the distribution of sodium and potassium inside and outside the nerve cells. If this balance/becomes disturbed, so too will the functioning of the nervous system. And, in fact, a number of studies (e.g. Shaw 1966, Coppen 1967) have indicated that psychotic depression is often accompanied by abnormally high sodium levels and that these levels tend to return to their normal state after recovery. Furthermore Coppen (1967) has shown that lithium salts, which on many occasions have been used successfully in the treatment of affective disorders, may achieve their effects by reducing the patient's sodium levels.

(3) A final biochemical hypothesis has to do with changing levels of amines, a type of body chemical. It is widely believed that two groups of amines the catecholamines and the indolamines, both of which facilitate the transmission of impulses between nerve fibers-play a role in the etiology of depressive illness. According to the "catecholamine hypothesis", depression is caused by a deficiency and mania by an excess of catecholamines and particularly of one catecholamine known as norepinephrine (Schild Krant 1965). More specifically this theory holds that too much nor epinephrine results in over stimulated nerve Fibres and consequently in the over excitability of mania. Conversely too little norepinephrine leads to under stimulated nerve Fibres and hence to under excitability of depression.

Integrative view of Affective Disorder : While Psychoanalytic, Learning, Biological, Biochemical, Humanistic etc. theories can explain some aspects of the affective disturbances, no one approach seems complete enough to account for the variety of observed-patterns.

For example, some depressions are clearly caused by life stresses such as the death of a loved one, but there are other depressive episodes for which there seems to be no identifiable psychosocial or environmental cause. In an attempt to overcome these and other problems brought about by the limitations of the single-factor paradigms, researchers such as Akishkal and Mckinney (1973,1975) and Anisman and Zacharko (1982) have proposed integrative models of affective disorders.

In Akishkal and Mckinney's integrative model depression is defined as the outcome of an interaction among three levels of function: the experiential, the biochemical, and the behavioural. As seen in Figure 11.2, severe affective symptoms are seen as a biological final common pathway reflection a variety of interacting experiences and events. As Figure 11.3 shows, the initial cause of an affective disturbance may be biological and/or psychosocial. For instance, \psychosocial stress in the form of adult object loss, physical disease, learned helplessness, and the like can begin the process of depression. Also, however, these same symptoms can begin as a result of a genetic predisposition to develop the disorder. Even with their different sources, Aksihkal and Mckinney note that once depressive reactions have begun, they are biologically mediated in the same way. Hence, deficits in nor epinephrine and abnormal levels of serotonin are Kkely to be present whether a particular depression is physiologically, psychosocially, environmentally, or genetically based. In another interactive view of affective disturbance, Anisman and Zacharko have integrated the biological and systems views. They agree with Akishkal and Mckinney that neurotransmitter dysfunctions are a final common pathway for affective symptoms. They state further that these neurochemical problems are produced by the effects of stressful life events on neurobiochemistry.

Figure 11.2 : Multilevel causes of Depression which include experimental, chemical and behavioural factors

Experimental	Chemical	Behavioural
Nonrelatedness Anhedonia hopelessness loss of control	Alteration in functional level catechotamines and indoleamines. Electrolyte disturbance.	Disturbance in sleep or appetite. Psychomotor dysfunction (slowing or agitation)

Figure 11.3: Depression : An Integrated View

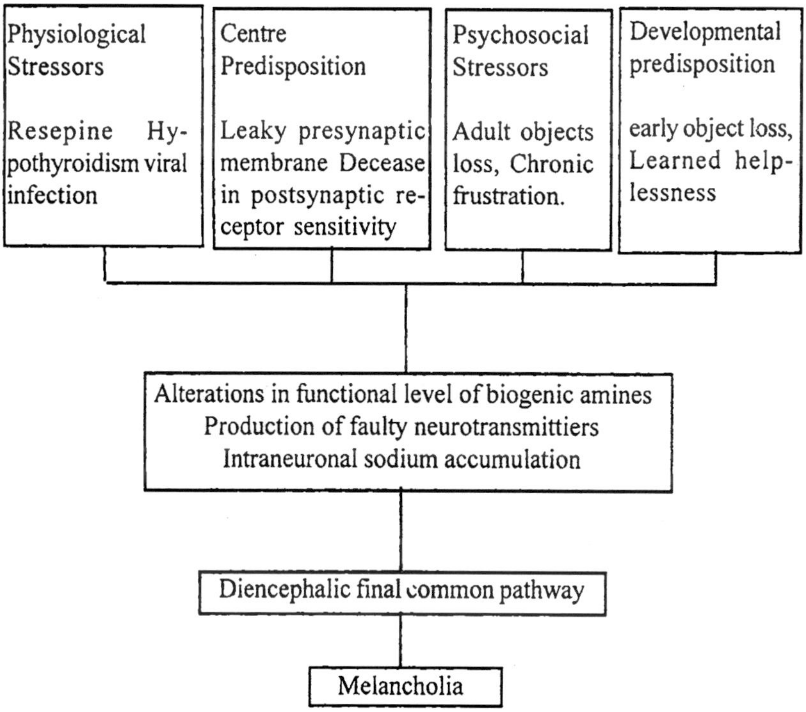

Physiological Stressors	Centre Predisposition	Psychosocial Stressors	Developmental predisposition
Resepine Hypothyroidism viral infection	Leaky presynaptic membrane Decease in postsynaptic receptor sensitivity	Adult objects loss, Chronic frustration.	early object loss, Learned helplessness

Alterations in functional level of biogenic amines
Production of faulty neurotransmittiers
Intraneuronal sodium accumulation

Diencephalic final common pathway

Melancholia

Affective disorders can be treated with a wide variety of therapeutic approaches ranging from medical electro convulsive therapy (ECT) to chemotherapy to psychodynamic and behavioural approaches and psychotherapy. Generally, today the biological, behavioural and psychological approaches are combined together to alleviate depression,

I. Biological Theraples

(a) **Electro Convulsive Therapy (ECT) :** Among the Biological treatments ECT and Drug treatment are the most common and effective. We will study more about the ECT in the last chapter which is solely devoted to the therapeutic aspect of abnormal behaviour. Briefly speaking, ECT has a long history of use in Psychological disorders. It was originally developed to treat Schizophrenic disorders because it was discovered that the incidence of Schizophrenia is less in individuals having epileptic disorders. Hence it was reasoned that if epileptic seizures *ate* produced artificially (by giving ECT) Schizophrenic disorder will disappear, the ECT works well not only with Schizophrenic patient but also with affective disorders. It has been used very frequently with good results, with severely depressed individuals, who have suicidal thoughts, and with uncontrollable aggressive manics, having homicidal tendencies. The precise therapeutic mechanism of ECT is not known, all that is known is that it works. Recently Avery and Winokur (1976-1978) too, noted that ECT reduces the risk of suicide in depressed patients. However, ECT has been severely criticized as the barbaric form of treatment. Many have criticized this technique for producing temporary memory loss and other side-effects. However, in spite of its drawbacks, its clinical use is very frequent. It has been noted by many that properly administered ECT is associated with very low morbidity and mortality. The success rate is quoted by some as greater than 90%.

(b) **Drug therapy** : Medication has proved to be very useful in the treatment of severe depression. The anti-depressant drugs alleviate mood and shorten the duration of the depressive episode in the majority of the cases. The effective, use of medication is dependent upon the diagnostic precision of the disorder. A major depression is treated differently as compared to bipolar depression. For example; in major depression only antidepressant will suffice whereas in bipolar disorder a combination of lithum and antidepressant is used.

The two most important antidepressants are the Tricyclic antidepressants 3, and Monoamine Oxidose Inhibitors (MAOI). The tricycles are the favorite and most common drugs to be used, the most common tricyclic being imipramine and amitriptyline. These drugs have to be started gradually and it takes lime to be effective. Full therapeutic effectiveness usually is seen after two to six weeks of treatment. Tricyclics do not provide immediate relief, hence for immediate relief ECT is used. Many of these drugs have potent anticholinergic effects like dryness of mouth, blurred vision, dizziness,-urinary retention, sedation, gastroinicstinal disturbances, constipation and involuntary tremors.

Besides tricyclic antidepressants, Monoamine Oxidose Inhibitors (MAOI) are sometimes used to treat depression. However, these medications (MAOI) are complicated to prescribe because their toxic effects are dangerous as compared to tricyclics. MAOI potentates sympathomimetic agents, in the diet and interact with numerous other medication. Hence, they have to be used carefully and with certain restrictions.

Lithum carbonate is used in the treatment of manic disorders of Bipolar disorders. Recently Fiene (1971) pointed out that lithum salt is highly effective in reducing the exaggerated mood of mania in 80 per cent or the persons who take it. Again, this drug should be used very carefully because it has dangerous side- effects which range from nausea and vomiting to seijure, coma and even death.

Many stimulants are also available which can easily alleviate depression. However, they are not recommended by physicians because "tolerance" develops quickly and side effects at high doses are numerous.

II. Psychotherapeutic Approaches:

Psychological approaches are quite diverse and are generally used in combination with biological therapies. The right type of psychological approach to be used depends upon the characteristics of the patient and the depth of depression. The type or psychological approach selected to alleviate affective disorder also depends upon the theoretical orientation of the clinician.

(a) **Psycho-dynamic approaches :** Psycho dynamically – oriented. therapists have long worked with depressed patients, in fact, they were the First to devise approaches to deal with affective disorders. Calhoun et.al. (1977) have suggested that in general, psychodynamic treatment of the affective disorder have three goals.

(1) First, the therapist attempts to bring the patient to a fuller consciousness of the stressful periods of early childhood during which the patient presumably experienced a loss of a love object.

(2) Second, the patient is encouraged to explore his evaluation of himself. and to remember the conditions that led to his diminished self-esteem. If the patient can recall and work through these early repressed childhood difficulties, then presumably, 'he may begin to respond to the present situation in a more adequate fashion.

(3) Finally, working on the "anger in" premise, the therapist will also try to make the patient aware of his own capacity for anger and will encourage him to express his hostile feelings rather than turn them inward. This unleashing of

depressed aggression, presumably liberates the individual from his depressive self-punishment.

(b) **Behaviour Therapy:** Among behaviour therapists Lewinsohn and Shatter (1971) and Iiberman and Raskin (1971) have devised methods for treating depressed patients. They place great emphasis on teaching patients "more effective coping behaviours". Behaviour therapists insist that patient's relatives participate actively in any therapeutic programme. They believe that it is especially important for patient's family to avoid reinforcing depressive behaviours.

Lewinsohn views depression as caused by a low rate of response contingent positive reinforcement. His treatment approach is, therefore, directed at increasing the patient's participation in pleasant, positively reinforcing activities.

Lazanis (1968) has developed another behavioural treatment strategy for depression which is very similar to systematic desensitization. In systematic desensitization therapists evoke responses that are incompatible with anxiety. Here such responses are evoked that arc incompatible with depression. The technique for depression is based on the premise that "anger or the deliberate stimulation of amusement, affection, sexual excitement or anxiety tends to break the depressive cycle".

(c) **Cognitive Therapy** : It is one variation of behaviour therapeutic technique which generally centres its attention on thought processes. Cognitive therapy attempts to change one's thought processes and helps one to verbalize rationally and think logically. Aaron Beck is one of the leading proponents of the cognitive therapy as applied to depressed patients.

Cognitive therapy is structured, directive, generally short-term and has been used most successfully with mild to moderate depressive disorders. Beck views depression as caused by maladaptive or irrational cognitions or beliefs. The major goal of therapy is to modify these negative cognitive patterns and to replace them with realistic and positive ones. Beck reports that his approach effectively relieves depression. Shaw (1977) compared Beck's cognitive therapy and Lewinsohn's behavioural treatment of depression in terms of clinical effectiveness. Results of a study treating depressed college students indicated that both treatment techniques alleviated depression more, as measured by self-report and objective clinical ratings then did no treatment of a control group. However, the cognitive modification therapy group improved significantly more than the behaviour therapy group. Similarly, the work of Kovacs et.al. (1981) which compared the effectiveness of cognitive therapy and chemotherapy, pointed out that cognitive therapy worked more rapidly and resulted in greater reduction of self-reported depression than chemotherapy.

Conclusions about Therapy : The following are the brief points to be noted with regard to treatment of affective disorders :

(1) ECT and Pharmacological treatment i.e. Drug therapy is the only choice for patients showing very severe affective disorder.

(2) For those showing moderate to severe affective disorder a combination of psychological approaches and medication works best.

(3) And for those showing milder form of affective disorder psychological approach alone is sufficient.

(4) Manic disorders are best treated with lithum carbonate.

PREVENTION OF SUICIDE

In recent years, many suicide prevention centres have been established throughout the United States, Europe and even in India to attempt to aid an individual during a suicidal crisis. The main goal of these centres is to help the 'individual who is contemplating suicide to cope with the immediate life situation triggering these thoughts and wishes. As noted earlier, the great majority of suicidal persons are ambivalent about taking their own lives. Attempts are therefore, made to try to convince these persons that they have some reason for staying alive, and to persuade them to postpone the act until the immediate crisis passes and the decision can be evaluated more objectively. The hope is that the person can be dissuaded from committing suicide and convinced to get involved in some form of therapy or assistance so that he or she can work through the problems that are causing this desire to die.

Most suicide prevention centres operate a 24hour a-day "hot line," staffed by psychiatrists, psychologists, social workers, or other trained personnel and volunteers, available for telephone contact. These centres also provide therapy for suicidal individuals or a referral service to direct these individuals to other mental health .organizations that will provide more intensive and long-term assistance. Although it is difficult to assess precisely the success of these centers in reducing suicides, there have been some preliminary data suggesting that they are having an effective impact (Coleman 1976).

In many suicide prevention centres, the staffs use demographic factors in . determining how great the suicidal risk is for a particular individual. Usually a checklist is employed to help guide the staff member's questioning of each hotline collar. For example, characteristic factors associated with high-risk suicidal persons point to middle-aged or older males who are divorced or separated and living alone and who have a previous history of suicidal attempts. These demographic variables, in combination with the suicidal person's expression of an intense sense of hopelessness, are usually quite predictive of actual suicide attempts.

Investigators are continuing to search for factors that will allow them to better predict suicide. Researchers like Kiev (1974) has identified three factors that may help us to take steps to avoid or prevent suicide. These three factors are as follows:

(1) Degree of interpersonal conflict.

(2) Presence or symptom distress, and

(3) the social setting of the suicide attempt (e.g. proximity of others and the individual's inclination not to seek help afterwards).

A routine psychological assessment of depressed individuals is also made, at many places, to screen out potential suicide victims and to help them to overcome suicidal ideation and attempts.

DEPRESSION IN CHILDHOOD AND ADOLESCENCE

Kraepelin (1896), a trailblazer in the classification of mental disorder, observed that the prime time for onset of the first attack of a bipolar disorder was in the age period of 15 to 20 *years.* He noted that it was rare to find such cases in children younger than 13. However, according to Winotair and his colleagues (1969) and more recently Toolan (1981), Call and Bland (1979), and Akiskal and Webb (1983) have reported cases of affective psychosis in children and adolescents.

Toolan (1981) suggested that one possible reason for believing that depression did not occur in younger children was *"be* assumption that mood disturbances in youngsters would take the same form as they do in adults. However, if we assume that normal emotional reactions of 5-year olds and 50-year olds differ significantly, then we can assume that abnormal reactions may differ as well. This pathoplastic effect of age, (the pathoplastic effect of age refers to the fact that the same disorder will be manifested indifferent ways in different age-groups. For example, symptom pathoplasty is exemplified in a disease like chicken pox which, in infants, is typically a mild disease, but which, in adults, can be quite serious and painful) leads us to accept the possibility that a "depressed" child might act differently from a "depressed" adult. Toolan (1981) notes further that it may not be until age 20 that depression in young people takes on adult form.

While childbed affective disorders were seen infrequently because we Used adult symptoms to diagnose children, some researchers believe that the rarity of affective disorders in adolescents may be due to other factors. For example, Bowden and Sarabia (1980) concluded that affective disorders tended to be under diagnosed among teenagers. Whereas researchers find actual prevalence of schizophemia and affective disorders in teenagers equal to that of adults, the diagnosis of schizophrenia is used up to nine limes more frequently for adolescents. Bowden and Sarabia believe that this overuse of the schizophrenia diagnosis may be due to hesitancy in applying the affective diagnosis because of a continuing belief that while schizophrenia occurs in young people, affective disorders do not.

POSTMORTEM DEPRESSION

In addition to there being special forms of depression associated with childhood, there are also specific patterns which occur in conjunction with new motherhood. Called Postmortem depression, a moderate to severe affective disturbance can follow the birth of a child. During this period of time when many mothers experience a mild case of the "blues", some may have problems severe enough, to require psychiatric intervention. Penfold (1981) notes that greater attention paid to what she terms the "fourth trimester of pregnancy" could have significant impact on reducing postmortem reactions. 0'Haraet.al. (1982) found that many postmortem depression could be prevented given greater sensitivity to the special stresses experienced by expectant and new mothers.

10

Organic Brain Disorders

Not much attention is devoted towards the study of organic brain disorders, by the students of psychology in general and clinical psychology in particular. The organic disorders of brain differ from other disorders discussed in the earlier chapters of this book, in that they are definitely biogenic in nature. The symptoms of organic brain disorder, very often overlaps with symptoms of other nonorganic brain disorders. A good diagnostician can easily arrive at the right diagnosis, through psychological tests and other available procedures.

There are five major symptoms of organic brain disorders. These are impairment (i) of orientation, (ii) of memory, (iii) of general intellectual functioning, (iv) of judgement, and (v) of control over affect.

DSM-III describes three main group of disorders in which brain malformation, disruption or damage are a primary cause of observed symptoms. These groups are

(a) The age-disease or injury based organic mental disorder,

(b) The substance induced organic mental disorder, and

(c) Mental retardation.

In this chapter we will first discuss what are organic brain syndromes or organic brain disorders its classification and major symptoms seen in these disorders.

Following this we will distinguish between delirium and dementia-as these two represent the major brain syndromes.

We would then discuss the various organic brain disorders, its symptomatology and etiology.

Epilepsy has attracted a great deal of interest not only among researchers and clinicians but also among general public. It is very common organic mental disorder. It is an enigma for researchers because for epilepsy, there is often no known cause. Epilepsy victims experience unpredictable seizures, where they lose consciousness. While some seizures may be produced by directly identifiable tumors, inflamatton or 'trauma in brain, about 75 per cent of epileptic disorders are termed ideopathic, i.e. are of unknown origin. We would discuss the different types of epileptic disorders.

We would then discuss the treatment of these various organic brain disorders.

ORGANIC BRAIN DISORDERS

Organic brain disorders re also called as organic brain syndrome or organic dysfunction and refers to a mental disorder in which intellectual, emotional and behavioural functioning are impaired because of pathological brain dysfunction. The dysfunction can be, organic or biochemical in nature.

The organic brain syndromes are symptom patterns reflecting temporary or permanent disruption of brain function regardless of cause. They can be either acute (reversible with rapid onset) or chronic (mostly irreversible and with slower, more insidious onset), but in either case, they may be characterized by

both phvsical and mental disturbances. Generallv. brain syndromes arc marked by difficulties in orientation, memory, perception, judgement, intellect, and emotion. Thus, people may not always know where or who they are and may not be able to remember recent activities and experiences. They may have difficulty in reproducing on paper visually presented stimuli or may be unable to plan future behaviour or make sound decisions. Finally, they may be incapable of retrieving and using facts and information and may show inappropriate emotional reactions. Rarely are all these general characteristics of brain syndromes present in any single case; more typically, the actual pattern of deficit varies as a function of the specific type of brain syndrome in question.

The major symptoms of organic brain disorder may be summarized as follows:

1. **Impairment of orientation:** The person may be confused as to who he or she is, where, what the date is, and so forth.

2. **Impairment of memory**: The person may forget events of the distant past or, more typically, of the very recent past and may invent stories to fill in these memory gaps. (Memory impairment may be the most common symptom of brain disorder).

3. **Impairment of other intellectual functions** such as comprehension, calculation, knowledge, and learning. The person may be unable to define simple words, do ordinary addition and subtraction, name the President of the United States, and the like.

4. **Impairment of judgement**: The person ceases lo be able to make appropriate decisions cannot decide what to have for lunch, when to keep clothes on and when to take them off, and so forth.

5. **Liability or shallowness of affect**: The person passes quickly and inappropriately from apathy to hostility or from laughing to weeping. From the above symptoms, we see that the symptoms of organic brain disorders heavily overlaps with the symptoms of functional disorders like schizophrenia and affective disorder. Differential diagnosis is an important aspect of the job of a clinician to rule out any organic disorder when the above symptoms are present.

CLASSIFICATION OF ORGANIC BRAIN SYNDROMES

DSM-III describes the major brain syndromes of delirium, dementia, intoxication, and withdrawal, as well as a group of less frequently occurring patterns involving amnesia, hallucinations, delusions, and affective and personality changes.

Besides the DSM-HI classification, clinicians classify organic Brain Syndromes as either actue or chronic.

In Acute brain syndrome onset is sudden and often the syndrome is reversible. Generally speaking, such an organic brain syndrome is induced by nutritional inadequacies or associated with drugs, alcohol or poisons.

Chronic Brain Syndromes are taught to have a gradual onset and brain damage that is typically permanent and/or irreversible.

Bootzin and Accocella have classified organic Brain Syndromes on the basis Or etiology as follows:

I Cereberal Infection

(a) Cereberal abscess

(b) Encephalitis

(c) Neurosyphilis.

II. Brain Trauma

(a) Concussion

(b) Contusions

(c) Lacerations

III. Vascular Accidents

(a) Cereberal Thrombosis

(b) Hemorrhage.

IV. Brain Tumors

V. Degenerative Disorders

(a) Presenile degenerative disorders

(i) Huntington's chorea

(ii) Parkinson's disease.

(iii) Pick's disease.

(iv) Aizheimer's disease.

(b) Senile degenerative disorders

(i) Senile dementia

(ii) Multi-infarct dementia.

VI. Nutritional Deficiency

(a) Korsakoffs Psychosis

(b) Pellagra

(c) BeriBeri.

VII. Endocrine disorders

(a) Thyroid syndromes

(b) Adrenal syndromes

VII. Toxic Disorders.

Delirium and dementia are the two important symptoms of organic brain syndrome that may result due to a large variety of disorders. We would discuss delirium rod dementia in brief.

DELIRIUM

The basic feature of delirium is a "clouded state of consciousness... manifested by difficulty in sustaining attention...sensory misperceptions and a disordered stream of thought" (American Psychiatric Association). The symptoms may vary in severity, but in all cases they begin quickly and last a relatively short time. Formally called acute brain syndrome, in delirium people may have difficulty attending to conversations or, when speaking, may shift from topic to topic. Frequently, they also misinterpret sensations; for example the backfiring of a car may be mistaken for a rifle shot. People with delirium can experience symptoms ranging from simple drowsiness to stuporus or comatose states and from simple hyperactivity to severe agitation an insomia. While delirium can occur at any age (especially if it is substance-induced), the syndrome occurs most frequently in association with physical diseases in children and in adults overage 60-(Strub&Black,1981).

DEMENTIA

While delirium is usually short-lived and primarily affects consciousness, dementia includes more permanent deterioration of intellectual abilities, especially in the realm of memory. Memory difficulties may range from forgetting of things that one is about to do to an inability to remember names of close relatives, birthdays, or even one's own name or occupation. People with dementia may show impaired judgement and poor impulse control and if the dementia continues will become increasingly "different" and "not like themselves." For example, they may show an increasing frequency of poor social and business decisions.

The rate of onset and duration of symptoms of dementia will vary with its cause. If caused by accidental brain damage, then the loss of intellectual abilities is rapid but does not progressively worsen. On the other hand, in-cases of degenerative nerve diseases the pattern may develop more slowly but progressively intensify. Finally, when dementia is caused by brain tumors or chemical poisoning, its symptoms may be reversible if appropriate medical treatment is applied (Joynt & Shoulson, 1985). As people become aware of losing their intellectual abilities and of their difficulties in compensating for these losses, they often become frustrated and depressed.

Table 12.1 & 12.2 briefly summarizes the clinical differentiation and causes of delirium and dementia.

Table 12.1 Clinical Differentiation of Delirium and Dementia

	Dellrium	Dementia
Onset	Acute	Usually insidious, if acute, preceded by coma or delirium
Duration	Usually less than 1 month	At least 1 month, usually much longer
Orientation	Faulty, at least for a time; tendency to mistake unfamiliar for familiar place, person.	Many be correct in mild cases.
Thinking	Disorganized	Impoverished.
Memory	Recent impaired	Both recent and remote impaired
Attention	Invariably disturbed	May be intact
Awareness	Always reduced, tends to fluctuate during daytime and be worse at night.	Usually intact
Alertness	Increased or decreased	Normal or decreased
Perception	Misperceptions often present	Misperceptions often absent
Sleep-wakeful cycle	Always disrupted	Usually normal for age

Table 12.2 Some causes of Delirium and Dementia

Delirium: Alcohol, inhalation of gasoline, glue, or solvents, lack of oxygen; endocrine disorders; systemic infections, intercranial infections; head injuries; espilepsy; migraine headaches; tumors; exposure to extremes of temperature; food allergy.

Dementia: Degenerative disease like Alzheimer's and Pick's diseases; senility; multiple heart attacks; metabolic disorder; head trauma; epilepsy;

meningitis; encephalitis; heat stroke; electric injury; multiple sclerosis.

CEREBAL INFECTION

Viral and bacterial infection to brain tissues can result in cerebral infection which may result in varying forms of behaviours disorders. There are three major categories of cerebral infection. These are as follows:

(a) Cerebral Abscess

(b) Encephalitis, and

(c) Neurosyphilis

We would discuss these three in brief

(a) **Cerebral Abscess:** A cerebral abscess, like an abscess in any other part of the body, is an infection that becomes encapsulated by connective tissues so that it cannot drain and heal like an infection on the outside of the body but simply continues to grow inside the body. Brain abscesses can result when an infection in some other part of the body travels to the brain or when some foreign object (e.g., a bullet, a piece of shrapnel) enters in the brain, introducing germs.

Symptoms of cerebral abscess vary widely. In the early stages of the infection, the patient may experience chills, fever, stiffness of the neck, loss of appetite, and sometimes convulsions as well. However, once the infection becomes closed off by the connective tissue, the symptom picture changes. As the abscess grows within the tissue, it presses against neighbouring brain structures and interferes with their functioning, in much the same way as a brain tumor. Hence the later symptoms of brain abscess are similar to those of brain tumor; headache, nausea, vomiting, problems with vision, and in some cases marked personality changes. As the pressure in the brain continues to build, it may produce extreme lethargy and eventually stupor, in which the patient becomes mute and motionless.

The usual treatment for cerebral abscess consists of surgical drainage or removal of the abscess and administration of antibiotic drugs. However, even after this treatment, the patient may continue to have behavioural problems. The nature and severity of the problems will depend on the size and location of the abscess and on the age of the patient at the time of the infection.

(b) **Encephalitis**: The term encephalitis means an inflammation of the brain tissue. There are a number of different varieties of this viral disease.

(i) One form, epidemic encephalitis (also called von Economo's disease, after the Viennese physician who first identified it), was particularly widespread following World War 1. Its most striking symptoms were profound lethargy and prolonged periods of sleep, often for days or even weeks at a time. For this reason, the disease was often called "sleeping sickness". In their periods of wakefulness, however, patients might become extremely hyperactive, irritable, and then breathless and unable to sleep. Other symptoms included convulsive seizures and delirium a state of excitement and disorientation marked by incoherent speech, restless activity, and often hallucination. Furthermore, striking psychological after effects could be observed in victims who survived the disease, especially in children, who are more susceptible to it than are adults. After an episode of epidemic encephalitis, a primordially cheerful and affable child might demonstrate a marked moral deterioration, including such offensive behaviours as lying, cheating, cruelty, and sexual aggression. In short, such children came to resemble young sociopath a condition that often persisted into adulthood.

The virus responsible for epidemic encephalitis, while still active in certain areas of Asia and Africa, LI now virtually unknown in Europe and America.

(ii) Besides epidemic encephalitis; there remain scores of other viruses that can cause different types of encephalitis, most of which are grouped under the general heading of *unspecified encephalitis.* Typically transmitted by such animals as mosquitoes, ticks, and horses, these viruses induce many of the same symptoms that we have described as typical of epidemic encephalitis: Lethargy, irritability, convulsion and the like.

(iii) A final variety of encephalitis is *meningitis,* an acute inflammation of the meningitis, the membrous covering of the brain and spinal cord. Meningitis may be caused by bacteria, viruses, protozoa, or fungi. As in cerebral abscess, these foreign bodies may be introduced into the brain either through an infection elsewhere in the body or by an exogenous agent such as a bullet. Among the psychological symptoms usually observed in-the various forms of meningitis are drowsiness, confusion, irritability, inability to concentrate, memory defects, and , sensory impairments. In milder cases the primary infection may be effectively eradicated, but residua] effects such as motor and sensory impairments and, in infants, mental retardation are not uncommon. In more severe cases, meningitis progresses rapidly from drowiness to come to death. Autopsies in such cases generally reveal that the brain is swollen and covered with pus and that the pressure from the swelling has caused the gyri (i.e., the convolutions in the surface of the brain) to flatten against the inside of the skull.

(c) **Nenrosyphilis**: Neurosyphilis, the deterioration of brain tissue as a result of syphilis, was once more common than any of the forms of encephalitis.

Throughout the previous centuries syphilis had raged unchecked through Europe, taking a fantastic toll in infant morality, blindness, madness and death. Among its more famous victims were Henry VIII, along with most of his many wives, and probably Columbus. Indeed, it is thought that the disease was first introduced into Europe by Columbus's crew, who were apparently infected by the natives of the West Indies (Kemole, 1936). Nearer our own times. Lord Randolph Churchill, father of Einston Churchill, and Al Capone both suffered gruesome deaths from neurosyphilis.

Syphilis begins when the spirochetc known as Treponema pallidum invades the victim's body through tiny skin lesions or, more commonly, through the mucous membranes in the mouth or gential areas. The transmission almost invariably occurs during sexual intercourse (genital or anal) or oral-genital contact with a syphilitic sexual partner. Once contracted, the disease runs a well-defined course:

Stage one: About ten-to twenty days after the disease has been contracted, a chancre, or sore, appears at the site of the infection be it the genitals, the mouth, or the anus. Unfortunately, the chancer is often painless and .disappears without treatment, the result being that many people either do not recognize this early warning sign or conclude that they are cured once the chancer disappears.

Stage two: About three to six weeks after the appearance of the chancer, the victim develops a copper-coloured rash that covers the body and may be accompanied by fever, headaches, and other indispositions. However, this symptom also passes quickly, after which cither the spirochetes may eventually be eliminated from the body, or in less fortunate individuals, the spirochetes simply multiply, carrying the individual into the decisive third and fourth stages of the disease.

Stage three-In this stage, called the latent stage, which may last anywhere from ten to thirty *years,* the spirochetes slowly and insidiously invade the vital organs of the body.

Stage four: Whatever damage has been done during the latent period *now* becomes apparent, in any one of a wide variety of organ failures, including heart attack, blindness, or if the spirochetes have infiltrated the brain-general paresis.

General paresis develops in approximately 3 per cent of untreated syphilitics. Its onset is usually marked by a vague but pervasive slovenliness of behaviour. The person begins to show up later for work, ignores the feelings of others, dispenses casual insults, loses interest in his or her appearance, evades responsibilities, arid so forth. As the disease becomes more advanced, a number of better-defined symptoms make their appearance, including tremors, slurring of speech, deterioration of hand writing, a shuffling gait, and, almost invariably, disturbance of vision. One very common indication is the so-called Argyll Robertson symptom, in which the pupil of the eye makes an accommodation to distance but not to light.

This physical deterioration is accompanied by an equally have deterioration of the personality, in which the individual becomes increasingly sloppy, indifferent, and callous. Memory losses begin to appear. At the same time the individual may became severely depressed or, on the other hand, expansive, delusional, and euphoric. When the disease has progressed to this stage, the only possible treatment is custodial. In the final stage preceding death, both body and mind are virtually non-functional. The individual is paralyzed, inarticulate, cut off from reality, and subject to frequent convulsive seizures.

While syphilis is normally contracted through sexual acts, it may also be transmitted by a syphilitic mother to her unborn child as blood in this case containing the syphilitic spirochetes passes from one of the other across the placenta. If the child lives (many syphilitic fetuses are still born), he or she stands a good chance of developing juvenile paresis, the childhood form of general paresis. While the juvenile paretic may seem normal at birth, the same symptoms of intellectual and physical deterioration seen in general paresis generally appear sometime between the ages of Five and twenty. As in the case of general paresis, juvenile paresis is irreversible, usually resulting in death approximately five years after the onset of symptoms.

With the development of such early-detection procedures as the Wassermann test and with the advent of penicillin, the incidence of syphilis decreased dramatically in the late 1940s and the 1950&. The reward of this conquest is that at present general paresis accounts for less than I percent of all first admission to mental hospitals in the United States.

BRAIN TRAUMA

Brain injuries or traumas can result into a wide variety of behaviour disorders.

Brain injury or trauma can lead to behaviour disorders that may range from l\mild to the debilitating. In brain trauma, brain tissues is jarred, bruised or cut by some exogenous source.

Although automobile accidents are the most frequent cause of brain trauma, alcoholics and epileptics are particularly prone to bead injuries due to falls. However, any extreme physical force suddenly applied to the head, whether from an automobile windshield or an ill-aimed baseball bat, may result in brain damage. Brain trauma is subdivided into three categories : (a) concussions, (b) contusions, and (c) lacerations.

(a) **Concussions:** In the case of a concussion, the blow to the head simply jars the brain, momentarily disrupting its functioning. The result is a temporary loss of consciousness, often lasting for only a few minutes, after which the individual is typically unable to remember the events immediately preceding the injury. A familiar example of a concussion is a knockout in a boxing match. The fighter loses consciousness, falls to the floor of the ring (probably hitting his head a second time), and may then show some reflexive twitching of the arms or legs.

Soon he is up again and ready to retaliate.

Nonetheless, concussions may involve posttraumatic symptoms lasting for as long as several weeks. (In general, the longer the person remains unconscious after the blow, the more severe the postraumatic symptoms and the longer they will last). In addition to headaches and dizziness, the person may display apathy, general memory difficulties, inability to concentrate, insomnia, irritability, fatigue, and a decreased tolerance for noise, light, heat, alcohol, and exertion. In most cases, however, these symptoms also pass, leaving no residual damage.

(b) **Contusions:** In a contusion the trauma is severe enough so that the brain is not simply jarred; it is actually shifted out of its normal position and pressed against one side of the skull, thus brushing the sensitive neural tissue. The results of a contusion are correspondingly more severe than those of a concussion. The person typically lapses into a coma lasting for several hours or even days, and afterward he or she may suffer convulsions and/or a temporary speech loss. Furthermore, on awakening from the coma, the person may fall into a state of disorientation called traumatic delirium, in which, for example, he or she may imagine that the hospital staff are enemies or kidnappers. Other patients may simply wander away if they are not carefully watched. These symptoms generally disappear within a week or so, but a very severe contusion or repeated contusions (such as are often suffered by boxers) can result in permanent emotional instability and intellecual impairment. Again, the length of the period of unconsciousness is a good predictor of the severity and duration of the postraumatic symptoms.

(c) **Lacerations:** Lacerations, in which a foregin object, such as a bullet or a piece of metal, enters the skull and directly ruptures and destroys brain tissue, constitute the most serious form of brain trauma. The effects of a brain laceration depend greatly on the exact site of the damage. Lacerations in certain areas of the brain result in death or in extremely debilitating impairments of intellectual, sensory, or motor functioning-, damage to other sites may lead to only relatively minor consequences. Periodically the newspapers will report a case in which a person, after being shot in the head, simply resumes normal functioning after the external wounds have healed and goes about daily business with a bullet or two lodged in the brain. Such cases, however, are exceedingly rare, Normally, a cerebral laceration results in some form of physical impairment or personality change, whether major or minor.

VASCULAR ACCIDENTS
Or
CEREBRAL THROMBOSIS AND CEREBRAL HEMORRAGE

Endogenous vascular accidents can also lead to organic brain syndrones. In vascular accident there is a blockage or breaking of cranial blood vessels which results in injury to the brain tissue. Vascular accidents fall into two categories

(i) Cerebral thrombosis, and

(ii) Cerebral hemorrhage.

We will discuss these two types of vascular accidents in brief.

(i) **Cerebral thrombosis:** The major cause of aphasia, apraxia, and agnosia is cerebral thrombosis, in which a blood clot forms in one of the bloody vessels feeding the brain and thus cuts off the circulation in that vessel. The result is that the portion of the brain served by that blood vessel cannot longer take in nourishment or dispose of chemical wastes and consequently cannot function properly. An occurrence of cerebral thrombosis is technically labeled a cerebrovascular accident (CVA), though it is known in the popular vocabulary simply as a "stroke."

The most common form of organic brain disorder, CVAs are found in 25 per cent of routine autopsies. This does not mean that the CVA was necessarily the cause of death. Many people apparently have what are called "silent strokes"- small CVAs that occur in less critical regions of the brain and thus have less noticeable effect on behaviour. In other cases, CVAs are immediately fatal. And in still other cases, the patient lives, but with a variety of aftereffects, the most common being aphasia, agnosia, apraxia, and paralysis, usually of one limb or of one half of the body.

These disabilities (whether they result from CVAs or from any other organic brain disorder) are almost invariably accompanied by some degree of disturbance, partly organic and partly a functional response to the new impairment. One possible reaction is emotional liability; the patient may, pass from laughing to weeping in an instant. Another response that is sometimes seen is a catastrophic reaction (Goldstein, 1948), in which the patient, utterly bewildered by his or her inability to perform elementary tasks long since taken for granted walking across a room, forming a sentence, reading a magazine reacts, understandably, with disorganization and sometimes violent fury. Later, as a means of coping with the impairment, patients may develop seemingly odd habits. For example, to compensate for memory losses, some people may make elaborate inventories of their belongings and may react with anger if something is moved from its proper place. Again, the response depends greatly on the premorbid personality. People with compulsive tendencies are generally intolerant of any reduction in their mental acuity and may become depressed in response. Likewise, people with suspicious natures, exacerbated by their sudden helplessness, may develop paranoid symptoms, accusing others of making fun of them, of stealing their belongings, and so forth. The symptomatology, then, is not just the result of a specific disorder in a specific part of the brain, but of this disorder working on a specific personality.

Some of the behavioural impairments resulting from CVAs may disappear spontaneously, while some others can be remedied through rehabilitation therapy. And as the disability is remedied, so in most cases is the attendant emotional disturbance. In some cases CVA patients recover completely, but more often they continue to labour under some form of impairment for the rest of their lives. In general, the younger the patient and the smaller the area of brain damage, the better the chance of recovery.

(ii) **Cerebral Hemorrhage:** Unlike cerebral thrombosis, in which the affected part of the vascular system remains intact (although useless because of blockage), cerebral hemorrhage involves an actual rupture of the vessel wall. Vessel breakage most commonly occurs when a weak part of the vessel wall balloons out into what is called an aneurysm and eventually ruptures as a result of the pressure exerted by the bloodstream. Other common causes of vessel rupture are trauma, hypertension, tumors, drug usage, and bacterial infection (Yarnell and Stears, 1974). Whatever the cause of the ruptures, the result is that blood spills out the vein and onto the brain tissue, damaging or destroying it.

As with other brain disorders, the specific effects of cerebral hemorrhage depend on the location and extent of the damage. Usually the patient lapses into a coma, sometimes accompanied by convulsions. Victims of extensive hemorrhaging usually die within two to fourteen days. Those who survive the hemorrhage generally suffer paralysis, speech difficulties, and/or severe psychological impairment, such as confusion or loss of memory.

BRAIN TUMORS

Although the actual cause of tumors, both bening (noncancerous) and malignant (cancerous), has not yet been determined, the clinical course of a brain tumor is clear. For some reason, a few cells begin to grow at an abnormally rapid rate, destroying the surrounding healthy brain tissue and resulting in a wide variety of psychological symptoms. Because of the inexplicable cellular growth, brain tumors arc referred to technically as intracranial neoplasms that is, new growths within the brain.

In most cases, the first signs of brain tumor are subtle and insidious headaches, visual problems, neglect of personal hygiene, in difference to previously valued activities, and failures of judgement and foresight. With the progressive destruction of brain tissue, the patient eventually develops at least one of the more obvious symptoms: abnormal reflexes, blunting of affect, poor memory and concentration, double Vision, and jerky motor coordination. The kind and severity of symptoms are directly related to the location of the tumor in the brain the functions controlled by that section will probably be impaired earlier and more severely than other functions. However, as the tumor grows, pressing against other sections, their functioning too will be affected.

Malignant tumors are much more likely to bring on any of these symptoms than are benign tumors. Nevertheless, any tumor that continues to grow undetected and untreated in the brain will eventually cause extreme physical distress (splitting headaches, vomiting, seizures), along with personality changes that may reach psychotic proportions. Prior to death, the patient may become overtly psychotic and finally lapse into a coma.

Tumors can be removed surgically and in many cases they are. However, since the surgery itself can cause permanent brain damage, the physician may choose to avoid it. Surgeons are especially reluctant to operate on the language areas and on the major motor areas (for the obvious reason). In such cases, radiation treatment is used, though this too may destroy brain tissue. In other cases, surgery and radiation are used in combination, the former to remove the growth and the latter to prevent future growths.

(C) **Nutritional Deficiency and Organic Brain Syndromes:** Malnutrition or, specifically, insufficient intake of one or more essential vitamin scan result in neurological damage and consequently in psychological disturbances. The most common conditions of this kind arc (i) Korsakoffs psychosis, *(ii)* pellagra, and *(iii)* beriberi.

(i) **Korsakoffs Psychosis:** In cases of Korsakoffs psychosis, considered irreversible, patients invariably show a history of alcoholism. Alcoholics have notoriously bad diets, and it is generally agreed that the primary pathology in this disorder is due to a deficiency of vitamin B or thiamine (Redlich and Freedman, 1966; Brion, 1969).

There are two classic behavioural signs of Korsakoffs psychosis, anterograde amnesia and confabulation. Anierograde amnesia is the loss of memory for immediately preceding events, and confabulation is the tendency to fill in these memory gaps with invented stories. For example, in response to questioning, patients may placidly offer an utterly outrageous account of why they arc in the hospital, if indeed they even admit that the place is a hospital. Such patients usually seem calm and affable, while at the same time their total unawareness of the fantastic quality of their stories reveals a psychotic impairment of judgement. This impairment gradually spreads to other aspects of psychological functioning and many include disorientation.

(ii) **Pellagra:** Pellagra, caused by a severe deficiency of the Vitamin B - niacin, is most common in geographical areas where the population subsists primarily on corn meal. In the early 1900s, pellagra accounted for about 10 per cent of all admissions to state mental hospitals in some areas of the United States, 'particularly the South (Millon,1969), but since that time improvements in the average American's diet have virtually eliminated this syndrome in our society. the early physical symtoms of pellagra are skin rash and diarrhea. These are generally accompanied by depression, anxiety and eventually delirium and hallucinations prior to death. Massive vitamin therapy, if instituted in time, can halt the progress of the disease.

(iii) **Beriberi:** Like Korsakoffs psychosis, beriberi is due to thiamine deficiency. -It often appears in association with other disorders, such as chronic alcoholism, pellagra, pernicious anemia, or diabetes. The most prominent clinical signs of beriberi include lack of appetite, insomnia, disturbances in memory and concentration, irritability, and above all, extreme lassitude. (The name of the disease comes from the Singhalese word Beri, meaning "weakness"). This disorder has been a particular problem in areas such as the Far East, where polished rice constitutes a major portion of the diet.

ENDOCRINE DISORDERS

The endocrine glands are responsible for the production of hormones. When released into the bloodstream, these hormones affect various bodily mechanisms, such as sexual functions, physical growth and development, and the availability of energy. Disturbances in the endocrine system, and particularly in the thyriod and adrenal glands, can give rise to a variety of psychological disorders.

Thyroid Syndromes: Over activity of the thyroid gland a condition called hyperthyroidism, or Graves disease-involves an excessive secretion of the hormone thyroxin, which in turn gives rise to a variety of physical and psychological difficulties. Psychological symptoms accompanying the disorder may include severe apprehension and agitation, hallucinations, excessive motor activity, sweating, and other symptoms suggestive of anxiety.

Opposite in both cause and effect is hypothyroidism, sometimes referred to as myxedema, in which- under activity of the thyroid gland results in deficient production of thyroxin. Hypothyroidism may be due to iodine deficiency, a problem that has become much less common in the United States since the advent of iodized table salt. Individuals suffering from hypothyroidism are frequently sluggish, have difficulties with memory and concentration, and appear to be lethargic and depressed. Again, however, symptomatology depends greatly on premorbid personality. (The same is true of hyperthyroidism).

Another condition resulting from thyroid deficiency is cretinism, in which the thyroid has not developed, has been injured, or has undergone degeneration. When the deficiency occurs during the prenatal or prenatal period, the unwelcome result is mental retardation. Cretinism has become relatively rare as a result of public health measures involving prevention, early detection, and treatment. With early treatment, normal intellectual and personality functioning can usually be restored.

Adrenal Syndromes The adrenal glands are a pair of ductless glands located above the kidneys and consisting of an outer layer called the cortex and an internal portion called the medulla. Chronic under activity of the adrenal cortex gives rise to Addison's disease, which involves both physical and psychological changes. Again, the psychological symptoms vary considerably according to the individual's premorbid adjustment. Some patients simply appear moderately depressed and withdrawn; others experience debilitating extremes of depression, anxiety, irritability, and invalidism. Appropriate medical therapy can alleviate the symptoms of even a severe case of Addison's disease, restoring the individual to normal functioning. Such was the case with President John F. Kennedy, who suffered from Addison's (Lasky, 1966).

When the adrenal cortex is excessively active, several disorders may arise, one of which is Gushing's syndrome. This relatively rare disorder usually affects young women. As with the other endocrine disorders, Cushing's syndrome involves both physical symptoms in this case, obesity and muscle Weakness and psychological difficulties, especially extreme emotional liability, with fluctuations in mood ranging from total indifference to violent hostility.

TOXIC DISORDERS

Various plants, gases, drugs and metals, when ingested or absorbed through the skin, can have a toxic or poisonous effect on the brain. Depending on the individual, the toxic substance, and the amount ingested, the results of such brain poisoning range from temporary physical and emotional distress to psychosis and death. However, one sign that is almost always present in the toxic, disorders is delirium.

Mushroom Toxins: The ingestion of certain species of mushrooms can cause extreme physical illness as well as a number of psychological symptoms. For example, most mushrooms of the genus Amanita cause hallucinations, delirium, and periods of extreme excitement alternating with periods of sleeps Such symptoms are typically transitory. However, certain members of this genus, along with the genus Galerina, can be fatal.

Lead: Much more common than mushroom poisoning is lead poisoning. The excessive ingestion of lead causes a condition called lead encephalopathy, in which fluid accumulates in the brain, causing extreme pressure. Early symptoms include abdominal pains, constipation, facial pallor, and sometimes convulsions and bizarre behaviours such as hair pulling. In severe cases; the symptom may be similar to those of psychosis, including delirium and hallucinations. The most common victims of lead poisoning are children, who may become menially retarded as a result.

In recent years, consumer advocacy groups have identified a number of sources of lead contamination, including old lead-lined water pipes, lead-based paint on children's toys and furniture, old plaster walls, candles with lead-core wicks, certain electric tea kettles that release lead from soft solder joints when heated, pottery glazes from which acetic foods (e.g., grape juice) can leach lead, exhaust from automobiles burning, leaded gasoline, and industrial pollution. As may be seen from this list, the issue of metal poisoning often involves a conflict between the needs of industry and the needs of the individual. An illustrative case is the community of Kellogg, Idaho, whose primary industry is a lead-smelting plant which, at the same time that it provides the economic support for most of the people of Kellogg, is probably damaging the brains of many of these people's children with the lead dust that it released daily into the air.

Other Heavy Metal Toxins: The "industry vs. the Individuals" conflict also crops up in two of the more common varieties of heavy-metal poisoning, mercury and manganese poisoning. Victims of these toxin disorders are usually those whose jobs bring them into close daily contact with mercury and manganese. However, other victims are simply unwitting citizens whose food or air has been contaminated by industrial wastes containing metallic toxins. One notorious source of such poisoning is fish taken from water polluted by mercury wastes from nearby factories. In Japan, for example, thousands of people have been permanently paralyzed and brain damaged as a result of eating mercury-contaminated fish (Kurland et. al., 1960)

Early signs of brain damage due to mercury poisoning arc memory, loss, irritability, and difficulty in concentration. As the disease develops, the individual typically develops tunnel vision (that is, loss of peripheral vision), faulty motor coordination, and difficulty in speaking and hearing. In extreme cases, these symptoms lead to paralysis, coma, and death. Manganese poisoning is manifested in motor and speech impairments, restlessness, and emotional instability. In the case of both types of poisoning, some clinicians believe that personality changes are often simply pathological exaggerations of the individual's premorbid personality traits.

Psychoactive Drugs: Abuse of psychoactive drugs such as alcohol, narcotics, and amphetamines can cause severe psychological disturbances. Other drugs have also been implicated in organic brain damage. In recent years, for example the inhalation of aerosol gases and fumes of certain glues has become a popular means of getting "high" among adolescents. Unfortunately, the toxins in these gases and fumes tend to accumulate in the vital organs and may cause permanent damage not only to the liver and kidney but also to the brain, which in turn may result in severe psychological deterioration and, in extreme cases, death.

Another example of drug-induced brain disorder is bromide psychosis. Many popular nonprescription sleeping pills consist of compounds containing bromides, despite the fact that bromides are not particularly useful in producing sleep. Chronic insomniacs may take so many of these, pills that they inadvertently ingest a toxic dose of bromides, which may result in permanent brain damage if appropriate medical treatment is not instituted quickly. Depending on the dose ingested, the symptoms of bromide overdose range from simple intoxication to what is called "bromide schizophrenia," involving hallucinations, withdrawal, and extreme suspiciousness (Levin, 1948).

Carbon Monoxide: Carbon monoxide, an odorless, tasteless, and invisible gas usually inhaled from automobile .exhaust fumes, combines with the hemoglobin in the blood in such a way as to prevent the blood from absorbing oxygen. The usual result of this process is a swift and rather painless death, which makes carbon monoxide inhalation a favored means of suicide. Patients who survive, however, will suffer a number of psychological consequences, typically .including apathy, confusion, and memory defects. While these symptoms may clear up within two years, some patients suffer permanent mental impairment (Kolb,1973).

DEGENERATIVE DISORDERS

Degenerative disorders are those organic brain syndromes in which intellectual, emotional, and mortor functioning appear to deteriorate as a function of advancing age. This is not to say that such disorders are part of normal aging; most people grow old without any sign of pathological brain deterioration. Nevertheless, when the degenerative disorders strike, they more often strike the middleaged and the elderly.

Degenerative disorders are subdivided into two groups: (1) The presenile forms, generally affecting the forty-to-sixty age group, and (II) the senile forms, generally affecting those over sixty.

(1) **Presenile Degenerative Disorders**-The presenile degenerative disorders, involving deterioration of the brain and central nervous system, are both uncommon and poorly understood. We shall study four syndromes: (a) Huntington's chorea, (b) Parkinson's disease, (c) Pick's disease, and (d) Aizheimer's disease, each named for the physician who first described it.

(a) **Huntington's Chorea:** Huntington's chorea is one of the very few psychological disorders definitely known to be transmitted genetically. Passed on by a dominant gene from either parent to both male and female children, Huntington' s cannot be detected at birth. Indeed, whether or not a person Ins been unlucky enough to inherit Huntington's cannot usually be determined until after the age of thirty, when the symptoms typically appear. At present, there are 7,000 to 10,000 Americans showing overt symptoms of Huntington's chorea (Boll et. al., 1974).

The primary site of damage in Huntington's is the basal ganglia, clusters of never-cell bodies located deep within the cerebral hemispheres and responsible primarily for posture, muscle tonus, and motor coordination. However the first signs of the disease are not so much motor impairments as vague behavioural and emotional changes. The patient may become slovenly and indifferent to every day social amenities. Furthermore, his or her moods may become in predictable and inconsistent, running the gamut from obstinacy, passivity, and depression to inexplicable euphoria. Intellectual functions, particularly memory and judgement, are also disrupted. As the disease progresses, delusions, hallucinations, and suicidal tendencies commonly appear (Boll et. al 1974).

In addition to these psychological problems, the patient will eventually begin to show the characteristic motor symptoms that is, involuntary spasmodic jerking of the limbs to which the term "chorea" (from the Greek word choreia, "dance") refers. This sign appears to indicate irreversible brain damage (James ct. al., 1969). The victim's behaviour becomes increasingly bizarre; the person may smack tongue and lips involuntarily, spit bark out words (often obscenities) explosively, and walk with a jerky or shuffling gait. Eventually the victim of Huntington's live for ten to twenty years before dying. Such was the case with folksinger Woody Guthrie. And at present his son Arlo Guthrie must live with the knowledge that along with his father's talent, he may have inherited his father's disease thought it is still several years before he will know for sure whether he carries the fateful gene.

(b) **Parkinson's Disease**: Parkinson's disease, first described in 1871 by James Parkinson (who also suffered from it), also involves damage to the basal ganglia. The cause of this condition is unknown, although it has been attributed to a variety of sources, including encephalitis, heredity, viruses, toxins, and

deficient brain metabolism. The illness occurs most frequently to persons between the ages of fifty and seventy.

The primary symptom of Parkinson's is tremor, occurring at a rate of about four to eight movements per second. The tremors are usually present during rest periods, but tend to diminish or cease when the patient is sleeping. Interestingly, patients can often abruptly stop the tremors, at least temporarily, if someone orders them to do so, and for a short time they may even be able to perform motor activities requiring very Fine muscular coordination. However, such remissions are always temporary, and the patient once again lapses into the typical rhythmic jerking of arms, hands, jaws, and/or head.

Another highly characteristic physical sign of Parkinson's is an expressionless, mask like countenance, probably due to deterioration of muscle tonus resulting from damage to the basal ganglia.

Parkinson's patients also tend to walk, when they can walk, with a distinctive slow, stiff gait, usually accompanied by a slight crouch.

Psychological disturbances associated with Parkinson's disease area memory deficit, withdrawal from social contact, difficulty in concentration and apathy. In more severe cases there may be highly systematized delusions and severe depression, including suicidal tendencies. However, ills difficult to determine whether these symptoms are due directly to the brain pathology or simply to the patient's distress over his or her physical helplessness.

Parkinson's is unusual among the presenile degenerative disorders in that it can be treated with some success. L-dopa, a drug that increases the amount of the neurotransmitter dopamine, can in most cases control the tremor and other motor symptoms, though it cannot cure the disease. Antipsychotic drugs such as chlorpromazine deplete the brain of dopamine, which has led some researchers to propose that Parkinson's disease and schizophrenia are complementary malfunction of the dopamine system, one resulting from too little and the other from too much dopamine (Paul,1977).

(c) **Piek's Disease:** Pick's disease is an extremely rare disorder in which the frontal and temporal lobes of the brain gradually show atrophy. The disorder usually appears between the ages of forty-five and sixty and results in death four to seven years later.

Initial symptoms very from difficulty with simple reasoning and memory tasks to confusion, indifference, and occasionally, suspiciousness. Interestingly, victims of Pick's disease may exhibit either marked under activity or marked hyperactivity in their cognitive, emotional, and motor functions. Extremely hyperactive patients may at times become explosively violent and destructive.

As the disease advances, intellectual abilities slowly deteriorate, resulting in distractibility, concrete thinking and aphasias. Eventually the person is reduced to vegetative state, which may last for several years before death.

(d) **Alzheimer's Disease:** Like Pick's disease, Alzheimer's disease results from an atrophy of the brain, though in the case of Alzheimer's the damage is more diffuse, involving the entire cerebral cortex, along with the sub cortical structures. The characteristic early signs are irritability and difficulties in concentration and memory (Miller, 1973). As the disease progresses, a wide array of further deteriorative symptoms appear, including facial paralysis, involuntary movements and convulsions, physical aggression, hallucinations and delusions, and a strikingly rapid intellectual decline, involving aphasia, apraxia, and agnosia. The course of the fatala disease averages approximately four years.

The differential diagnosis of Pick's disease and Alzheimer's disease is sometimes difficult because the two syndromes strike the same age group, those in their forties and fifties, and share many of the same clinical signs. A general difference is that the deterioration of functioning is more widespread and occurs more rapidly in the more common Alzheimer's disease. A rule of thumb sometimes used is that victims of Pick's disease are typically indifferent, whereas patients with Alzheimer's disease generally appear quite anxious. Furthermore, clinicians suggest that people suffering from Pick's disease are more likely to show motor under activity. However, there are numerous exceptions to these, rules, and in practice the decision as to whether a patient is suffering from Pick's or Alzheimer's usually depends on biopsy or, ultimately, on autopsy.

(II) Senile Degenerative Disorders: Almost all old people experience some psychological changes simply as a function of ageing. Though the precise biochemical processes involved are still not clear, it seems that all behaviour mediated by the central nervous system slows down as the body ages (Birten, 1974). Old people in general show a slowing of motor reactions, a lessened capacity to process complex information, and a decreased efficiency in memory and in learning new materials. These changes, however, are part of the normal process of aging; they are no more pathological than wrinkles and gray hair. By contrast, the two major senile degenerative disorders, senile dementia and multi-infarct dementia, are pathological; they are the direct result of a severe organic deterioration of the brain.

The differential diagnosis of these two syndromes is often extremely complicated, since they have many of the same clinical signs. To make matters even more complicated, it is not uncommon for both of these syndromes-senile dementia and multi-infaret dementia to appear together in the same patient. A final source of diagnostic confusion is one that we have mentioned earlier, the symptoms in any individual case of organic brain disorder have everything to do with the patient's premorbid personality and psychosocial history, the availability of outside supports, and any number of other intangible factors. Of all the organic brain disorders, this is perhaps most true of the senile dengerative disorders. Thus, it is not rare for a proper diagnosis to be arrived at only after postmortem examination.

(a) **Senile Dementia**: Autopsies of victims of senile dementia commonly reveal extensive atrophy of brain tissue. This atrophy is identical to that seen in Alzheimer's disease. Precisely why this condition leads to the bizarre habits and intellectual incapacity's typical of senile dementia has not been fully explained. When the link is discovered, some kind of rehabilitation may enable many old people to live out their lives, with greater emotional and intellectual fulfillment.

In terms of symptoms, victims *of* senile dementia show a gradual increase in general behavioural problems. They' may neglect personal hygiene, going for days without bathing or changing their clothes. Oblivious to themselves and to those around them, they may explode in bursts of impulsive behaviour, such as ordering a houseful of new furniture when they can barely afford their monthly rent, or they may take a sudden interest in unusual activities atypical of their premorbid personalities.

As the disease progresses, cognitive defects particularly loss of memory for recent events become increasingly severe, further isolating the person from reality. Many patients, for example, may be able to give you the lineup of their favourite baseball team sixty years ago, complete with bating averages and runs batted in, but will not remember what they arc for lunch. (In some cases, there is permanent memory loss for distant events as well). Some patients mutter in unusual verbal patterns, stringing together the same jumbled phrases over and over again a condition called logorrhea. Other typical symptoms include emotional lability and a pronounced hatred of anything new.

(b) **Multi-infarct Dementia:** When an area of the brain ceases to function because a blood clot has cut off its blood supply in other words, because the person has suffered a CVA that area is called an infarct. And as the name indicates, multi-infarct dementia is the cumulative effect of multiple small strokes, eventually closing down many of the brain's faculties. Multi-infarct dementia used to be called cerebral arteriosclerosis. This, however, was a misnomer. Cerebral arteriosclerosis is a hardening of the walls in the blood vessels of the brain a condition that simply slows down blood flow through out the brain. By contrast, the disorder we arc considering is due to discrete blood clots (i.e., CVAs) cutting off circulation of blood altogether to discrete parts of the brain.

There are certain physiological signs blackouts, heart problems, symptoms of kidney failure, hypertension, and retinal sclerosis (a scarring of the retina of the eye) that suggest to the physician that multi-infarct dementia is the proper diagnosis. The prominent psychological symptoms are similar to those of senile dementia: confusion, memory defects, emotional lability, a declining interest in hygiene. However, according to Rothschild (1956), if the psychological manifestations are complex and are marked by alternating periods of lucidity and confusion, the patient is more likely to be suffering from multi-infarct than from senile dementia. Another specific indication of multi-infarct dementia is a fluctuation in the ability to recall distant events, which may be remembered in exquisite detail on one day and totally forgotten the next day. By contrast, memory deficits in senile dementia are constant and permanent.

EPILEPSY

Epilepsy is a Greek word that means "Seizure". Most forms of epilepsy are associated with a period of unconsciousness and involuntary movements.

Epilepsy is also associated with various forms of organic brain syndromes.

Epilepsy is actually a generic term covering a variety of organic disorders characterized by irregularly occurring disturbances in consciousness, in the form of seizures or convulsions. These seizures appear to be due to a disruption in the electrical and physiological activity of the discharging cells of the brain. About 85 per cent of epileptics manifest brain-wave abnormalities in EEG recordings. However, the remaining 15 per cent of epileptics have normal EEGs a fact that suggests that the abnormal discharges may occur too infrequently for detection by this instrument or that the disturbance arises from deeper with in the brain and consequently is not detectable by surface electrodes.

In most cases, epilepsy, regardless of its type, can be controlled with medication. However, in some very severe cases, surgery may be considered in order to remove the portion of the brain responsible for the seizures. In such cases the affected area can often be localized by EEG studies (Rasmussen and Branch, 1962).

Types of Epilepsy

Historically, epilepsy has been classified into four main types. These are

as follows:

1. Grand ma] epilepsy.
2. Petit mal epilepssy.
3. Jacksonian epilepsy.
4. Psychomotor epilepsy.

We will discuss these four types in brief

1. **Grand Mol Epilepsy** is the most dramatic, best known and most prevalent. Grand mal (literally, "great illness"), involves a generalized seizure, throughout the brain. There are thought to be four stages of grand mal, the first of which is the aura phase, in which may or may not occur. The second stage is the tonic phase, in which the person's body becomes very rigid with arms flexed, legs outstretched, add fists clenched and undergoes strong muscular contractions. During this phase, which may last for as long as a minute, breathing ceases. In the third stage, or clonic phase, breathing resumes and the muscles begin to contract and relax in a rhythmic way, causing the body to jerk in violent and rapid generalized spasms. In this stage there is some danger that the patient may be injured because of the violent jerking movements. The clonic phase also lasts about a minute, after which the convulsions dissipate. In the last stage, the

coma, results the muscles slowly relax while the patient remains unconscious. When the patient regains consciousness, he or she typically is somewhat confused, has a headache and feels quite exhausted and sleepy. In severe cases, such attacks may occur as often as several times a Jay. Historically, epilepsy has been classified according to four main types: (a) petit mal, (b) jacksonian (c) psychomotor, and (d) grand mal.

2. **Petit Mal:** Petit mal (literally, "small illness") the seizure generally lasts for Only a few seconds and involves only a brief, and not necessarily total loss of consciousness. During the attack the individual remains immobile, becomes completely unaware of his or her surroundings, and simply stares straight ahead. A loss of muscle tone may or may not accompany the seizure. After the attack the individual, unaware that anything has happened, simply resumes whatever he or she was doing prior to the attack. Such attacks can occur as often as a hundred times a day, but usually their occurrence is much less frequent, in which case the individual may not even require treatment.

3. **.Jacksonlan Epilepsy**: Jacksonian epilepsy, first described by the neurologist Hughlings Jackson, begins with a muscular twitching or a tingling in the hands and feet, which may then spread to other parts of the body. The part of the brain from which the seizure originates is thought to be quite localized, and treatment sometimes involves removing that portion of the brain. The Jacksonian seizure is often a preluded to a full-scale grand mal seizure, a type that we will examine shortly.

4. **Psychomotor Epilepsy**: In psychomotor epilepsy (now sometimes called "partial-complex" epilepsy), the attack, preceded by an aura, usually involves nothing more dramatic than a loss of contact with reality lasting anywhere from a few seconds to several minutes. During this time the person may appear quite normal and may engage in some rather mechanical activity. After the attack has passed, the person will resume his or her former business and will be amnesic for the episode.

Psychomotor attacks are unique among the epilepsics in two respects. 'First, during attacks, psychomotor epileptics may show bizarre, schizophrenic-like behaviour, such as public disturbing and urination, hallucinations and paranoid delusions and possibly violent aggression as well (Standage, 1973). Second, in very rare instances a person will commit a crime or an act of violence during a psychomotor seizure. Turner and Merlis (1962), for example, reported that 5 out of the' 337 epileptics included in their study had engaged in illegal activities during a seizure. Part of the unsuccessful defense of Jack Ruby, who killed Lee Harvey Oswald, the alleged assassin of President Kennedy, was that A Ruby had carried out Oswald's murder during a psychomotor seizure.

Causes of Epilepsy

Although epileptic seizures are due to disorganized, relatively spontaneous firings of groups of neurons, the basic, causal mechanism for the disorganized action of the neurons is still unclear. One widely considered possibility is that these neurons are biochemically hypersensitive to stimulation (Pinkus & Tucker, 1978). They are more irritable than normal. In some cases, such hypersensitivity may be a result of a prior injury. Individuals who have experienced a physical trauma to the brain are more likely to develop a seizure disorder than those who have not experienced brain damage. This is such a common phenomenon that individuals who have suffered brain injury or undergone brain surgery are often placed on anti seizure medication as a routine precaution.

A large proportion of people with epilepsy have no signs of brain damage other than their seizure disorder or an abnormal EEG, or electroencephalogram. Why do these individuals have hypersensitive neurons? Some studies have indicated that some forms of epilepsy, particularly the psychomotor type, may have a genetic component (Dejong & Sugar, 1972). Perhaps, in these cases, some biochemical defect is transmitted from parent to child. Yet in most cases of epilepsy of all types, no history of the disorder is found in the family prior to the involved individual, or in the affected individual's children. We still do not understand all the factors that can result in the development of neural hyperactivity and epilepsy.

TREATMENTS FOR BRAIN SYNDROMES AND EPILEPSY

The person who manifests and organic mental disorder often inquires a variety of treatment approaches. Since the damage is organic, medical interventions may be required. However, many of the problems in organic mental disorder are due to psychological reactions to the loss of previous abilities, and are responsive to non medical interventions such as psychotherapy or behaviour therapy and other environmental modifications. In this section, we will examine the contributions of both medicine and psychology to the treatment of these disorders.

Medical Intervention: A major focus of medical intervention in organic mental disorder is on the identification of the underlying pathology. This is a critical activity, since rapid diagnosis may allow effective treatment of some conditions. In Table 12.3 some examples of organic mental disorder, typical underlying pathology, and common .medical treatments are given. However, effective medical treatment of underlying pathology (such as a brain tumor) often does not "cure" the organic mental disorder. The underlying pathology may be treated and cured, but because of the extent of residua] brain damage, the individual may continue to have a chronic brain syndrome. Medical treatment can have a range of effects:

1. The underlying pathology may be successfully treated and the organic mental disorder may also remit. Delirium is a prime example an organic brail syndrome that is very likely to clear up if the underlying Pathology is treated. Other than syndromes, such as those caused by some toxins or metabolic disturbances, may also respond well to medical treatment.

2. The underlying pathology may be successfully treated, but permanent damage to the brain may result in an ongoing organic mental disorder. Such an outcome may include successfully removed tumors, neurosyphilis, and multi-infarct dementia.

3. The underlying pathology may be so severe that medical treatment is infective, or the disorder may have no known treatment. The primary examples of this outcome are the degenerative disorders of presenile and senile dementia.

Chronic organic mental disorder is a major health care problem, especially among the elderly. Although the degenerative dementias cannot be reversed, many medical researchers are looking for treatments to reduce the impairment of senile dementia. Some researchers are studying the effects of a chemical called physostigmine on memory deficits in degenerative dementia. This drug appears to slightly increase memory performance in animals and normal humans. However, its effects are only temporary. The memory enhancement lasts only while the drug is being given intravenously, and decreases after about 15 minutes of continuous medication (Christile ct al., 1981).

Unfortunately, physostigmine is not a useful treatment for memory disorder in degenerative dementia. Medical researchers will, however, continue to search for more effective, longer-lasting treatments for these disorders. Perhaps some aspects of dementia will be medically treatable in years to come (Wells, 1978).

Rehabilitation: Most body tissue regenerates when injured. If a finger is cut or scratched, new cells form during the healing process, and only a slight scar or no scar will remain. Brain cells, in contrast, do not regenerate. Once dead or destroyed, they arc gone forever. However, when a part of the brain is damaged or destroyed other parts of the brain may be able to take over some functions of the destroyed section. Some functions, once lost, can never be regained (e.g., loss of judgement because of frontal lobe damage does not appear to be relearnable).

The functions that appear most likely to be reclaimed include motor coordination, speech, and bowel and bladder control. A victim of a major stroke often has deficits in these areas, but the potential for long-term recovery of at least a portion of these abilities is good. The relearing is unlikely to be spontaneous. Brain-damaged persons require many months, even years, of structured practice in order to regain some of their predamage ability. The rehabilitation process can be frustrating and even physically painful, but if the training and practice do not occur, the functions may be lost permanently (C.B. Stevens, 1974).

Psychotherapy and behaviour therapy: The verbal psychotherapies have been used to help organically damaged individuals. Emotional and motivational problems such as anger, depression, and despair may be alleviated through the process of sharing feeling and receiving understanding and summit. The recognition that all physical disorders have a psychological component has led to a much wider availability of psychological treatment for individuals with chronic brain syndrome (and other chronic physical illness).

Behavioural therapy, like verbal psychotherapy, may assist the individual in making a better adjustment to the organic damage that has been suffered. Behaviour therapy can also maximize the potential of individuals with degenerative-disorders. When reinforces are made contingent upon appropriate behaviour, certain behaviours which are often presumed to be due to the deterioration of the brain can be changed. Bowel and bladder control may be reinstituted, hygiene improved, and some bizarre behaviours reduced. The implementation of a token economy can have broad effects on the functioning of' wards of geriatric patients. Lest this give too optimistic an impression, we must remember that progressive brain deterioration will wipe out these gains in the long run. In addition, some organic deficits prevent effective learning. The individual with presenile or senile dementia who cannot store memories may never learn (remember) that keeping tidy results in reinforcement.

Even if not associated with specific reinforcers, some general environmental changes can help maximize the functioning of brain-damaged individuals. For example, individuals who have memory problems can be helped if calendars are available and others remind them what to do and where to be. Problems in speech comprehension may be alleviated if people talk slowly and clearly to the individual. Books with large print and large printed signs may help people read and find their way about. Patient and caring helpers can assist in reducing the psychological trauma of organic mental disorders. Too often, some modifiable aspects of brain-damaged individual's behaviour are attributed to the organic damage and are left unchanged.

The following table summarizes the common organic mental disorders and their respective medical treatment approaches.

Table 123. Organic mental disorder, underlying pathology, and common medkal treatments

Organic mental disorder	Example of underlying Pathology	Medical treatment
Delirium	Fever due to pneumonia	Antibiotics; sedative for moderate agitation. .
Amnestic syndrome	Thiamine deficiency and chronic alcohol use	Vitamin therapy.
	Tumor	Surgery
Organic affective syndrome	Hypothyroidism	Thyroid medication.
Organic personality. syndrome	Benign frontal lobe tumor	Surgery
Dementia	Strokes due to high blood pressure Malignant tumor	Treatment of high blood pressure Surgery, radiation, or chemotherapy

11

Disorders Of Childhood And Adolescence

Disorders *at* childhood and adolescence has not received much attention as the adult disorders have received. Unlike the troubled adults, children and adolescence with psychological problems cannot seek help for themselves. Often, they cannot be helped without the consent and cooperation of their parents. Childhood psychological disorders, when they are not disabling, often go unlabelled and untreated.

The disorders observed in children cover a broad spectrum varying in symptom content, severity, and duration. Some disorders are less severe such as developmental deviations anxiety disorders and hyperactivity, others are more severe, pervasive developmental disorders, also called as childhood schizophrenia or psychosis, autism etc.

We would first discuss the eating and elimination disorders of children. Among the eating disorders; we will discuss the eating disorders of obesity and anorexia nervosa. These disorders generally appear in late childhood and early adolescence. Among the elimination disorders the two disorders of significance are enuresis and encopresis.

We would then discuss speech disorders and certain disorders associated with masculature like tics, tourette's syndrome etc. in the form of short notes.

School phobia and anxiety disorders are also commonly seem in many young children. These two disorders can interfere with a wide variety of normal everyday life activities and may also lead to various other developmental disorders. We would discuss these two disorders in brief.

Attention deficit disorder, some times also called as Hyperactivity is one of the most common disorder seen in child guidance clinic. This particular disorder is not only troublesome for parents but it also interferes with normal school functioning. We will examine this disorder in detail.

Following this we would discuss some pervasive developmental disorders, these disorders are of serious attention as they resist any treatment intervention and cause a great deal of disturbance not only to an individual but also to his family members. The two most widely studied pervasive developmental disorders are childhood schizophrenia and autism. We would discuss these two in detail.

Adolescence is rightly remarked as a period of 'stress and strain Adolescence calls for new expectations, new roles, new demands and more better adjustment. Adolescence is also a period where sexual changes, identity crisis, career choice etc, are taking place. All these and many more changes lead to great deal of stress and strain on the child.

Among the most common disorders of adolescence are the eating disorders of anorexia nervosa, and Bulimia we would discuss these two disorders in detail.

We will then discuss the conduct disorder and its types as listed in DSM-III. Children with conduct disorders are cause for grave social concern; for all parents, teachers, lawmakers, social workers, police etc.

We would then end this chapter with a few short notes.

EATING AND ELIMINATION DISORDERS IN CHILDREN

Eating Disorders, especially among the children are of great concern to mental health experts. Since the time of Freud, feeding has been regarded as a crucial aspect of development. Young children, for food, depend upon others, their experiences during feeding are likely to have a major influence on future interpersonal relationships. Feeding is also associated very often, in many individuals, with anxiety, conflict and dissatisfaction. The most important disorders of feeding are obesity, anorexia nervosa and bulimia. We will discuss obesity and anorexia nervosa.

It has been estimated that 25 percent of children have a recognized eating problem.

Obesity: In children, as in adults, is defined as an excessive amount of fatress on the body. Most investigators consider a child as obese if his/her weight is 40 percent higher than the median weight for children of the same height.

Hilde Bruch has classified obesity into 3 type (a) normal (b) developmental and (c) reactive.

A child may become obese not because of any emotional problem, but because overeating is the "normal" thing to do in his ',' her family and ethnic group. This is "normal" obesity.

In the second "developmental pattern" obesity may occur as a function of family problems, especially marital problems between the parents. When parents are in conflict with each other, they often attempt to satisfy their own needs through their children. The response of the mother, in particular, may be to overprotect and overfeed the child. As a result, the child becomes obese and remains so by overeating, whenever he/she is subject to stress and frustration. In the third or the "reactive" pattern, obesity may develop in response to some acute emotional stress (e.g. the death of a parent or the birth of a sibling) and, overeating may function as a form of consolation and reassurance.

Obese children suffer from a number of emotional and adjustment problems. They are made a target of fun. Guilt, rejection, self contempt and exclusion from peer group activities then becomes a further source of stress; causing such children to overeat even more than before.

Anorexia Nervosa - is another very common disorder, mostly seen among young adolescent. About 95 percent of anorexia are girls and in most cases onset is between the ages of 12 and 18.

Predictably the most dramatic physical sign of anorexics is the weight loss.

Anorexic is defined as one who looses 25 percent of his/her body weight. The weight loss is normally accompanied by amenorrhea, suspension of menstrual period, and by other physical signs.

In behavioral terms, the anorexic usually follows one of two patterns: cither she simply refuses to cat, or she eats (sometimes voraciously) and then cither vomits spontaneously or induces vomiting. Some patients report that they are so repelled by food that they never experience normal sensations of hunger, but they are the exceptions. Most anorexics clearly have normal appetites, at least in the early stages of the disorder (Broh, 1973). Indeed, they may become quite preoccupied with food, collecting cookbooks, preparing elaborate meals for others, and going through sporadic episodes of bulimia, or uncontrolled binge

eating, followed by self-induced vomiting. Whatever else they do with food, however, they do not allow themselves to digest it in any reasonable quantity for fear of becoming obese.

Anorexia is notoriously difficult to treat. Time and again, investigators b8ve reported cases in which hospitalized patients responded to treatment but then relapsed, especially upon discharge from the hospital. One problem in treatment is that once malnutrition has progressed to a certain point, whatever appetite the patient had does disappear; in addition, she may be too weak to cat, However, the major impediments to treatment are the anorexic's distorted body image and her iron determination to correct this situation by refusing to eat. Long-term follow-up studies indicate that about one-fifth of anorexics literally starve themselves to death (Halini et. al., 1975). For the others, prognosis ranges from complete recovery to lifelong maladjustment, with persistent eating problems. Somewhere between 25 and 50 percent of patients have recurrent bouts of the disorder (Moldofsky and Garfinkel, 1974).

The cause of anorexics is attributed to two factors:

(a) **Suppression of sexuality:** Anorexia is interpreted by some clinicians as a strategem for avoiding the adult sexual role and especially for avoiding the possibility of pregnancy. "The fact that amenorrhea often precedes the weight loss and is thus presumably psychogenic rather than the consequence of malnutrition, lends some support to this hypothesis. Besides amenorrhea sex derive commonly disappears and the "figure" of the person also changes and appears to be less sexually appealing.

(b) **Family warfare** - is another suspected cause of anorexia. The child uses self-starvation as a weapon against parents. Disturbed parent child relationship is usually found among those who have this disorder.

Elimination Disorders: Like feeding, toilet training may be an arena of intense conflict. This is the first time that children are forced to comply with demands that run counter to their natural impulses. And sometimes these demands can be extreme, for our society places great emphasis on the achieving of eliminative control at an early age. Failure to pass this developmental milestone is classified as either enuresis or encopresis, depending on whether it is bladder control or bowel control that is lacking.

Enuresis: Enuresis is usually defined as a lack of bladder control past the age when such control is usually achieved. In other words Enuresis is defined as the occurrence of "persistent" bed-wetting after the age of 5. The most important point to keep in mind before labelling a child enuretic is that the definition of enuresis depends to a great extent on the child's age. Infants and very young children, for instance, wet their beds, yet are not enuretic. Thus, far, bed-wetting is the only reaction that occurs normally up to a certain age and thereafter is considered abnormal. Care must be taken before this label and subsequent treatment are applied.

Another point is whether the child has ever had bladder control. If a 5- or 6-year-old has displayed bladder control for, say, two or three years and then relapses, the label can be applied. On the other hand, labelling by itself does no good, it could even be harmful. The purpose in specifying that a problem exists is so that intervention methods can be started immediately.

Bed-wetting should be taken seriously. Bailer (1975) tells us that bed-wetters often feel very guilty, think they are deviant and odd, and thus hold a low view of themselves. He cites evidence of changes in self-concept after successful treatment.

Causes: The etiological theories explaining enuresis are numerous; a few of the more popular ones are that it is an inherited defect; that it is a result of poor toilet-training; and that it is a symptom of an underlying problem, that is, it is emotionally induced.

(a) **Organic Viewpoint:** There are two organic viewpoints :

(i) The first view suggests that enuretics have an organic impairment or infection in the urinary tract, that is, a defect in the bladder, urethra, or kidneys. The preponderance of male enuretics (about three to two) is often used as evidence for this organic defect view. The observation that drugs may have some effect in lessening bed wetting also used to support the organic view. In this connection, the drug of choice has been imipramine, and antidepressant that has been shown to be effective in certain cases. Why is an antidepressant effective? According to few theorists, the reason is that the drug reduces anxiety. In one etiological view, conflict (anxiety) is thought to play some role in bed-wetting.

(ii) Another organic or hereditary theory states that enuresis tends to "run in the family." Young (1963), for example, found that approximately 50 percent of a sample of 320 enuretic children had relatives who were also enuretic. Bakwin and Bakwin (1972) cite studies conducted in Israel and twin studies that strongly imply, that heredity plays a part in enuresis.

(b) Learning viewpoint: The second view claims that. enuresis is learned. Or, more specifically, that it is unwittingly "taught" by the parents. Bailer remarks that "a high percentage of bed-wetting can accurately be attributed directly and exclusively lo a child's being 'taught' to urinate while asleep. To further explain this interesting view. Bailer remarks that many parents keep up the practice of placing the child on the toilet while he or she is still asleep. Obviously this procedure is intended to help the child learn to urinate in the appropriate places. But what appears on the surface to be good parenting actually trains the child to urinate while he or she is still drowsy. Rather than taking sleeping child to be bathroom, he or she should be awakened before being gotten out of bed.

(c) **Emotional factors and Enuresis:** The third theory states that enuresis is emotionally induced. Stated differently, this position suggests that enureis is a symbolic expression of some underlying conflict. Psychoanalysts have traditionally taken this point of view. They contend that bed-wetting is a symtom of repressed desires or conflict. The repressed desire, it is thought, involves repressed sexual material; bed-wetting has been called a symbolic form of masturbation. The psychoanalytic view also states that bet-wetting may represent an expression of hostility o; aggression; analytically inclined theorists have called it "revenge wetting". Finally, it has been suggested that bed-wetting is simply a consequence of being depressed and unhappy. Sperling (1974) quotes the remarks of a persistently enuretic 5-year-old who said, "People sometimes do these things because they are unhappy. They do it to make themselves feel happy".

The psychoaftalytic view, in short, does not view enuresis as an organic defect or an accident of learning, but as a symbol of some unconscious wish. Treatment based on this model therefore aims at uncovering the unconscious motivation, not at alleviating the symptom.

Treatment-An effective treatment based on learning theory was developed by Morwrer and Mowrer (1933,1938). The Mowrer procedure was the prototype for conditioning treatments of enuresis. The apparatus used in this "bell-and-blanket" method consists of a liquid-sensitive gauze on which the child sleep. When the discharge of urine contacts the liquid-sensitive gauze, an alarm (a bell) is sounded that arouses the child. How this procedure teachers the child to wake up before he or she urinates is still a matter of some dispute. Mowrer asserted that bladder distention, a stimulus, occurs prior to the alarm; after many pairings with the alarm, bladder distention takes on the awakening qualities of the aversive sound. A contrasting view claims that the child learns to wake up in order to a avoid the alarm. Regardless of why or how the child learns to wake up prior to bed-wetting, the method is very effective.

Encopresiss- When toilet-training failure involves a lack of bowel control rather than of bladder control, the pattern is called encopresis. In some ways encopresis resembles enuresis. It too is classified as either primary (in which control is never achieved) or secondary (in which control is mastered and then lost). It too may have an organic basis, in the primary form. It too is more common in males than in female". Finally, even more than enuresis, encopresis can earn a child mockery from peers and wrath from parents, compounding whatever problems he or she has.

In other respects, encopresis differs from enuresis. It is much less common, occurring in approximately I percent of the general population (DSM -III, 1980). And it is regarded as a much more serious disturbance. While wetting one's pants can be considered (and is often called) an "accident" defecating in one's pants is generally viewed as an antisocial act. Thus most psychologists interpret encopresis as a clear sign of psychological distress, possibly in reaction to family conflict. This is especially the case with secondary encopresis, since the primary form may be due in some cases simply to haphazard toilet training.

SPEECH DISORDERS

Though there are many different childhood speech disorders, psychological disturbance appears to be implicated in only two of these conditions delayed speech and stuttering.

(i) **Delayed speech**: Most children say their first words within a few months after their first birthday. And between eighteen and twenty-four months, they usually begin to formulate two or three-word sentences. There are wide individual differences in this schedule, and a few months' delay in developing normal speech is rarely thought to have any diagnostic significance. Some normal children begin to speak much later than others: Albert Einstein, for example, did not utter his first words until he was fully three years old. However, a prolonged delay in speaking is usally taken very seriously, as a possible indication of an organic or functional disorder.

In some cases, failure to speak is an early sign of autism, deafness, mental retardation, or some other, more specific form of brain damage. Often, however, there is more. manageable, functional cause-lack of encouragement or verbal stimulation from the parents, a trauma such as hospitalization or any long separation from the parents, or a discouragement of the child's independence on the part of the parents.

(ii) **Stuttering**: Stuttering refers to the interruption of speech fluency through blocked, prolonged, or repeated words, syllables, or sounds. Many people stutter on occasion, and speech hesitation in young children is a very common phenomenon. Consequently, with stuttering as with so many other childhood disorders, it is often difficult to decide what is a serious condition and what is not. Persistent stuttering occurs in approximately I percent of the population, males outnumbering females four to one. The disorder is not likely to appear either between two and three-and-a-half years or between Five and seven years. In any case, the onset is almost always before age twelve (DMS-III, 1980).

Causes1- As usually, the etiological theories of stuttering are divided between biogenic or psychogenic causes. The biogenic view suggests that stuttering results from organic impairment hi the central nervous system. Support for this position again comes from the overrepresentation of males among stutterers (three to eight times more prevalent than females). In addition, it is often noted that stuttering is seen uniformly throughout the world, implying that culture makes little difference (Sheehan 1975).

The psychogpnic position maintains that stuttering is learned behaviour. One particular learning theory model was proposed by Bloodstein (1975): the anticipatory struggle hypothesis. This hypothesis proposes that the stutterer . behaves as though he or she has "acquired a belief in the difficulty of speech...." For example, the child takes for granted that he or she will fail in speaking. Bloodstein further notes that stuttering occurs primarily in social situations and "becomes intensified when (he or she feels) socially ill at case, tense, insecure, or uncomfortable...." Since the stutterer can, in certain situations, speak rather fluently, it is the anticipation of failure and the struggle not to fail (anticipatory Struggle) that undermines normal speaking. As Polow (1975) remarks, the person does not stutter so much when he or she feels confident. The harder the person tries, the more likely he or she is to fail.

Bloodstein offers several antecedent environmental conditions that may cause a child to develop a poor self-concept and a belief in his or her inability to speak. Parents often demand perfection, or they may seem over concerned about their child's speech. All these factors lead to stuttering or other speech difficulties.

Treatment: Treatment based on the anticipatory struggle hypothesis involves counseling with the parents to lessen environmental pressures. Other essentials of treatment are (1) desired speech patterns should be reinforced; (2) the child's anxiety about stuttering should be reduced by bringing the problem out in the open; (3) the child should recognize that other persons do not always speak perfectly; (4) the child should not avoid the opportunity to speak. Sheehan (1975) similarly suggests that the key element in therapy is "avoidance-reduction," That is, the stutterer should not try to avoid speaking, but should make every effort to speak when it is appropriate to do so. The stutterer should, therefore, talk more, not avoid activities because of the possibility that he or she will stutter.

TICS AND MOTOR HABITS

A tic is a meaningless, repetitive, involuntary motor activity. They usually include such motor activities as persistent eye-blinking, twitching, shrugging the shoulders, grimacing, and so on. One question always raised is whether the tic is the main problem or merely represents some underlying difficulty. Kessler (1972) suggests that persistent tic-like behaviours usually indicate emotional difficulties.

A distinction is normally made between transient tics and chronic tics. the diagnostic cut-off point being a duration of one year. Transient tics are often thought to be reactions to situational pressure or perhaps to a generally stressful period in the child's life. Chronic tics, on the other hand, are often interpreted as an indication of serious anxiety. Chronic tics may persis for years in about 6 percent of cases, they actually continue into adulthood. Normally they disappear to diminish considerably during adolescence (Bakwin and Bakwin, 1972).

Closely related to tics are motor habits, repetitive and nonfunctional patterns of motor behaviour that, like tics, seem to occur in response lo stress. These are sometimes called "nervous habits", sometimes "tensional outlasts," They include nail biting, tongue sucking, hair pulling (i.e. pulling out one's own hair), and numerous other habits all of them irritating to parents but by far the most common is thumb sucking.

Causes: Specific etiological theories about tics include learning theory positions and a psychoanalytic position.

(a) The tension-reduction hypothesis, one learning viewpoint, implies that tics reduce tension or anxiety and so are continued. According to Bandura (1969), tics can be acquired by accident; that is, under stress, certain responses may be made by chance and be found to reduce tension. This position, however, appears to overlook the initial stressors that produce the "random" motor activity.

(b) Another learning theory dealing with tics is modelling. This notion suggests simply that tics are learned by watching or imitating others. This view is circular, because it docs not tell us how the "model" developed the tic.

(c) Finally, the psychoanalytic position is an elaboration of Kessler's position that tics are emotionally induced symbolic activities expressing some underlying wish or conflict. The explanation is virtually identical to the one given for bed-wetting both actions arc thought to release either repressed sexual or distinctive impulses.

Treatment: Treatment of a tic depends chiefly on the orientation of the clinician. The behaviorist might use massed practice (also referred to as negative practice), in which the tic is performed intentionally for a long time. For instance, a child with a shoulder-shrugging tic would be instructed to practice shrugging his or her shoulders for one hour without stopping. Massed practice is perhaps the most effective treatment approach.

Psychoanalysts, on the other hand, argue that eliminating the symptom without getting the underlying cause will not help the child in the long run. Treating the symptom alone (the behavioural approach) only shifts the "energy" to some other activity or symptom. This is referred to as symptom substitution.

Although this argument sounds plausible, Bandura (1969) cites numerous studies to refute the symptom substitution idea. Nevertheless, psychoanalytic therapy involves uncovering repressed material that is thought to provide the motivation for the tic.

TOURETTE'S SYNDROME

Tourette's syndrome is a disorder characterized by recurrent, involuntary, repetitive, rapid, purposeless motor movements (tics) and multiply vocal tics. The vocal tics may involve verbal utterances in the form of swearing, epithets, and obscenities. These verbalizations are at times accompanied by spitting, blowing, and barking sounds. Such behaviour, termed coprolalia (faces speech), is present is about 60 percent of all patients; it typically occurs without warning (Silver, 1980). Tourette's disease is very rare, occurring in about I out of every 12,500 cases presented in psychiatric clinics. Of the 250 cases of this disorder studied over the past decade, there are more females than males at a ratio of about 3 to I (Hajal and Leach, 1981). A rare case of Tourette's in twins is also found.

Although the etiology of Tourette's remains unknown, the biological paradigm may be the best guide to its ultimate discovery. While there is no clear support for a biological cause, Tourette's has been found to be associated with a higher incidence of minimal brain dysfunction, abnormal clectro-encephalograms, and left handedness (Silver, 1980). While there is no connection between an cffcctive physical treatment and a physical cause, it is at least consistent with biologically based paradigmatic explanations, that drug treatment, specifically haloperidol, significantly reduces Tourette's symptoms (Shapin, et. al Shapiro ct al 1973).

SCHOOL PHOBIA

A phobia is an intense but unwarranted fear of some object or situation. Somatic symptoms such as nausea, refusal to eat, vomiting, and abdominal pains may accompany the fear or anxiety. While children may develop animal phobias and transportation phobias (Kessler 1966), school phobia is the most common.

Specifically, a school phobia consists of anxiety, panic, and often abdominal pains that develop when the child is faced with having to go to school. Bakwin and Bakwin (1972) remark that the fear is usually related to a particular teacher, classmate, or anticipation of an exam.

Causes: The hypothesized causes of school phobia are rather simple learning theorists, for instance, hold that the phobia has been acquired because it is reinforcing to avoid school. Stated differently, the school setting is perceived as aversive; any behaviour that keeps the child from the dreaded situation will be reinforced or strengthened. Somatic complaints (such as nausea) are also thought to be learned, for they reduce the likelihood that the child will have to go to school. Another etiological thesis states that going to school is feared because the child has not learned to "separate" from his or her mother. The child is

pathologically attached to her, and the prospect of separation engenders anxiety and panic.

ANXIETY DISORDERS

Children with diagnosis of anxiety disorder arc characterized by fear and apprehension associated with varying factors. Children with anxiety disorders are often unable to pay, go to school, attend special events, or take part in many of the everyday activities of childhood.

Forms of Anxiety Disorders In Children

Childhood anxiety may manifest itself in several forms. Among these are (a) separation anxiety, (b) avoidant disorder, and (c) overanxious disorder.

(a) **In Separation Anxiety,** children show "exaggerated distress at the separation from parent, home, or familiar surroundings" (DSM-III). They may ruminate about their parents becoming ill, injured, or killed. In *some* cases these worries may include fantasies about being kind napped or banned when they are separated from their parents. Fears are shown by "expressing discomfort about leaving home, engaging in solitary activities and continuing to use the mothering figure as a helper in buying clothes and entering social and ***recreational*** activities"(Werkman, 1980). Anxiety increases during transitions such as among going to and from school, changing schools, or moving away from home.

(b) **Avoident Disorder-As** with most of the anxiety related disorders, in avoidant disorders children also have difficulties making, transition. While usually fine at home, youngsters with avoidant disorders shrink from interaction , and show embarrassment, timidity, and withdrawal when forced to come in contact with strangers. Timidity is a great roadblock to the building of normal peer relationships and to the experiencing of interpersonal activities necessary to growth and maturity. Avoidant youngsters, though not usually participating in many activities, do seem to want to be accepted by peers and to be competitive, in academic and athletic situations. However, should their initial efforts meet with failure, they typically stop trying and quickly withdraw from the activity.

(c) Over anxious Disorder: While rumination can be part of all anxiety disorders, it is the major symptom in the overanxious disorder. These youths ruminate about things such examinations, possible future events, and past difficulties. Interested in pleasing others and usually quite conforming, overanxious children also are prone to gain attention by exaggerating their pains or illnesses and having more than their share of accidents. Their sleep is often disturbed because night time appears to bean especially favourable time to ruminate about the past day's events.

Treatment of Anxiety Disorders

Most of the interventions for children with anxiety-related disorders have been derived from the psychosocial paradigm. They can be subsumed under the main headings of play therapy and behavioural therapy. While play therapy was derived specifically for children, the behavioural methods are a subset of the more general behavioural therapies applied to adults as well.

Play Therapy: Play therapists take advantage of the fact that children often can express themselves better in play than in talking. The approach can be used to treat less severely disturbed children, but it is especially useful with children who have limited verbal ability.

In psychoanalytic play therapy, the therapists role is to identify problems in psychosexual development and to attempt to understand the symbolic nature of the child's play behaviour. Through "corrective" play and interpretation, insights and behaviour change may occur as the child is placed back on the normal track of psychic development. By skillful interpretation of the use of play materials, the psychoanalytic therapist can gain an understanding of the child and can direct the efforts towards more developmentally appropriate play objects. If a child smears finger paints for a long time, a therapist may try to help the child to use crayons, a more controlled mode of emotional expression. It is assumed that this more controlled mode of expression will generalize to situations outside the playroom.

Instead of trying to redirect deviant psychosexual development, therapists espousing nondirective play therapy (Axling, 1964) provide an atmosphere of acceptance that will help the child work out problems with a minimum of direction and guidance.

Behavior Therapies: Rather than focusing on the relationship between child and therapist, therapists using behavioral techniques emphasize procedures derived from learning theory. In token-reinforcement methods, tokens are given to children when they perform acceptable behaviour. Teachers have long used "tokens" like stars and smiling face stickers to reward positive performance of their students. A token is any object that has acquired value because it can be traded for something else of value. For example, a nickle is a "token" that can be "traded" for some gum. In token-reinforcement system, tokens are given for desirable behaviour and can be used to obtain other valued items. Ten stars may enable a child to get a candy bar. Perhaps they receive one star every time they clean their room. Thus, each star represents one-tenth of a candy bar.

In a typical application of a token reinforcement system, parents, child and therapist all agree on target behaviors, or behaviors that need to be altered. Target behaviors may include "dos" like homework and cleaning up rooms, or "dont's" like not poking baby brother or talking with a full mouth. There are various ways to keep track of the children's positive behavior. In one application children arc presented with a pictorial representation of a road that has 10 "toll booths" or "gates" with 10 stars or tokens required for passage through a gate. At the very end of the road is a representation of a previously agreed upon reinforces (toy or a similar desirable object) that the child may obtain only by traversing the "road". Behaviors that will result in the awarding of a token are clearly set forth for the child. At each lO-token gate, a smaller reinforces (a candy bar or comic book) may be given to the child. These intermediate reinforces ensure the maintenance of behavior from the beginning of the program to the final reward which may be as many as 100 tokens down the road. Using the token-reinforcement star road, such behaviors as school avoidance, lying, irritating a. younger sibling, and refusing to do homework may be effectively changed and replaced with more acceptable behaviors.

Some professionals have suggested using progressive relaxation training for children who have high levels of tension or identifiable fears (e.g.,0'Bannon, 1981). Procedures may have to be modified for treating children. They need to be rewarded for complying with the instructions and their sessions should be much shorter, probably about 15 minutes in length. However, it appears that therapists may be too creative in adapting desensitization procedures for children (Hatzenbuehler and Schroeder, 1978) to the extent that there is little evidence for particular repeatable interventions (Rickard and Elkins, 1983).

ATTENTION DEFICIT DISORDER WITH HYPERACTIVITY

Attention Deficit Disorder with Hyperactivity is extremely widespread. It is the most common behaviour disorder seen by child Psychologist/Psychiatrist and the most common cause of childhood referral to mental health clinics. According to conservative estimates, it affects at least 5 percent of the elementary school population, with boys outnumbering girls ten to one.

Its most salient features are incessant restlessness and an extremely poor attention span, leading in turn to impulsive and disorganised behaviour. These handicaps affect almost every area of child's functioning.

The inability to focus attention has a ruinous effect on the academic progress. Hyperactive children have great difficulty following instructions and finishing tasks; often they cannot even remember what they set out to do. Consequently, while often intelligent, they have severe learning problems. They are also extremely disruptive in the class-room, interrupting, darting here and there, and making incessant demands for attention.

Hyperactive children also show poor social adjustment They knock over other children's blocks, disrupt games, get into fights, refuse to play fair, and throw temper tantrums when they do not get their ways. They do this not out of aggressiveness but due to low frustration tolerance.

Attention deficit with hyperactivity are usually variable. The child may seem greatly improved one week and then much worse the next week. The disorder .also varies situationally. In many cases, hyperactive children function adequately on a one-to-one basis but fall apart in group situations; hence they may do well at home but not at school.

Hyperactive children seem to be driven, easily distractible, and readily excited. One moment they may be frustrated and tearful because they cannot find their pencil, while at the next moment they will be laughing loudly because one of the other children made a strange noise. They arc described by their parents as frequent criers, very active and erratic caters and sleepers (Laufer & Shetty, 1980).

Although attempts have been made, no paradigm has generated an acceptable theory for the origins of hyperactivity. Some investigators with biological perspectives have implicated defects in cortical arousal(Rosenthal & Alien, 1978; Hastings & Barkley, 1978), environmental toxins such as lead poisoning or food additives (Feingold, 1975), and minimal brain dysfunction (Me Glannon,1975) in causing hyperactivity. The wide variety of possible causes suggests that there may be more than one way to become hyperactive.

The proponents of psychosocial and biological paradigms have clashed over the correct ways to treat hyperactivity. For example, drugs that usually stimulate the brain and energize behavior, like amphetamines and caffeine, paradoxically calm hyperactive children (Goodman & Oilman, 1982; Safer & Alien, 1973). Others have pointed out that prolonged use of anti activity drugs like Dexedrine and Ritalin may result in a number of serious side effects such as liver disorders and suppressed growth (Laufer & Shetty, 1980). However, those opposed to drug treatment for hyperactivity have suggested the use of psychosocially based programmed learning procedures and, in some instances, cognitive behavioral techniques that combine positive reinforcement with verbal self instructions (e.g., Kendall & Finch, 1978; Meichenbaum & Goodman, 1971).

Long-term follow-up of hyperactive children shows that they fall further and further behind their peers academically. The resulting loss of self-esteem compounds their personal problems and they may become isolated or delinquent in their later years. (Minde et. al 1971; Pelham, 1978; Solomon, 1972).

Discuss childhood psychosis, its symptomatology and its classification.

Or

Distinguish between Infantile antism and childhood schizophrenia.

Childhood psychosis is a general term used to refer to pervasive developmental disorder which are more serious and which resist most interventions.

Although DSM-III has classified most forms of childhood psychoses under the rubric of pervasive developmental disorders, the theory, research, and therapy for severe disturbances of childhood continue to reflect the existence of two major patterns childhood schizophrenia and autism.

Childhood Psychosis* or *Schizophrenia

Many investigators have found a common cluster of symptoms characterizing psychotic children. Perhaps the most widely cited set of criteria was given by Creak (1961) and his co-workers in England. This group listed nine basic symptoms of childhood psychosis; Goldfarb also has confirmed them in the children he observed in the United States:

1. Gross and sustained impairment of emotional relationships with people.
2. Apparent unawareness of personal identity.
3. Pathological preoccupation with the attachment to particular objects.
4. Resistance to any change in the environment.
5. Abnormal perceptual experiences, even though sensory functions are almost normal.
6. Acute, excessive, and illogical anxiety.
7. Speech defects and arrests, or failure to use language appropriately.
8. Distorted movements or bizarre stereotyped behaviors-twirling, toe-walking, hand-flapping.
9. A history of serious retardation, yet with some unusual or near normal abilities in certain areas.

This list is intended to be comprehensive; only rarely will a single psychotic child manifest all these symptoms. Nevertheless, three of them are considered particularly important for the current and future adjustment of the child and are likely to appear in any child diagnosed as psychotic. These are (1) disturbed social relationship; (2) speech impairment; and (3) bizarre motor behavior.

Sometimes identified as the cardinal trait of childhood psychosis, the disturbance in social relationships may take the form of total withdrawal, or at the other extreme, of obsessive attachment, either to the mother or in some cases to an inanimate object such as a vacuum cleaner, a garden house, or something equally unlikely. In short, the psychotic child cither fails to respond to his or her social environment or responds in an inappropriate manner.

No doubt closely linked to the impaired social skills of psychotic children is their equally severe impairment of speech. Many psychotic children are actually mute, in which case they merely babble, shine or howl like a three-to six-month-old infant. When speech is present, it is marked by a number of peculiarities and may be used cither in a totally no communicative fashion or for the communication of bizarre or incoherent ideas.

To the observers, however, the most striking oddity of psychotic children is their bizzare motor behavior. These behaviors can vary considerably, ranging from a total lack of movement (catatonia) to wild tantrums, self-induced vomiting, and faces smearing. Most typical, however, is the psychotic child with a limited repertoire of movements that he or she repeats endlessly, in stereotypic fashion, with no observable goals. These self-stimulatory responses may involve fine or gross motor movements of the hands, face, arms, and/or trunk, in combination or in isolation. Examples include twirling, toe walking (a sort of prolonged tiptoeing), hand flapping, rocking, and tensing of various parts of the body. If left to themselves, psychotic children, especially those in institutions are likely to spend up to 90 percent of their waking hours engaged in these apparently nonfunctional behaviours (Lovaas et. al., 1971a).

Infantile Autism

For many years it was generally believed that childhood psychosis was in fact a single disorder. Then in 1943 Leo Kanner described eleven cases in which an inability to relate to others, an obsession with sameness, and impaired speech were shown to appear in very early childhood. Kanner proposed that these children suffered from an inborn disorder that could be differentiated from other psychotic disturbances of childhood. Since the primary symptom seemed to be an inability, apparent from infancy, to relate to anything beyond the self, Kanner named the new syndrome early infantile autism, from the Greek word autos, meaning "self."

Kanner's distinction is not universally accepted. Certain investigators (e.g., Bender, 1969) still hold to the view that autism and childhood schizophrenia are simply earlier and later manifestations of the *same* childhood psychosis. Perhaps the major research support for this position is a study showing that by the time some autistic children reach later childhood, their symptom picture has changed in such a way as to fit the diagnostic criteria for childhood schizophrenia (Brown and Reiser, 1963). Nevertheless, most specialists in childhood psychosis now accept the distinction between autism and childhood schizophrenia (though some of them favor different names for childhood schizophrenia). And this distinction is currently reflected in the major systems for classifying childhood psychosis (Rutter et al.,1969; GAP, 1966), including DSM-III (1980). Under "pervasive developmental disorders," DSM-III (1980) list tow disorders: infantile autism and a syndrome called "childhood Onset pervasive developmental disolder," roughly synonymous with what others call childhood schizophrenia.

According to those who recognize the distinction, the two syndromes differ in th following respects (Rimland, 1964; Rutter, 1968,1972; Wing, 1972):

I. **Age at onset:** The symptoms of autism invariably appear before the age (two and a half years, whereas schizophrenia becomes apparent later, usually at age s or older.

2. **Premorbid adjustment:** The autistic child appears to be disturbed from birt while schizophrenic children often experience a period of normal or near-normal deve opment, after which they regress.

3. **Autistic aloneness:** While autistic children are severely withdrawn, schiz phrenic children do respond, however inappropriately, to their social environment ai to physical contact.

4. **Preservation of sameness**: The obsession with the preservation of samene in the physical environment is extremely typical of the autistic child whereas it may may not appear in the schizophrenic child.

5. **Perception of environment:** While schizophrenic children have a distort perception of their environment, autistic children seem to be "Over selective" in th perceptions. That is, they seem to have a kind of tunnel vision in which they a attentive only to very restricted portions of their environment.

6. **Hallucinations:** While hallucinations are not common in childhood psych sis, they have been reported in schizophrenic children, but not in autistic children.

7. **Language:** Autistic children who can speak, use their speech in non comn nicative ways, whereas schizophrenic children use speech to communicate biza thoughts.

8. **Intellectual abilities:** Autistic children are more likely than Schizophre children to have IQs indicating severe retardation.

9. **Family history of mental disorder:** The incidence of psychological disord in close relatives is higher than average in the case of the schizophrenic child, but in the case of the autistic child.

10. **Sex ratio:** While the incidence of autism in males is approximately three tir higher than in females, there is no sex differences in the case of childhood schizoph nia.

Thus it does appear that there is some justification for classifying auti children separately from schizophrenic children.

The table 13.1 summarizes the different characteristic of autism and childh psychosis.

Table 13.1 Comparison of Early Infantile Autism and Childhood Schizophrenia

Characteristics	Autism	Schizophrenics
Onset and course	Present from beginning of life	Disordered behaviour follows period of normal development
Health and appearance	Excellent health, well formed, good-looking	Poor health from birth; somatic problems in all body systems
EEG	Normal	Over 80% have abnormal EEGs
Physical responsiveness	Do not adapt to being held; are stiff and unresponsive	"Mold" to parents-clinging
Alones	Withdrawn; demand isolation	Seem isolated, but wish contact and care
Preservation of sameness	Go to any length to keep things exactly as they are	Do not care about sameness; will throw things into disarray
Hallucinations	No hallucinations or delusions	Frequent delusions and visual and auditory experiences
Motor performance	Excellent	Poor coordination, balance, and locomotion
Language	Do not use the word/until age 7 or order, repetitious	Often incoherent, but use the words/ and yes early in life
Personal orientation	Unoriented, detached, oblivious to environment; do not wish to relate	Disoriented and confused; try to relate but can't
Condition ability	Difficult to condition classically	Easy to condition classically
Parent's background	Highly educated, higher class, intellectual	Poorly educated, lower class, not intellectual
Family history disturbance	Low incidence of disorders in relatives	Higher rate of disorders in families
Development	Arrested	Regressed
Fascination with mechanical objects	Fascinated by mechanical objects	Not fascinated by mechanical objects
Thoughts	Inhibition of thoughts	Confusion of thoughts
Spinning of objects	Deft spinning of objects	Clumsy spinning of objects

Childhood Schizophrenia, its symptomatology etiology and treatment

Early infantile autism is an exceedingly rare psychopathology. An initial epidemiological survey conducted in Middlesex (England) found that approximately four children in every 10,000 were diagnosed as autistic; a Danish study showed the same incidence. American reports, too, generally agree: Schreibman and Koefel (1975) place the incidence at four in 10,000; Oppenheim states that the incidence is between two to five cases per 10,000.

Another component of the incidence of early infantile autism is its sex ratio: males outnumber females 3 or 4 to I (Rimland 1964; RuHer 1968; DSM-III 1978).

Kanner (1943) noted that autistic children are usually males (4 to 1) who during the first 10 weeks of life, are described as exceptionally healthy and precious. The earliest and reliable sign of autism occurs is at 6 months of age when parents notice that the child doesn't make the typical anticipatory movements that normal children to before they are picked up. Between 6 and 18 months of age, the additional sings of autism may appear; head-banging, apathy toward people and playthings, highly repetitive and situational play, unusual language patterns, and an insistence upon being left along. What Kanner called autistic aloneness", the child's insistence on being left alone, leads the autistic child to withdraw into a world of inner fantasy, devoid of people, by the age 2.

Symptomatology of Infantile Autism

The term Autism was coined initially by the Swiss psychiatrist Eugen k Blueler and was used by him to describe the characteristic withdrawn nature of adult schizophrenics. Kanner proposed four cardinal symptoms of early infantile autism. For the most part, these symptoms represent some of the current criteria for diagnosing this syndrome:

1. Social aloofness and indifference to people.
2. Resistance to changes in certain environment of the child (maintenance of sameness).
3. Failure to adopt normal language usage (particularly speech).
4. Preoccupation with manipulation of various sorts of objects (stones radios, electric motors, etc.)

In addition to these cardinal features, Kanner also proposed that these children were paradoxically endowed with good intelligence as well as "strikingly intelligent physiognomies".

Since Kanner's publication of these cardinal features, other clinicians and researchers have confirmed most of his findings. Disagreement has focused principally on Kanner's declaration that autistic children typically are intelligent and look bright (Rutter 1968; Rutter and Bartak 1971; Wing 1972). For example, many assert that in terms of intelligence, autistic children may either be normal, retarded, or gifted.

Modem diagnostic systems are based mainly on clinical findings, but traces of Kanner's cardinal features are still evident. DSM-II, the 1968 version, contained no description of early infantile autism. The new DSM-III docs contain information about this syndrome, giving five operation criteria for infantile autism:

1. Onset usually prior to 30 months but up to 42 months.

2. Lack of responsiveness to other human beings ("autism").

3 Gross deficits in language development.

4. If speech is present, peculiar speech patterns such as immediate and delayed echolalia, and pronoun reversals.

5. Peculiar interest or attachments to animate or inanimate objects.

Bootzin and Acocella have discussed the following symptoms found in autistic children in detail.

(i) **Social Isolation**: The social withdrawal of the autistic child what has been called "extreme autistic aloneness is usually evident in the first or second year of the child's life. Parents often recall that their autistic children were "good babies." That is, they didn't pester adults for attention; in fact, they seemed happier when left alone. Furthermore, they were very difficult to hold and cuddle, because unlike normal babies, who instinctively mold to the body of an adult who is holding them, they stiffened (or in some cases, went limp) when picked up. As autistic infants grow up, this recoil from personal contact becomes even more marked. They avoid looking anyone in the eye and treat people as if they simply didn't exist. If they form any attachments at all, it is to-inanimate objects.

(ii) **Speech Deficits**: The social isolation of autistic children is increased by their failure to communicate through the use of language. Many autistic children are mute. The speech of others is limited to echolalia, in which the child merely repeats words or phrases that he or she has hear snatches of songs, television commercials, and the like. These words arc echoed not in any apparent attempt to communicate, but simply aimlessly, without any concern for their meaning. If any actual communicative speech does develop in the autistic-child, it is accompanied by problems of pronoun reversal (i.e., a boy might refer

to himself not as "I" but as "you" or "he", or by his proper name), extreme literalness, and repetitiveness. Where an autistic child falls on this scale of speech deficits, there seems to be an excellent indicator of prognosis: it has been shown that the child most likely to benefit from almost any attempt at treatment is the one who has developed some meaningful speech by age five (Ruller et al., 1967).

(iii) **Preservation of Sameness**: Another distinguishing characteristic of the autistic child is an anxiously obsessive desire to maintain sameness in the environment. Toys must always be placed in the same position on the same shelves. At breakfast the egg must be eaten first: then the vitamin pill, then the toast. In the bath, the face must be washed first, then the arms, and so on. If any items in this intricate order is disturbed, a tantrum may ensue. Interestingly enough, a similar concern for sameness is also commonly observe in the normal child at about age two-and-a half, thus raising the possibility that the autistic child's development is stalled at this point.

(iv) **Ritualistic Motor Activity**: The autistic child frequently has a number of other problems as well. As we have noted, tantrums are common and self mutilation sometimes occurs. Almost universal is the total absorption in some endlessly repetitive movement such as spinning, rocking, or hand flapping, or in the manipulation of some object. Such activities often take preference to food, and as a result the child may eat only sporadically. One study, for example found that when engaged in ritualistic movements, a group of autistic children who had not eaten for twenty-four hours cither would not respond or would delay their responses to an auditory signal indicating that food was available. The remarkable finding was that these same children would immediately respond to the same signal when they were not engaged in such movements. Thus they knew very well what the signal meant, but even though they had gone without food for a whole day, they were still more interested in their repetitive motor activities than in eating (Lovaas, Koegel, and Schreibman, 1978; Lovaas et al., 1971a).

Symptomatology of Childhood Schizophrenia

Generally the symptoms of childhood schizophrenia include gross impairment of relationships, unawareness of personal identity, increased or decreased sensitivities to perceptual experiences, auditory and visual hallucinations, age inappropriate speech, clumsy or rigid physical movements, and a history of serious psychological difficulties reaching a peak after 10 years of age.

It is very difficult to estimate the prevalence of childhood schizophrenia because of childhood confusion with the classification of autism. However, Dawson and Mesibov (1983) conclude that the prevalence is less than 4 cases in 100,000 with about three times as many boys as girls. Most of the children did not manifest symptoms of childhood schizophrenia until age 7. Eggers (1978) found that children who showed signs of this disorder before the age of 10 tended to develop a chronic rather than an acute course.

In general, a child is diagnosed as schizophrenic if, after two-and-a-half years or more of normal or near-normal development, his or her reality contact and social adjustment begin to show a severe decline. Specific symptoms include social withdrawal, disorientation, disorted sensory perception, speech disintegration, and intellectual retardation. In addition, schizophrenic children, usually show peculiar motor behavior, such as agitated hyperactivity, catatonic non activity, or the ritualistic movements that we have discussed in relation to the autistic child.

The specific areas in which childhood schizophrenia differs from autism have been listed earlier. In general, it may be said that-childhood schizophrenia manifests itself in symptoms that are somehow more familiar, albeit no easier to treat, than those of autism. Though schizophrenic children may also spend hours exploring their bodies and engaging in repetitive and nonfunctional motor behaviors, they are much less likely than autistic children to mutilate themselves. Though their behavior is bizarre, it is less obsessive than autistic behavior. And finally, though often withdrawn, the schizophrenic child lacks the seemingly impenetrable aloofness of the autistic child.

Having drawn these general distinctions, we must point out once again that in actual cases the differential diagnosis of autism and childhood schizophrenia is often difficult to make on the basis of current behaviour alone. In many if not most instances the crucial variable is the child's level of adjustment before the onset of symptoms (Eisenberg and Kanner, 1956; Ward, 1970). In a diagnostic decision between autism and childhood schizophrenia, the child who once functioned adequately is labelled schizophrenic the child who never functioned adequately is labelled autistic.

Etiology of Infantile Autism and Childhood Schizophrenia

Different theorists have given differing view with respect to the development of these two different but related disorders.

(a) **Psychodynamic Theorists** views childhood psychosis as a failure in ego development. Psychodynamic theorists are fairly unanimous in blaming disturbed parent-child interactions for this failure, particularly in the case of autism. For years it was widely assumed that children became autistic through being raised by cold, detached, intellectual parents. "Emotional refrigerators," in the words of Kanner and Eisenberg (1955). This ideas that pathological family relationships are the primary cause of childhood psychosis has been explored by many researchers (Kanner and Eisenberg, 1955; Eisenberg and Kanner, 1956; Singer and Wynne, 1963), including some who have no allegiance to psychodynamic theory (Rimland, 1964).

However, the foremost publicist of the family theory has been the psychodynamic psychologist Bruno Bettelheim. Bettelheim's theory, which applies specifically to autism, is laid out in detail in his book. The Empty Fortress" (1967). Autism, Bettelheim argues, is a child's response lo an extreme situation in which parents\reject him or her and fail to respond to the child's slightest attempts to influence the environment. Particularly crucial is the parents' failure to provide stimulation during the earliest period of life, when object relationships develop (birth to six months) and when language and locomotion begin to emerge (six to nine months). As a result of this lack of stimulation, the child has no basis on which to form emotional attachments or to develop proper speech and motor skills. Most important of all, because of the parents' unresponsiveness, the child feels Unable to control the external world in any way. Hence, be or she withdraws into a private fantasy world, while attempting to impose some order and constancy through the insistence on sameness.

This position Has been questioned by many other investigators, particularly because siblings of autistic children arc usually normal. Recent research does not support the notion that parents *of* autistic children are cold and aloof (Kolvin et al., 1971; Rutter et al., 1971; Cox et al., 1975). Furthermore, those studies that have found that autistic children are dealt with by their parents differently from normal children are still subject to the chicken-and-egg question. That is, while it is possible that unresponsive parents give rise to autistic children, it is equally possible that autistic children give rise to unresponsive parents. A study by Goldfarb and his colleagues (1973), though, it dealt with schizophrenic children, will serve to illustrate our point. In this experiment the investigators compared the communications between mothers and their schizophrenic children with communications between mothers and their normal children. The main finding was that in general, when the mother of a schizophrenic child was asked to describe to her child an object he or she was to pick up from among a number of objects, she conveyed less information, was more ambiguous, and was less supportive than the mother of normal child. From this the investigators concluded that childhood schizophrenia might be rooted in deficient mother-child communications. It is equally likely, however, that the inadequate mother-child communications in the schizophrenic sample were the result rather than the cause of the children's condition. After years of having their words ignored or misunderstood, these mothers might understandably lack the motivation to, communicate clearly with their children.

(b) **Behavioral Theorists** attributes the development of infantile autism and childhood schizophrenia to learning, environmental factors, faulty reinforcement and parent child interactions.

In the opinion of one leading behaviorist, Ferster (1961), childhood psychosis, like any other behaviour pattern, is learned. Ferster agrees with the psychodynamic theorists that the basic cause of psychosis in children is unresponsiveness in their parents, but instead of analyzing this process in subjective terms, he limits himself, in classic behavioral style to external stimulus-and-response patterns. According to Ferster, the reason the child fails to develop appropriate language skills, social responses, and cognitive abilities is that when he or she directs appropriate responses at parents, they either ignore the child or deliver feedback only intermittently. Hence these responses eventually extinguish. The child may then resort to some kind of violent and inappropriate behavior, such as head banging or a tantrum, and find that unlike the appropriate behavior, this does get attention. In other words, essential adaptive responses are not reinforced, while extremely maladaptive responses are reinforced. The result is what we call a psychotic child.

This theory has not found wide acceptance, even among behaviorists. There is, now, considerable evidence that autism at least is due in part to organic causes, and many behaviortists have come to feel that these organic causes may outweigh the role of learning, hence, these investigators have devoted their research efforts not so much to the causes as to the treatment of childhood psychosis.

(c) **Humanistic-Existential Writers** had more to say about the psychosis of adulthood than about those of childhood, a general humanistic-existential conceptualization of childhood psychosis is that, it results from interplay between, on the one hand, the child's drive to adapt lo his or her psychosocial environment, and on the other, the demands made by that environment. While the child, attempts to make some sense of the environment and adapt it to his or her need, this drive is frustrated by the environment itself, which is constantly asking the child to be something else. Thus Laing's (1967) theory of schizophrenia would apply to children as well as to adults: the psychotic break is a retreat away from the world and into the mind a retreat that may ultimately prove productive and therapeutic if allowed to run its course.

The role of the social environment in the development of childhood psychosis is a matter that has been taken up not only by humanistic and existential psychologists but also by the theologists Niko and Lies Tinbergen, whose views on the subject are consistent with the humanistic-existential approach. According to the Tinbergens (1974), autism, which they define very broadly as failed socialization', is on the rise because environmental changes are occurring too fast for genetic evolution. These rapid changes place on the organism a constant pressure to adapt and readapt. Most children manage to withstand such stress. They explore their environment and interact with it, becoming more confident and competent with each additional experience. In short, they become socialized. In certain other children, however, this environmental stress gives rise to an intense motivational conflict. These children naturally desire to interact with and adapt to their world, but the very instability of that world makes them apprehensive. While they are starved for social contact) their fears prevent them from responding to others. Likewise, language fails to develop not because these children cannot talk, but because they are too afraid to engage in the kind of social interactions that would lead to speech. The result is a general failure to respond to the environment in other words, autism.

(d) **Cognitive view-All the etiological** theories of childhood psychosis that we have discussed so far have two things in common, *(i)* First, they all view the primary defect as a disturbance in the child's relationship with other people, usually with parents, *(ii)* Second, there is very little empirical evidence to support any of these theories, and it is only because of subjective reports of some success in treatments based on these theories that we continue to relay on them. In contrast, the cognitive perspective sees the primary defect in the autistic child not as a disturbance in social relationships per se, but in the way information about the environment is processed. Adherents of this perspective do not deny that the autistic child has severe problems in relating to people or that these problems contribute heavily to the child's distress. But they maintain that the social maladjustment is not the root cause; the root cause is organic dysfunction, of which social maladjustment is simply one of many unwelcome results.

Cognitive theorists have concentrated almost exclusively on autism. Their basic position is that autism is due to an impairment of the child's organic equipment for perceiving and interpreting the environment. As for the nature of that impairment, there are several competing theories.

Ruller (1968, 1971) claims that in autism the basic defect is an impaired comprehension of sounds, (It is not that the autislic child cannot hear or see as well as normal child; the autistic child's brain does not seem to interpret or integrate data from the sense in the same way as a normal child's). Thus autism is seen as comparable to other disorders of language (e.g., aphasia, the loss or impairment of speech as a result of brain damage), differing from these only in that the autistic child's defective comprehension of sound is accompanied by other perceptual problems as well. In support of this view, Rutter points out that retarded speech has an early onset in the autistic child and is one of the most important defining symptoms. In addition, autistic children show a number of signs of improper sound comprehension: they are often suspected of being deaf; they either don't respond to sounds at all or they respond inappropriately-for example, ignoring a loud, startling sound and then responding to a soft sound; they aren't easily distracted; and they tend to echo words and reverse pronouns. A primary language impairment is also suggested by the pattern of cognitive abilities typically seen in autistic children the fact that they perform far better in visual motor and rote memory tasks than in verbal and conceptual tasks. Finally, one of the strongest arguments in support of Rutter's hypothesis is the fact, noted earlier, that it is language ability that is the best predictor of the autistic child's chances of benefiting from treatment.

Another cognitive hypothesis, put forth by Lovaas and his colleagues *(1978),* is that the basic impairment in autistic children is that they are over selective in their attention that they because of perceptual defect any can only process, and thus respond to, one stimulus at a time, be it tactile or visual or whatever. Such an impairment (which has also been proposed as the basis of adult schizophrenia) could easily account for the social and intellectual retardation of the autistic child. Much of a child's intellectual and emotional development is based on the association of paired stimuli, through the process of respondent conditioning. Thus as a child's mother comes to be paired in his or her mind with food and with holding, the mother comes to be loved. If, however, when a child is being fed or held, this or her perceptual faculties can only process the stimulus of the food or of the holding and not of the mother's presence as well, the mother fails to take on any positive meaning. Furthermore, it is possible that with limited processing abilities, the child will select irrelevant aspects of the environment on which to base responses. One autistic child, for example-appeared to base his identification of his father on the father's eyeglasses. When the father was wearing his glasses, the child was extremely responsive to him. But when the father did not have his glasses on, the child ignored him completely.

Other cognitive theorists (e.g., Wing, 1969,1972) argue that autism is the product not of a single, fundamental perceptual defect, but of a cluster of perceptual defects. This new line of investigation has led to some interesting treatment approaches designed to circumvent the child's supposed cognitive defects. For example, some behavior therapists have taught autistic children sign language, thus taking advantage of their sensitivity to touch and movement and getting around their insensitivity to spoken language (Webster et al., 1973). Other researchers have tried to develop reinforcers more effective than auditory stimuli, such as the therapists' saying, "Good", For example, Newsom and his colleagues (1974) found that lights flashing on and off after a correct response were surprisingly effective reinforcers more effective even than food, to say nothing of verbal praise. The treatments that arc emerging from such experimentation treatments based on a combination of cognitive and behavioral theory appear promising, at least for autistic children. No such encouraging results have as yet emerged from the use of such therapy with schizophrenic children.

(e) **The Biological Viewpoint:** There are two biological viewpoints concerning the etiology of autism and childhood schizophrenia.

(i) Rimland (1964) has written perhaps the most thorough text on early infantile autism. After having reviewed all the hypothesized causes of this disorder and staling that the psychogenic views were "pernicious", he postulated that autism is -a consequence of neuralgic impairment in the brain stem. This hypothesized defect yields a child who cannot "relate new stimuli to remembered experience".

Specifically, Rimland (1964) status that the reticular formation-a center in the brain that is thought to regulate consciousness, attention, and alertness has been damaged because of an hereditary susceptibility to oxygen injury. He presents data to support his conclusion showing that a high proportion of these children were administered medical oxygen soon after birth. Rimland says, "Oxygen in excess of an infant's tolerance can in some cases produce or stimulate infantile autism".

(ii) Another very popular biological viewpoint is that proposed by Deslauriers and Carlson. They propose that autism is caused by an inborn organic imbalance existing in the arousal system. According to these writers, normal people have two states of arousal, but no imbalance between them. Autistic children, on the other hand, have an inborn imbalance. The two-arousal hypothesis was first proposed by Ruttenberg (1966, 1968) as a model of how the brain arouses and activates the neocortex. Without such activation or arousal, learning and memory would not be adequate.

Arousal system I is an "activating-drive energy" system. Arousal system II is a "reward-positive incentive" system, the first system motivates or moves the organism; the second provides for the feelings of pleasure, pain and, reinforcement in general. Structurally, system I is the reticular formation; system II is the limbic area. According to Deslauriers and Carlson (1969), system I and system II are in disequilibrium in the autistic child, reflecting an imbalance between reticular and limbic areas.

Basically two conditions of disequilibrium can exist; System I can be too high, thus suppressing system II. When this occurs, very little learning can take place, but because of a high energy level, aimless, repetitive, and stereotyped responses prevail. It is noteworthy that many clinicians suggest the existence of two varieties of early infantile autism: the hyperactive/hypersensitive variety, and the hyperactive /hypersensitive variety that is thought to be caused by high arousal of system I and the suppression of system II. System II can be higher than system 1. In this case a hypoactive/ hyposensitive autistic infant exists.

***Biochemical* abnormalities**

Although structural anomalies have yet to be detected in the brains of autistic children, biochemical abnormalities have been recently reported. , Goldstein, Mahanand, and Lee (1976) found low levels of dopamine (a neurotransmitter) in a sample of autistic children. Lake, Slegler, and Murphy (1977) subsequently confirmed the Goldstein findings. Investigators have also reported imbalances in other neurotransmitter substances such as serotonin. But it is possible that these chemical anomalies may be effects rather than causes of autism.

Treatment of infantile autism and childhood schizophrenia varies from different perspective. We will discuss the treatments according to different perspective.

(a) **Psychodynamic treatment:** Generally requires that the child be removed from the home situation and placed in a residential treatment facility. Here he or she is provided with a counselor who is constantly available and sympathetic a steady, reliable image which the child can internalize. The basis of this treatment is constant responsiveness to the child's needs on the part of the counselor and the staff. Thus, in an example cited by Sanders (1974), when a new child was being shown around the school and said mashed potatoes during the visit to the kitchen, the kitchen staff responded by giving him a special serving of mashed potatoes at every meal.

In this way the child learns what, according to psychodynamic theory, he or she could not learn at home : that by communicating through speech and movement, he or she can influence the environment. Once this foundation is laid, the child can begin to develop emotional attachments and to build a stable personality.

A major problem in evaluating psychodynamic treatments is the general lack of concrete suggestions for actual therapy (Wieland, 1971). Ruttenberg (1971) has made an attempt to dispel this vagueness by offering a highly specific outline of treatment procedures, based on the Freudian theory of psychosexual development. Ruttenberg sees the autistic child as being fixated at a preoral period, with the result that the child is totally absorbed in autoerotic and auto aggressive behaviors at an extremely primitive sensor motor level. Treatment is therefore aimed at reactivating the stalled developmental processes by furnishing optimal gratification through a consistent, positive, and accepting "mother". The "mother" (i.e. the therapist) must meet the needs of the child at his or her primitive level of sensorimotor functioning. Treatment consist of holding, cudding, rocking, singing, feeding, and so forth in an attempt to provide the child with necessary tactile-kinesthetic, visual, and aural contact. Once an object . relationship has been established with the mothering figure, social, motor, perceputal, and cognitive skills can be developed through (1) imitation of the child's behaviors and vocalizations; (2) verbalization of affect; (3) naming and

conceptual verbalization of activities, functions, body parts, and objects that the child encounters; and (4) gradual introduction of expectations for self-care, impulse control, and problem solving. The result of this gradual treatment is a progression through a sequence of lesser psychotic states. That is, the child becomes symboitic, then oral omnipotent, then anal sadomasochisfic, and so on until he or she finally arrives at the appropriate stage of psychosexual development.

As yet there is no truly firm evidence of the effectiveness of these psychodynamic therapies.

(b) **Behavioural Treatment Techniques:** In keeping with their theoretical background, behaviorists do not claim that they "Cure" the "condition" of childhood psychosis. Rather, they analyze behavior patterns in terms of deficits and excesses, and then attempt to modify them. In the case of psychotic child, the deficits include an impoverished repertoire of social, verbal, and cognitive responses, while the excesses include inappropriate and violent behaviors such as repetitive mannerisms, tantrums, and self-mutilation. In many instances, behavioral therapist have been successful in correcting these deficits

and excesses.

The major techniques of behavioral therapy for psychotic children are direct reinforcement (e.g., giving the child a cookie if he or she refrains from engaging in the undesirable behaviour engages in a desirable behavior), extinction (e.g., withdrawing attention in response to undesirable behavior), and punishment (e.g., administering a spanking in response to unacceptable behavior). Thus, in a reversal of the process described by Ferster, adaptive behaviors are reinorced while maladaptive behaviors are either punished or simply allowed to extinguish.

Role of Extinction: Reports indicate that all of these techniques are effective but that their effectiveness depends greatly on what behavior is being eliminated. For example, self-mutilating responses such as head banging will eventually extinguish if social attention is withdrawn when the head banging occurs. In one case, however, it took nearly eight days and 1,800 head bangs before the response dropped out (Simmons and Lovaas, 1969). Another problem with extinction procedures is that some behaviours seem to be maintained by internal rather than external rewards, in which case withdrawing social attention or food will have little if any effect. For example, psychotic children's ritualistic motor behaviours-which, as we have seen, they will prefer over food even when they are highly resistant to extinction through the withdrawal of food or attention (Renter et al., 1974), apparently because they satisfy an internal need for stimulation (Litrownik, 1969).

Role of Punishment: Of course, if extinction doesn't work, the therapist can resort to punishment, usually in the form of spankings or, in cases of extreme self-destructive behavior, electric shock etc. O.I. Lovaas has conducted research on the use of electric shock in treating autistic children, and as he point out, it is extremely effective in eliminating self-mutilating behavior: "seemingly independently of how badly the child is mutilating himself or how long he has been doing so, we can essentially remove the self-destructive behavior within the first minute" (1970). But even though this immediate effect may be desired in some cases – the case of self-mutilation, for example – moral, ethical, and legal concerns frequently limit the use of aversive procedures. Many people believe that punishing a psychotic child for undesirable behavior only compounds the problem (Bettelheim, 1967). In response, Lovaas argues that psychotic children are treated like people that is, rewarded, punished, and generally held d responsible for their Behavior rather than like patients. Lovaas has also pointed out that if self-destructive behavior is not eliminated by some kind of treatment, the child may spend long period of time tied down in restraints, unable to take part in any other kind of therapy.

Symptom Substitution: Another potential problem in eliminating appropriate behaviors is symptom substitution, the replacement of a suppressed maladaptive behavior by a new maladaptive behavior. Once a child's rocking behavior is eliminated, for example he or she may suddenly begin hyperventilating (Renter et al., 1974). What this seems to mean is that once we have eliminated a behavior in which a child has been engaging frequently and at long stretches, we can't expect the child simply to sit quitely and wait for someone to teach a new, appropriate behavior with which to fill the vacuum. Hence, with childhood psychosis as with drug addiction and sexual deviation, most behavioral treatment programs aim simultaneously at eliminating old, inappropriate behaviors and at fostering new, appropriate behaviors to take their place (e.g., Simmons and Lovaas, 1969; Wolf et al., 1964).

Development of Appropriate behaviour: Procedures for developing appropriate responses in psychotic children have first and foremost focused on establishing people as secondary reinforcers that is, the child must first see people as being important and valuable. This can often be accomplished through respondent conditioning, by pairing praise by the therapist (social reinforcement) with primary positive reinforcers such as food or with primary negative reinforcers such as pain relief (Lovaas et al., 1965). Next, through shaping and modeling with the use of social reinforcement as well as direct reinforcers such as food the child is taught new responses such as toileting, speaking, and playing with other children (Lovaas et al-,1966; Wolfet al., 1964). Once having teamed these basic skills, the child can be placed in a group learning situations (Kogel and Rincover, 1974), which will allow him or her to learn from observing others.

As in eliminating inappropriate behaviors, so in developing appropriate behaviors, there are problems in maintaining the change. Follow-up reports indicate that responses learned in the treatment laboratory often do not generalize to the school or the home (Nordquist and Wahler, 1973; Koegal and Rincover, 1977). And some children, especially those who are returned to institutions after their treatment, relapse completely. There is no question that institution foster such relapses, since in the usual institutional setting patients are expected to act in an inappropriate fashion and no rewards are given for acting otherwise. For example, one therapist who was visiting an institution decided to look up a child with whom he had worked with considerable success. He found her crouched in a corner, flapping her hand and making bizarre sounds. As soon as she saw the therapist, she got up, walked over, and said, "Hi, how are you?" She continued to talk and act appropriately while the therapist was there. After he left, she presumably returned to her corner. Recently efforts to go around this problem have involved keeping the child at home and directing treatment efforts at the parents as well as at the child. In this method the parents are actually trained to act as behavioral therapists. Such home therapy can apparently be very successful (Lovaas et al., 1973). Once the parents see the child improving as a result of their efforts, they are likely to try even harder, with the result that the child will make further gains. In general, behavior therapists have no illusions that they are transforming psychotic children into normal children (Margplies, 1977). Rather, their aim is to provide-these children with enough adaptive responses so that they can graduate from custodial care to a more useful and fulfilling existence, albeit in a "special" class. Critics of behavioral therapy for psychotic children have claimed that its products are no better than performing robots (Bettelheim, 1967), and in some instances this seem to be the case. For example, one psychotic child, when asked, "What did you have for breakfast?" she would tell you that she had, had "eggs, toast, jelly, juice, and milk" even on days when she hadn't had any breakfast at all. In short, she had no understanding off the concepts; she was simply responding with a programmed answer to a specific question. In many other instances, however, behavioral treatment has resulted in the development of responses that are spontaneous as well as appropriate. Substantial gains have been made in eliminating self-injuries and bizarre motor behavior and developing language, self-help, and social skills (Lovaas et al., 1973).

(c) **Humanistic Existential Treatment Technique**: According to Humanistic existential therapist Milieu therapy is the most preferred form of treatment technique for these two disorders.

The child is placed in a residential facility where his or her development is encouraged by an empathetic, warm staff, who provide the reassurance and structure necessary to calm the child's fears. In this way the child is freed to establish social relationships and to explore the world. Throughout the day, events such as eating, sleeping, dressing, and studying provide opportunities for human interaction and evoke behaviors to which the adults can respond on an individual basis, helping the child to become more self-confident and self-aware (Goldfarb, 1965).

Such treatment in many ways resembles that recommended by psychodynamic theorists such as Bettelheim. And as with the psychodynamic therapy, one problem with the humanistic milieu therapy is that actual day-to-day treatment procedures are not specified, and evaluations are vague and subjective. Hence, if such therapies are reported to be successful, it is difficult for others to initiate similar programms in an effort to replicate those results.

(d) **Biochemical Approach (Orthomolecular therapy)**-Because Rimland and several other theorists have proposed underlying biological or biochemical defect in autism, it follows that they would recommend biochemical efforts to manage autistic children. This is indeed the case. In his 1964 book, Rimland made some rather general statements about the potential benefit of oxygen, carbon dioxide, LSD, deanol, and nicotinic acid (vitamin B,). Since the publication of infantile Autism in 1964, Rimland and several other independent investigators have focused more sharply on megavitamin therapy, an approach often called or thomolecular therapy. Sagar (1974), paraphrasing the chemist Limus Pauling, defines orthomolecular therapy as "the treatment of mental illness by the provision of the optimum molecular composition of the brain". As a rule, orthomolecular therapy involves giving massive doses of specific vitamins to establish the optimum molecular composition of the nervous system.

In a 1969 publication, Rimland proposed that megavitamin supplements of nicotinic acid and vitamin C dramatically improved the behavior of approximately 80 percent of those taking the vitamins. But this investigation did have numerous methodological defects. Cott (1972) also reported impressive results with megavitamin treatment.

(c) **Multistrategy Approaches:** Two similar approaches are included in this category: those of Des lauriers and Carlson and of Oppenheim. Both methods use more than one .single guiding principle; they both employ behavior or learning theory procedures, as well as tactile and kinesthetic stimulation, affection, control, and rather standard teaching techniques.

Deslauriers and Carlson developed a treatment approach based on their hypothesis of imbalance in the two-arousal system. Generally, they contend that the affective system (system II) is too weak, resulting in sensory and affective deprivation. Again, this defect is "an inborn limitation." Since the autistic child cannot receive the sensory message or affective stimulation normally given by the environment, therapeutic strategy involves the application of "impactful affective stimulation," to activate system II (the reward area, or limbic system).

They describe two conditions under which an autistic child can learn: (1) learning can occur through "excessive repetition" or "repeated encounters with the same stimulus situation" (2) learning can occur if the thing to be learned is presented with a "strong affective" or emotional climate.

Aside from these two conditions, Deslauriers and Carlson also note that the hyperactive/hypersensitive child and the hypoactive/hyposensitive child are *to* be treated differently. The former must be presented with mild tactile, proprioceptive, and kinesthetic stimulation. Conversely, the hypoactive/hyposensitive child must be bombarded with high affective stimulation; that is, tactile, proprioceptive, and kinesthetic modalities (near-receptors) must be pelted, at the same time as stimuli are being repeated. That is, Deslauriers and Carlson believe that the best way to reach the autistic child is through sensory and preverbal modes. Only by beginning at this basic level can the affective barrier be surmounted. They claimed that their method was highly efficient, helping most of the children improve; but unfortunately, their research project had to be terminated for lack of funds (Oppenheim 1974). No others have reestablished their precise methods.

Rosalind Oppenheim (1974) began developing methods for treating autistic children because she had. a severely afflicted autistic son. After unsuccessful attempts to get help for her son, she began lo leach him herself Although she initially encountered seemingly insurmountable difficulties (he could not talk, would not look at her, etc.), she discovered that certain things did work.' Briefly, these arc the important points Oppenheim makes:

1. The crucial first step is the establishment of control. By this she means that the child must be required to perform the command or task you have shown him or her; e.g., if the child will not do what you command, physically show the child-"literally use his hands to put him through the activity."
2. The teacher must convey to the child that she or he is in control.
3. Much of the initial teaching must be conducted by touch.
4. The child must not be permitted to engage in autistic behaviors during the learning sessions.
5. The child must be required to attend to the lesson materials (Oppenheim explains in detail how to accomplish this goal).
6. Every activity during which the child engages in nonautistic behaviors must be praised and reinforced.
7. The physical setting should be quiet and relatively isolated.
8. The curriculum taught should resemble normal, school curriculum.
9. The autistic child must be required to repeat the same task over and over again drilling is a key feature. (Adapted from Oppenheim 1974).

Generally, Oppenheim's approach is behaviorally oriented, but it also makes use of touch, affection, drill, and standard teaching devices. Her program has been implemented at the Rimland School for Autistic Children (or which she is the director). She has presented clinical cases showing the effectiveness of her method in helping these children learn to speak, write, read, and develop important social skills.

EATING DISORDER

The Diagnostic and the Statistical Manual of Mental Disorder (DSM-III, 1980), has classified eating disorder into two types,

(a) anorexia nervosa and

(b) bulimia.

These two types of eating disorders are commonly found among college going adolescent female who is westernized and beauty conscious.

(a) **Anorexia Nervosa** is a life threatening disorder in which the individual, usually a female adolescent, has an intense fear of becoming obese, either eats very little or binges and then induces vomiting, loses at least a quarter of her body weight and feels fat even though emaciated.

There is the intense fear of becoming fat, a distorted body image and a sense of being obese despite conspicuous thinness, and a loss of 25 percent of body weight without any known physical illness. Anorexics exercise vigorously lo loose still more weight. They arc often perfectionists and are easily depressed when they cannot meet the standards that they have set for themselves.

Many different psychobiological and socio-cultural factors have been suggested as the cause of anorexia nervosa. It seems likely that both kinds contribute. On the biological side, there is a strong evidence that our physiques are determined to a very substantial degree by inheritance, on the socio-cultural side, there has been a recent growing emphasis on slimness as a requisite of beauty in women. Middle-class educated women, in particular, seem to have accepted this concept. Evidence for the existence of this emphasis are the models selected for advertisements and the highly publicised contestant in the so called "beauty pageants."

Anorexia is a life threatening disorder, because of the strict diet control that may create medical emergencies. The ratio of girls and women to boys and men with this disorder may be as high as twenty to one. Anorexia usually has its onset during adolescence, often shortly after the beginning of menstruation. The cessation of menstruation, or amenorrhea, may even precede noticeable weight loss. Like other sterned people, anorexics are preoccupied with food, but for them it takes the form of collecting recipes and planning and preparing meals for others.

The DSM-III gives these six criteria for identifying anorexia nervosa:

1. Refusal to maintain body weight over a minimal normal weight for age and height.

2 Weight loss of at least 25 percent of original body weight, or if under

eighteen years of age, weight loss from original body weight plus projected weight gain expected on pediatric growth charts may be combined to comprise, the 25 percent.

3. Disturbance of body image with inability to accurately perceive body size.

4. Intense fear of becoming obese. This fear does not diminish as weight loss progresses.

5. No known medical illness that would account for weight loss.

6. Amenorrhea (in Females).

Causes: The causes suggested for anorexia nervosa fall in two categories; psychogenic theories and biogenic theories. Psychogenic theories regarding anorexia are mainly psychoanalytic views. For example, one psychoanalytic theory contends that anorexia nervosa is a symptom of the child's refusal to grow up a type of protest. In this connection, some psychoanalytic theorists believe that adolescents having anorexia nervosa have much in common with borderline syndrome adolescents. In the borderline syndrome, pathological dependency and odd behaviors exist that resemble both neuroses and schizophrenia (thus the term "borderline"). Anorectic adolescents, then, have been viewed as highly dependent persons who fear separation and independence from parents. Further, both anorectic individuals and borderline individuals tend to be shy, tense, and hypochondriacally; it is often believed that they both have been overprotected.

Other analytic theories have approached this problem in a different ways. Because weight loss is profound, and is generally associated with undernourishment and death, a few clinicians have suggested that anorexia neivosa is really a form of sub intentional suicide. That is, they believe this behavior disorder to be motivated by self-destructive urges. Thus far, however, no empirical evidence exists to support *txy* of these theories.

By contrast, the biogenic positions contend that anorexia nervosa has a biological or genetic origin. Some evidence does show an association between certain abnormal chromosome patterns and anorexia in females(Korn et al. 1977). In particular, chromosome configuration XO (a condition called gonadal dysgenic or Turner's syndrome) is associated significantly with anorexia. Another investigation revealed that gonadal dysgenic individuals exhibit symptoms of positively, dependency, and, in the researcher's words, psycho infantilism (Kihibom 1969). Further research is required before a more complete understanding of the etiology of anorexia nervosa is achieved.

Treatment : Almost every technique imaginable has been tried with anorectic patients (Bliss 1975). Lobotomies, hormone injections, drugs isolation, electro convulsive therapy, behavior modification, hospitalization, insulin coma, and even "gentle reasoning" have been tried with these patients. In addition to physical methods, family therapy and individual psychotherapy (insight therapy) have been employed with varying degrees of success and failure. Perhaps no single therapy has emerged because there arc different causes of this disorder and different levels of severity.

(b) Bulimia has been described as the 'bingpurge" syndrome. It is a serious and spreading disorder marked by uncontrollable overeating, often followed by self-induced vomiting or overdose of laxatives to eliminate the caloric intake. Persons of normal weight, as well as those who are anorexics or obese, may be bulimics.

The bulimic- person attempts to counteract stress and depression by overeating but does so in an uncontrollable manner. The typical bulimic is a female in her twenties, white, middle-class, with some college education, and has been a binge cater for a number of years. It is difficult to know exactly how many people are afflicted with this disorder, but some experts estimate that one in Five college educated women have been or will be affected at some time in their lives. The incidence may be greatest in able, young working woman who are expected to have a career, to take care of a house, to raise children, and to retain the slim from that is highly admired in a male-dominated, sex conscious, achievement oriented society.

Reports indicate that some bulimics have consumed as many as 55,000 calories at a single-sitting. This would approximate sixteen pounds of food. More commonly, they consume 2000 to 5000 calories of pastries, bread, icecream, cookies etc; high calories of food are favoured by them. The recurrent pattern of heavy hinging and vomiting brings in its wake a number of devastating physical consequences; ulcers, gastric and dental problems, an acute disturbances in the chemicai balance of the blood which can cause heart-attacks. Other problems include sore throats, aching joints, feelings of weakness and dizziness and apathy.

Bulimic college students sometimes report that immediately before one of their caloric binges they feel depressed, angry and that vomiting may give them a pleasurable "high". Their problems, with eating and weight effect their social lives, their work, and their family relationships. Binge-purge caters may also have a history of over using such substances as alcohol, marijuana, amphetamines, diet pills and the barbiturates.

The DSM-in lists several operational criteria for bulima:

1. An episodic pattern of binge eating accompanied by (a) an awareness of disordered eating patterns, with a fear of not being able voluntarily to stop, eating, and (b) depressive moods and negative after-thoughts following the gorging.

2. The bulimic person must have at least three of the following symptoms:

a. Rapid consumption of food during the eating episode.

b. Ingestion of high caloric food during the episode.

c. Clandestine eating binges.

d. Following the binges, abdominal pain, sleep, social interruption, or self-induced vomiting.

e. Repeated efforts to lose weight-diets, cathartic vomiting.

f. Cyclical patterns of fasting.

Causes: Unfortunately no information is available concerning the possible causes of bulimia. Although a parent or sibling may be obese, no predisposing factors or stressors have been found, according to the DSM-III. It is not even known at this time whether, like obesity, bulimia is more common in lower social classes than in middle and upper classes; or whether, like anorexia nervosa, it is mainly a middle class disorder. To be sure, much more research is needed in connection with this problem.

Treatment: Since bulimia does not follow a pattern like that of simple overeating (obesity), it seems doubtful whether appetite reducing methods would be effective; many bulimic persons are not, infact, overweight. There seems to be no published evidence demonstrating a systematic and effective men as for dealing with this problem. While private clinicians may have dealt with some bulimics with success, these data have yet to be made public.

CONDUCTDISORDERS

While 5 to 15 percent of all adolescents shoe "occasional" acts of antisocial behavior (Meeks, 1980), the conduct disorders are characterized by more persistent displays of antisocial activity. Four types of conduct disorders share the DSM-III core description of repetitive and persistent patterns of antisocial behavior that violate the rights of others, beyond the ordinary mischief and pranks of children and adolescents.

(i) In the *conduct disorder of the aggressive and under socialized type,* youths shows a consistent disregard for the feelings of others, bully smaller children, have few, if any, same-age friends, and present serious school problems. They generally are. hostile, verbally abusive, defiant, and negativistic.

(ii) Though anger is also present to some degree, it is not as obvious in youngsters classified as *unaggressive conduct disorder, under socialized type.* While these youths are adapt at manipulating people for favours, they also share with their aggressive counterparts, a lack of concern for the feelings of others. Generally, they show one of two patterns of behavior. In the first pattern they are timid, unassertive, and shy, and often report feeling rejected and mistreated. At times they will be victimized, most often sexually. In a second pattern, the adolescents are less timid and more likely to exploit and manipulate others. Unlike their aggressive counterpart's response of uncontrolled anger when

frustrated, these youths are more likely to react to pressure with deviousness and guile.

(iii) Adolescents designated *as having socialized conduct disorders show* an ability to make friends with some of their peers. In aggressive conduct disorder, socialized type, youths commit violations of the basic rights of others usually by some combination of physical violence or robbery. While they do not seem to have feelings of guilt or remorse for their illegal activities, socialized aggressive adolescents have an ability to develop friendships and maintain them for 6 months or more. They will extend themselves to help those they call friends, even to the point of taking punishment rather than informing on them.

(iv) The final group of conduct disorders, the *unaggressive and socialized type, is* also marked by rebellion against authority, but lacks the physically aggressive quality of the aggressive and socialized pattern. Some of the behavior of the non-aggressive adolescents seems pranklike, but in actually they often end up in serious trouble with school and community authorities.

ADOLESCENT SUICIDE

The concept of suicide is not limited to self-murder. Some contend that suicide is simply the ultimate form of self-destructive behavior. This approach suggests, then, that there are degrees or levels of self-destructive behavior. The term life-threatening behavior (LTB) is used to represent a class of actions that are less lethal than suicide. Weisman (1976) lists these types of life-threatening behaviors:

1. **Self-injury and intoxication**: includes nonsuicidal overdoses of drugs, frequent alcohol abuse, and other repetitive acts that result in trauma.

2. Rash, regretted, incautious, or bizarre acts unskilled use of dangerous tools, instruments, and the automobile; where there is real danger, these people may show very poor judgment, which creates a death-related setting.

3. **Significant omissions**: omits medication, disregards medical or other professional advice.

4. **Significant excesses:** gross overeating, starvation diets, chronic alcoholism.

5. **Counter therapeutic behavior:** rebellions against rules, roles, and requirements during hospitalization.

In the late 1930s, in his book "Man Against Himself" Karl Menninger described how completed suicide, the ultimate act, is on a continuum with lesser self-destructive behaviors such as alcohol addiction, drug abuse, self-mutilation, polysurgery (exhibited by those who seek doctors who will operate on them), and other self-destructive acts. This profound point of Menninger's, that there exist degrees or symbolic acts of suicide, certainly seems to apply to particular adolescent actions.

Although suicide is not a leading cause of death for those between 10 and 14 year of age, between ages 15 and 19 it becomes the fourth leading cause of death, exceeded only by accidents, homicides, and malignant tumors (U.S. Public Health Service, National Center for Health Statistics, 1974). Of the approximately 25,000 suicides reported in one year, 4,000 were committed by the adolescent group. Another interesting statistic shows that in the last 20 years adolescent suicide has increased nearly 250 percent.

Symptoms of Adolescent Suicide

Although most of the clues to suicide have emerged from investigations of adult male suicides, a few of these conditions may also warn of adolescent suicide potential : (1) crippling physical disability; (2) early rejection by the father; (3) heavy drug use; (4) verbal statements about one's own worthlessness or the absence of hope or purpose in life; and (5) major setbacks or failures in social, academic, or family affairs.

(b) **Runaway**: Though many children and adolescents remain at home and act out their frustrations and anxieties aggressively, nearly I million youngsters per year run away. Involving nearly equal number of boys and girls, runaways have been characterized as insecure, unhappy, and impulsive (Jenkins and Stable, 1972), having low self-esteem (Beyer, 1974), and feeling out of control (Bartollas, 1975). The bulk of research on runaways shows them to be more disturbed than normal teenagers.

Disturbed parent-child relationships seems to be one of the most important reasons (e.g., Brandon 1974, Gottlieb and Chafetz, 1977), but runaways also have problems in school (Walker, 1976) seems to necd-to search for adventure and meaning (Wattemberg, 1956), and suffer from boredom (Tobias, 1970). Hoshino (1973) point out that the # entire family of a **runaway** may be under stress and each family member would, if given the opportunity, choose to run to runaways more often appear to be organized around punishment and negativism and seem unable to support one another in crises.

Occasionally, runaways end up in serious trouble, but the great majority of them return home safely. Unfortunately, they often return to home situations that have not changed, and they may have to face the very same problems that pushed them to run away in the first place. Hopefully, time away from the stressful family situation may give runaways an opportunity to reassess who they are and find new ways to deal with their difficulties. The laws in some states make running away a crime. When runaways return, they may face incarceration or they may be forced to see a counselor.

(c) **Identity Disorders of Adolescence**: DSM-III states that the major feature of this problematic reaction is the adolescent's uncertainly about his or her identity, and most important for diagnosis, severe subjective distress regarding this uncertainty. Identity is viewed in general terms in this disorder: identity deals with issues such as "Who am I?" "What am I going to do with my life?" "By what values and standards should I live?" and many similar issues.

William Glasser, a psychiatrist and founder of reality therapy, wrote a book called The Identity Society (1972) that deals with many identity issues' Glasser maintains that most young peopic in our society no longer strive for goals as younger people in past generations had. Rather, today "roles" are sought before "goals." To illustrate this contrast, Glasser says that "almost everyone is personally engaged in a search for acceptance as a person rather than as a performer of a task". Unfortunately for many of us, it is not "who we are" that counts, but rather 'what we do for a living'. Our identity is inordinately tied to our occupational role, a role that, to say the least, is vulnerable.

Thus, adolescents often experience profound distress over the task of making a career choice because there is uncertainty about what these careers are really like, and over whether or not they have access into educational prerequisites for these careers. The DSM-III says a problem may become "chronic" if the person is unable to establish a career commitment or if, on another dimension, he of she fails to form lasting emotional attachments because of shifts in jobs and interpersonal relationships.

12

Mental Retardation

Mental retardation has not received much attention either from psychologists, psychiatrists or from other mental health experts. It was only in the last few decades that mental retardation started receiving a great deal of research and rehabilitative attention as a result of the contribution of John F Kennedy, President of U.S.A and also as a result of joint efforts by a group of parents who started national association for the retarded children in U.SA

Mental retardation is one of the most common disorder of concern to parents, teachers, policy makers and mental health experts. Identification of a mentally retarded child and giving him/her special education has become an important task for educationists and teachers.

In this chapter we would define mental retardation and discuss whether mental retardation is a result of developmental delay or deficit. According to some researchers mental retardation is a result of developmental delay according to others it is due to some developmental defect. We would also discuss in detail, the various levels of mental retardation. There are four levels of mental retardation which include mild, moderate, severe and profound. We would discuss the characteristic behaviours associated with

each one of them.

Mental retardation has a wide variety of causes some of which are organic, whereas there are due to socio cultural factors. We would then discuss the organic or biological causes of mental retardation. The organic causes of mental retardation can be any one of the following (a) Genetic factors (b) Prenatal factors (c) Postnatal factors and (d) Factors of unknown etiology.

Psychologists and other mental health experts have also studied the environmental factors associated with mental retardation. These factors can be due to cultural, familial or environmental factors. Mental retardation arising out of these factors is also called as cultural familial retardation. We would discuss the nature and causes of such retardation also.

Following this we would then discuss the prevention treatment and management of mental retardation. This one of the most skillful and needed approach to mental retardation about which common man as well as experts are not much familiar with.

We would end this chapter with a few short notes.

Mental Retardation and discuss the various levels *of* mental retardation.

Mental retardation. Its various levels and discuss the controversy whether it is due to developmental delay or deficit :

DEFINITION OF MENTAL RETARDATION

Mental Retardation can be defined as significantly sub-average general intellectual functioning existing concurrently with deficits in adaptive behaviour and manifested during the developmental period. This definition given by American Association on Mental Retardation (AAMR) is also in accordance with the DSM-III definition of mental retardation. According to this definition, the essential feature of mental retardation are as follows:

1. Significantly sub-average general intellectual functioning.
2. Deficits in adaptive behaviour.
3. Deficits manifested in the developmental period i.e. onset of the condition during the developmental period i.e.' before the age of 18.

Mental retardation is diagnosed regardless of whether there is a coexisting mental or physical disorder. From the above definition, it is clear that not only are the mentally deficit people less intelligent but they are also socially inadequate. They cannot look after themselves. They cannot support themselves and their level is much lower than their age in almost every aspect of life.

Their drives and motives are not strong. They do not persist in what they undertake, their feelings are simple and primitive. According to David Wechsler, Mental Retardation is measured by measuring behaviours considered important in dealing with various aspects of life. Thus activity and abilities like verbal skills, arithmetical skills, concept formation skills and various motor tasks are very much helpful in determining the levels of Mental Retardation. From the above definition, it is very much clear that Mental Retardation not only refers to low

intelligence, but this low intelligence should lead to problems in adaptive behaviour. Mental retardation is not by definition irreversible. It designates to performance at a given time only.

LEVELS OF MENTAL RETARDATION

There are generally four levels of mental retardation. These include mild, moderate, severe and profound.

(1) **Mild retardation** is the most common form of mental retardation, approximately 90% of the mentally retarded individuals belongs to this group. The IQ of the individual having mild retardation range from 50 to 70. During the earlier period of development, except for a minor developmental delay everything else is normal. Early pie-school development of these individuals is not very much different from-that of many children of normal intelligence. Their intellectual impairment usually becomes more noticeable in their academic work. By late teens, an individual with mild mental retardation learns academic skills upto approximately 6th grade.

Intellectual deficit are noticed generally in the skilled academic learning experience of the primary course. The individual belonging to this group can be guided towards *social* conformity. They can develop social and communication skills and can usually achieve social and vocational skills upto minimum self support, but may need guidance and assistance under stressful social or economic condition. The most significant problem for some mild mentally retarded individual may be avoidance of socially appropriate behaviour. As adults, most of the individuals function in unskilled or semi-skilled occupation. Some requires some assistance or measure of supervision due to limited ability to foresee the consequence of their action.

(2) **Moderate retardation:** Roughly about 6% of the retarded individuals 'falls into this category of moderate retardation. These individuals have an IQ in the range of 35 to 49. These individuals have severe intellectual impairment which slows down their pre-school development. They have delayed develop-

mental milestones.

By the usual school age (5 to 6 years of age) moderately retarded individuals progress to a level more similar to a normal two or three years child. These children are unable to benefit from regular school curriculum. They can study only upto second grade. However, such individuals do learn the basic skills of self help. Such individuals develop minimum vocational skills. As adult, moderately retarded individuals can live semi-independent life. Many moderately mentally retarded persons have unusual mathematical or artistic abilities. One such case is that of 'idiot savant'. These individuals can live, as adults, semi-independent life in a protective environment, but independent functioning is impossible. Many behaviour problems are quite common in this group. Individuals in this group generally has an increased probability of suspected organic etiology.

(3) **Severe Mental Retardation**-Approximately 3% to 4% of the retarded people have severe mental retardation. The IQ of this group ranges between 20 to 34. The intellectual level of individuals in this category is so disabling that almost of the individuals belonging to this category spent most of their life in institution. There is a clear impaired development in infancy and in early childhood, usually there is a genetic or organic cause. There may be a physical defect, shortly before or after birth : There may also be physical disturbance in visual motor coordination. Infection and metabolic disorder is also common among this groups. Those who belong to this groups have rudimentary speech which may not develop until childhood and even as adults. Their vocabulary is limited. As adults, these individuals can communicate only at simple concrete level, that too, after rigorous training. In the area of self help skills and habits training they are very poor. Even in adulthood, socially adaptive skills are minimal, as a result of which they may face many problems; in social life.

(4) **Profound Retardation:** Profound retardation is a most disabling level of retardation. The measured IQ is below 29. Roughly about 1% of the retarded individuals fali into this category. Characteristic feature of profound mental retardation include almost no development of self care skills. Even if they survive in adulthood, at higher levels, individuals, of this group may be able to feed themselves with assistance. The speech is very rudimentary having a vocabulary of about 300 simple words. Individuals of this group usually have motor problems, especially visual motor co-ordination. Majority of the individuals have a high incidence of physical deformity. Most of them suffer from various diseases and die. Nursing care and supervision in most aspects of living is required through out their life.

The above mentioned different types of mental retardation is a part of the DSM-III classification of mental retardation. Educationists have classified mental retardation into slightly different category so as to devise appropriate educational programme for each category Table 14.1 gives a brief idea of classification of mental retardation by educational expectation.

Table 14.1

TERMINO-LOGY	APPROXIMATE IQ RANGE	EDUCATIONAL EXPECTATION
Dull-normal	75 or 80 to 90	Capable of competing in school in most areas except in the strictly academic areas where performance is below average. Social adjustment which is not noticeably difficult from the larger population although in the lower segment of adequate adjustment. Occupational performance satisfactory in Non-technical areas, with total self-support highly probable.
Educable	50 to 75 or 80	Second-to-fifth-grade achievement. in school academic areas. Social adjustment that will permit some degree of independence in the community. Occupational sufficiency that will permit partial or total support when an adult.
Trainable	20 to 49	Learning primarily in the areas of self-help skills, very limited achievement in areas considered academic. Social adjustment usually limited to home and closely surrounding areas. Occupational performance primarily in sheltered workshop or an institutional setting.
Custodial	Below20	Usually unable to achieve even sufficient skills lo care for basic needs. Will usually require nearly total care and supervision for duration of lifetime.

MENTAL RETARDATION: DEVELOPMENTAL DELAY OR DEFICIT

Some researchers are of the view that mental retardation is due to one or more specific cognitive defects which interfere with learning and memory. According to them, certain cognitive defects lead to mental retardation. On the other hand, some other scientists have opined that retardation is a result of slow development. These researchers are of the view that the retarded individual passes through the same stages as a person of normal intelligence, but reaches, a lower upper limit. There is a great deal of research evidence to support both these contrasting view points.

1. **Sacuzzo's Theory** According to Sacuzzo, mental retardation is a result of cognitive deficit or deficit of memory. According to this theory memorization occurs in several steps. Problems at any of these steps can lead to disturbed information processing which can create memory disturbances. Sacuzzo believes in the information processing theory of memory. According to the information processing theory of memory, memory passes through 3 stages. The first step is called as 'ionic stage' or sensory memory. The second stage is called as short-term memory and the third stage is called as long-term memory. According to Sacuzzo and other researchers, retarded individuals need longer period of time to put the information in the sensory memory. Retarded people according to this view, take longer period of time to get the information into the short-term memory than non-retarded individuals. Due to this longtime duration, stimulus information is likely to be forgotten rapidly in case of retarded individuals. As result, they face difficulties in terms of learning the material and associating the stimuli with each other. Thus, according to Sacuzzo's view, defects in Iconic memory' storage or in short term memory can lead to mental retardation.

2. **Zigler,s view** According to Zigier, mental retardation is due to a specific cognitive defect. According to him, mentally retarded individuals goes through the same basic stages of cognitive process as a normal individual docs but mentally retarded individual develops at a slower rate and with a lower upper limit. Zigler has taken this view after review of more than 30 studies and he has concluded that majority of the studies favour this formulation. This view of Zigler that the processing of cognitive, development is delayed in the retarded person is based on the theoretical views of Jean Piaget. Understanding mental retardation on the basis of Jean Piaget theory, Barbainhelder has pointed out that mentally retarded, especially sevre and profoundly retarded, function at a sensory motor stage. Moderately retarded adult function at the stage of preoperational thought and mildly retarded function at the stage of cognitive operation. This view has been supported by the work of Stephen and her associates. In her studies, Stephen and her associates observed the performance of the retarded and non-retarded individuals on a large variety of reasoning task. The research results pointed out that both retarded and non-retarded group devel-

oped increased reasoning abilities in a developmental consequences as stated by Piaget, but mentally retarded individuals mastered the reasoning, task more slowly than non-retarded individuals.

3. **Milgram's Theory:** Milgram has proposed that mentally retarded people suffer from specific cognitive defects. He has emphasized that retarded individuals failed to use cognitive mediators to associate words or concepts Normally children who need or want to associate two words such as table and book usually use cognitive mediator such as book is on the table. Retarded children fail to use such mediators and as a result they do poorly on such memory tasks. Milgram has further pointed out that when retarded children are provided with mediators, their performance improves.

Thus, we sec that Milgram and Sacuzzo are of the view that mental retardation is due to memory defects whereas Zigler and Piaget are of the view that menial retardation is a result of developmental delay. Research evidence supports both, the developmental delay and developmental defect positions. The work of Stephen and her colleagues give us some clues that both these positions may be partially correct.

ORGANIC CAUSES FOR MENTAL RETARDATION

The major organic causes of mental retardation can be classified into the following groups:

(1) Chromosomal abnormality and genetic defect.

(2) Pre-natal environment.

(3) Post-natal environment.

(4) Unknown .etiology.

1. **Chromosomal abnormality**: Chromosomal abnormality and genetic and organic causes are the main causes of mental retardation. The lower level of retardation is usually due to organic damage. Organic retardation makes up 25% of the population. Chromosomal and genetic factors are the most important. Among the Chromosomal abnormality Down's syndrome is the most common form of disorder that leads to mental retardation and among the genetic defect P.K.U is the most common. We would discuss these two in brief.

(i) **Down's Syndrome** is also called as mongolism or 'trisomy 21'. Down's syndrome occurs because of the presence of one extra chromosome. Usually in human beings there are 23 pairs of chromosomes (i.e. total 46 chromosomes). However, in Down baby, there are 47 chromosome, i.e. one extra chromosome, and this one extra chromosome is found in the 21st pair i.e. in the

21st pair instead of two chromosomes 3 chromosomes are present. Down's syndrome child has many physical abnormalities. Eyes are slanted upward, flat face and nose, fissured tongue, sturdy fingers and short stature. Because of abnormalities, individual also has defect in heart and other internal organs. The life expectancy of the people with Down syndrome is shorter. Intelligence of the Down baby is generally below 50. Yet a small proportion i.e. about 55 may have IQofabout70.

(ii) **Phenyiketonuria (P.K.U)**: In contrast to Down's syndrome which is caused by an extra chromosome, phenyiketonuria (PKU) is caused by a genetic error in which the enzyme responsible for the-metabolism of the. Biochemical phenyla-lanine is not present at birth. The result of this genetic error is that phenylaisninc can build to dangerous levels, producing severe brain damage and consequently mental retardation. Incidence of PKU has been found to range from I in every 6800 births to I in every 14,000 births (Murdock. 1 975). The average IQ of children with untreated PKU is about 50, placing the majority of them in the moderately to severely retarded range.

PKU was first described in 1934 by Folling (Robinson & Robinson, 1976), a veterinarian who developed an interest in a strange disorder present in a new born child of a relative. The child's mother complained to several physicians that there was a strange odour emanating from the child's urine; dissatisfied with the physicians' claims that there was nothing to worry about, Foiling went to study the problem and to discover the PKU defect.

Generally, the PKU child appears normal for the first few weeks of life, *but* usually motor problems appear around 6 months of age. The child may not be able to sit at age I, and may not walk by 4 years of age. About one-third of PKU children never learn to walk or to control defecation or urination, and about two-thirds never learn to talk. Unlike the usually friendly Down's syndrome children, typical PKU children may be wild, uncontrollable, and generally unpleasant to be around. Psychologically, they may be fearful, restless, and so hyperactive that they require restraint and institutionalization.

Fortunately, the effects of PKU arc preventable if the disorder is identified in the newborn infant. *A.* simple urine or blood test for PKU given at birth is now a requirement in most hospitals. When PKU is identified, the infant can be placed immediately on a special pheylalanine-free diet. If done in time, this early dietary restriction usually prevents severe retardation. Berman and Ford (1970) report that successfully treated PKU children tend to perform within the average range of intelligence. The Collaborative Study of Children treated for PKU (1975) reports that, in 95 percent of cases, neurological examinations are normal at ages 2 to 4, and that IQS are within the average range. Thus, simple control of diet can result in the avoidance of some of these devastating behavioral and intellectual deficits.

2. **Pre-natal Environment:** Many factors even before the birth of a child can also contribute towards the development of the mental retardation. Some of the factors that are responsible for the development of mental retardation during the pre-natal environment are:

(a) Maternal infections, (b) Blood RH factor, (c) Drugs (d) Birth complications.

(a) **Maternal infection:** A young infant is connected to mother through placenta. Many infectious illness of the mother do not cross the placenta to the blood supply of the foetus. However, some diseases do cross the placenta and effects the child which may lead to mental retardation. There are many such diseases. One well known disease, that is known to produce .mental retardation as a result of maternal infection is *rubella virus or German measles.* The danger is particularly great during the first three months of pregnancy. About half the infants of mothers, who have German measles during the first trimester (three month) of pregnancy become infected, and about one-third of them are born retarded (Chess 1978). There are vaccines to protect German mealses and the, incidence of this type of retardation now is much lower than in the past. Many of the maternal infection which can cause foetal retardation include untreated syphilis, herpes simplex and a protozoan infection called toxoplasmosis.

(b) **Blood RH factor:** If certain substances present in the blood of a foetus, which are not present in the mother's blood, problems may result. For example, foetus may inherit a substance from the father called RH factor. The foetus then has RH positive (RHP) blood. A mother who does not have this factor has RH negative (RH) blood. In such case, the mother will develop antibodies againsts the RH factor for the foetus blood. This usually does not cause a problem for the mother's first child. However second pregnancy can be complicated by the antibodies that remain in the mother's blood. In some cases. Mother's antibodies enter the blood stream of the foetus and destroy its red blood cells. The foetus then suffers oxygen deprivation and destruction of brain cells leading to mental relardation. Thus blood incompatibility between the mother's blood and infant's bloods can lead to mental retardation.

(c) **Drugs:** Certain prescribed drugs taken by the mother during the pregnancy can have a serious developmental effect on the foetus. These drugs taken by aspirin, thalidomide, certain illegal drugs such as Marijuana, Hashish, Mescaline, LSD can also effect child's intelligence.

(d) **Birth Complications:** Birth complication is another pre-natal factor, prematurity and anoxia (oxygen deprivation are to the main complication that can occur during the infant's delivery and lead to retardation and intellectual functioning.

3. **Postnatal Environment:** After child is born, many factors can lead to damage of brain tissue and cause mental retardation. Three major post-natal factors responsible for the mental retardation are is (a) infections (b) head trauma (c) poisoning.

4. **Unknown Etiology:** Many organic conditions that results in mental retardation remain mysterious. Some children for example manifest progressive destruction of the white matter of the brain for no known reason. We know that their retardation is due to the destruction of the brain issues. But, we do not known the cause of the retardation. Another important cause of this retardation is *anencephaly.* In this condition, an infant is born without most of the important structures of the brain and the flat bones of the skull. We know that mental retardation is due to destruction of the brain tissue, but we do not know its exact, etiology. These are just two of the many types of organic mental retardation of unknown etiology.

CULTURAL-FAMILIAL RETARDATION

Many individuals who fall in the category of mild retardation do not have any identifiable organic cause of retardation. To a lesser extent, some individuals in the moderate range of functioning also do not have identifiable physical etiology associated with their retarded intellectual functioning. These individuals come from disadvantage families and have parents or siblings who are mentally retarded. Such type of retardation present in these individuals is called as cultural familial retardation.

Thus cultural familial retardation means mild retardation which is non-organic in nature, and which is due to the combination of environment and hereditary factors. The individuals with cultural familial retardation have IQ usually about 50. Over the years psychologists have identified the various causes responsible for the development of cultural familial retardation, which has taken the shape of classical nature versus nurture controversy. This controversy, which originated in 1930s an~ 40s was partially resolved in 1950s and 1960s by taking an interactionist approach, some psychologists have argued that hereditary leads to lower intellectual functioning. Whereas, others have provided evidence to show that disturbed and impoverished environment is responsible for mental retardation. A great deal of research evidence has accumulated over the years to show that hereditary as well as environmental factors are both important. However, relative contribution of the two are difficult to assess. Scholars like H.J. Eysenck, Jensen and Cyril Burt have argued that hereditary plays an important role in the causation of lower intellectual functioning. Whereas, on the other hand classic experiments on impoverished environment carried out by Wayne Dennis on Lebanese orphange children and by Harry Harlow on rearing of monkey's in impoverished environment have shown the contribution of environment in the development of mental retardation. The largest segment of the retarded individual comes from Very low social and economic environment ànd arc largely a product of material **deprivation** and poverty. Malnutrition early in life has severe effect on the **developing** organism. Researchers have found that retardation is due to poverty and its bed effects like bad jiving conditions, inadequate food, poor medical care for both mother and child etc.

Special Education Programmes: For special education, retarded , people are usually classified into two groups, the educable mentally retarded (EMR) and the trainable mentally retarded (TMR). EMR people generally fall into the IQ range of 55 to 70. They may be expected to reach a level of anywhere between third and sixth grade by the time they finish school. Social adjustment and ability to take care of themselves are the primary objectives of their schooling. Special classes for EMR children generally are small and emphasize social competence and occupational skills rather than academic achievement There are special EMR classes and programs for people of different ages (Robinson and Robinson, 1976):

Infant Stimulation Class: For children from birth to 3 years of age, infant stimulation involves parents and teachers providing maximum healthy stimulation in the developing child.

Preschool Class: For children 3 to 6 years old with mental ages from 2 to 4 years, preschool classes introduce group experiences and continue healthy stimulation.

Elementary Primary Class: For EMR children 6 to 10 years of age with mental ages from 3 to 6 years, primary classes are generally preacademic. Experience such as those of a regular kindergarten are provided in hopes of building self confidence, early language development, and security in the school situation.

Elementary Intermediate Class: For EMR children 9 to 13 years of age with mental ages of 6 to 9 years, intermediate classes designed for children who cannot remain in regular classrooms due to inability to sit quietly and to exhibit other social skills necessary for regular schooling. Focus in class is one academic tools of reading, willing, and mathematics, as well as on practical everyday skills.

Secondary School Classes: For EMR children at junior and senior high school levels, secondly school classes emphasize vocational training and domestic skills. Students arc taught to apply basic tools to everyday problems such as use of money, reading of newspapers, application for jobs, and the like.

Postschool Programs: For persons who have completed formal schooling, postschool programs provide a place where continued vocational and educational guidance is available. Examples of such programs are sheltered workshops and rehabilitation agencies such as the Salvation Army and Goodwill Industries.

With few exception, TMR children arc more severely retarded than EMR children and present a different set of educational problems. TMR children have IQs in the range of 25 to 55 and may not be expected to achieve any more than the slightest mastery of academic skills. Primary goals for TMR children usually involve their being able to care for themselves and to sustain themselves in simple occupation endeavors.

The goal of the TMR class is to develop basic skills that normal and EMR children usually learn as they grow. TMR children must learn such "simple" tasks as washing themselves, eating properly, speaking, following simple directions, and the like. Instead of books, they must learn to read important signs: signs indicating "Danger" or "Stop" may be much more important to read than simple stories. Efforts to educate the TMR child can be frustrating.

Residential Placement: Residential placement of retarded people is different from education and psychotherapy in that it typically involves total control of the retarded person's life. Once known as institutionalization, residential placement involves removing retarded people from their homes and placing them in a setting where they may live either permanently or for some extended period of time although many moderately retarded individuals live in residential facilities, the majority of those who are institutionalized fall in the severely and profoundly retarded categories. In 1982, the number of retarded people in residential centers in the United States was about 250,000 (Hauber et al., 1984). Since about 7 to 9 million people in the United States may be considered mentally retarded, the number in permanent residential status is relatively small. This testifies to efforts to maintain retarded people in the community as part of the mainstream.

The decision to place a child in a residential facility is a stressful and emotional one for most parents. Yet there comes a time in the life of some families with a retarded child when this decision must be faced.

The decision to place a child in a residential facility is complex. An extensive study 'by Saenger (1960) of factors related to the decision to institutionalize a retarded child suggests several basic conclusions.

(i) First, the more severely retarded a child, the more likely it is that residential placement will be chosen. Nearly 9 our of 10 of Saenger's sample of profoundly retarded people were hospitalized as opposed lo I out of 10 of the moderately to midly retarded group. Saenger also noted that the presence of behavior problems outside the home was significantly related to institutionalization. A child who caused little or no trouble for parents was less likely to be placed in a hospital.

(ii) Another reason for institutionalization is that the retarded person causes unbearable stress and trouble at home.

(iii) Finally, the fact that outpatient care is not readily available to many lower socio-economic groups may leave institutionalization as the only recourse for the family of a poor retarded person. Many families probably would prefer to keep a retarded person at home, but when their choice is limited to no treatment, or residential treatment, they frequently are forced to decide in favour of the latter.

Residential treatment can take any of several form. There are the traditional state or private hospitals, as well as variety of residential programs that can provide positive experiences. One example of an alternative to the state hospital is the group home, a sort of boarding house in which a limited number of (perhaps 40) of retarded people live under the same roof with a staff of professionals. In this protected environment, home members can carry on simple vocational tasks, produce saleable items in sheltered workshops, take part in group therapy, and live as nearly normal a life as possible. The group home can avoid many of the detrimental aspects of the large institution and maintain many of the characteristics or a real "home" for the retarded person.

SEX CHROMOSOMAL DISORDER AND MENTAL RETARDATION

Many sex chromosomal disorders lead to mental sub normality and/or other defects. We would examine some of the sex chromosomal disorders which besides other disorders also lead to mental retardation. These are as follows:

(i) 47 **XXY Abnormality** This particular type of chromosomal abnormality is related with antisocial behaviour. In recent years this chromosomal abnormality has attracted great interest. People with this pattern are males, sometimes also referred to as "Super Males" because of the extra Y chromosomal. 47 XYY Males typically display certain characteristics which are as fol-

lows:

(a) most of them have a very bad facial can during adolescence,

(b) most of them are usually six feet tall at maturity, and

(c) most of them are rather dull mentally with an I.Q. between 70 to 95.

Some have epileptic like symptoms suggesting a brain dysfunction of some kind. Early studies of XYY males suggested that there was a higher frequency of this chromosomal abnormality among prison in males and mentally retarded patients. These findings were widely reported by the press, and throughout the world an image emerged of the XYY males as a tall individual of low I.Q., with strong tendencies towards aggression and violence. In nations far apart as Australia and France criminals with 47 XYY chromosomes were defended on the premise that they were helpless victims of their genetic inheritance and therefore could not beheld accountable for their offences. Many more recent studies have reported that the prevalence of XYY males among criminals is no higher than in general population and that most XYY men have no criminal tendencies.

In the scientific community the current view of the XYY male is much more cautious. Some researchers Still feel; that there might be a slight criminal propensity in such men but others do not. G.B. Hook has pointed out three reasons that why the incidence of 47 XXY is more in mental-Penal institutions:

(i) One explanation is that 47XYY males are born frequently than normal males into circumstances that lead to antisocial behaviour.

(ii) A second hypothesis is that the physical characteristics of these males makes social adaptations difficult and therefore lead to deviant adaptations,

(iii) The third hypothesis is that 47XYY chromosome pattern results in abnormal development of the nervous system, which in them tends to result in abnormal behaviour. No direct evidence favours any of these hypothesis.

(ii) **Turner's Syndrome :** Females who are born with only one X chromosome have a condition called as Turner syndrome. They have XO chromosome pattern as compared to normal XX pattern. These women arc short, have incompletely developed breasts and are sterile. They have Webbed neck and fail to develop sexually at puberty. Although usually of normal intelligence, they show some specific cognitive defect. They do poorly in arithmetic and on tests of visual form perception and spatial organization.

Since doses of the. hormone estrogen can induce the development of secondary sex characteristics such as pubic hair and breasts, estrogen therapy in adolescence can help women with Turner's Syndrome to have a normal appearance and to live relatively normal lives.

(iii) **Klinefelter's Syndrome** are individuals who arc males having an extra X choromosome i.e., they have XXY chromosome pattern. These XXY males are tall, thin and have long arms and legs. Their testicles are small and they arc usually sterile. These males have marked feminine characteristics. His breasts are large, testicles are small and do not produce sperms. Psychologically many have low l.Q, and show poor social adjustment. It is not known whether the individuals genetic make up or the social consequences of the genetic abnormality are to be blamed for this poor adjustment. This condition occurs one out of 900 births. Half of the persons so afflicted are mentally retarded.

(iv) Down's Syndrome is not a sex chromosome disorder but it is a genetic disorder that may lead to mental retardation.

Down's Syndrome is also called as Mongolism or Trisomy-21. This type of genetic abnormality leads to mental retardation. A person with the Down's Syndrome has the following characteristics:

(a) severe to moderate mental retardation (I.Q. is within the range of 20 to 69 where 100 is the normal),

(b) they have obliquely slanted eyes with an extra fold of skin over the eyelids (hence the name Mongolism),

(c) a round face.

(d) short stature,

(e) abnormalities of the skull bones and the jaw and

(f) short little fingers and other abnormalities of hand and feet.

"Down Babies" arc usually quiet and placid and their mortality rate during is high because so many of them succumb to respiratory infection and heart malformation. Chromosomal analysis of individuals with Down's Syndrome has shown that many of them have an extra chromosome in the 21st pair of the chromosome, *Le.,* in the twenty first pair instead of two, three arc often present, (thus it is also called as Trisomy-21).

In most of the cases presence of extra chromosome is lethal and miscarriage results. However some individuals survive, but have genetic abnormalities. Down's syndrome is unfortunately rather common. It occurs four birth per 10,(XX) among mothers under 30 years of age and its incidence is greater among older mothers, about one per I (X) for 40 years old mother and three per

100 for 45 years old mother. It is not known why the incidence is greater among older mother.

(b) **Disorder Associated with or leading to mental retardation.** There are many disorders that are associated with mental retardation. Some of these disorders that may lead to mental retardation are as follows :

(i) ***Tay Saches Disease:*** Near the end to the nineteenth century, two researchers, Warrent Tay and Bernard Sachs, described a new type of mental retardation observed during infancy. In this form of infantile retardation, which occurs predominantly in those of Jewish ancestry (at a rate of about one in every 5,000 births), neurological and ophthalmologic problems emerges by at least the sixth months of life, one of the first symptoms lobe noticed is extreme motor retardation; for example, the baby may be unable to raise its head or turn over. Furthermore, seizures are common, and by the end of the first year of life optic trophy, leading to blindness, has begun to develop. Accompanying these defects are gross intellectual retardation, emaciation, hearing loss, and paralysis. Berg (1974) points out that death usually occurs between the second and fourth year.

Tay-Sachs disease is often diagnosed by a "cherry-red" spot in the area of the retina. It may also be diagnosed before birth through amniocentesis. The cause of this variety of mental retardation is unknown, and at present no treatment can change its course (Brain and Watson 1969).

(ii) *Cretinism (Congenital Hypothyroidism)* For years, "cretin" has meant deformed idiot. Cretinism, as we know it today, refers to a type of mental retardation caused by impairment of thyroid functioning. For example, a pregnant woman whose diet is deficient in iodine may give birth to an infant with cretinism-congenital hypothyroidism. Although the infant with cretinism may appear normal shortly after birth, unless thyroid extract is given, the child's intellectual development will be retarded, and a number of other symptoms may emerge. If untreated, for instance, these infants usually become very apathetic and listless, and their bone development will also be severely delayed.

Mental and physical retardation associated with cretinism , can be ameliorated if therapy is started, very early, yet the prognosis for increments in intelligence vary considerably; that is, some respond with marked increased in mental ability while others do not.

(iii) *Hydrocephaly (Hydrocephalus)*Unlike several of the other organic forms of mental retardation, hydrocephaly is often recognizable at birth because of the enlargement of the baby's head and prominent scalps, veins, and turning? down of the eyes, 'rising sun sign' (Brain and Walton 1969). Hydro-

cephaly- meaning "water-head" or "water-brain is a rare form of mental retardation occurring when a blockage or failure in absorption prevents cerebrospinal fluid from flowing out of the ventricles located deep within the brain, or when fluid is trapped in the subarachnoid spaces surrounding the cortex. This interference with fluid circulation raises the pressure within the brain cavity, pushing the soft skull outward and often compressing the cortex.

In the infantile variety of hydrocephaly, symptoms usually include seizures, cerebral palsy, blindness, and sometimes gross mental retardation. Gradations of hydrocephaly do exist, producing various degrees of mental and physical impairment. For example, Tredgold and Soddy (1963) described two types of hydrocephaly, those who were severely retarded usually bedridden and untrainable and a less severe from. In some cases, excessive fluid may be drained or diverted from the cranial, cavity, preventing extensive retardation.

(iv) *Cat-cry Syndrome (Cri Du Chat).* One of the most severe forms of organic retardation is cri du chat, or the cat-cry syndrome. Infants with this variety of retardation, in addition to profound retardation, have a characteristic 'cat-like cry' caused by abnormalities of the larynx. This syndrome often has two additional physical characteristics, microcephaly (small head) and low-set ears There is no known treatment.

****